PHOTOMEDICINE - ADVANCES IN CLINICAL PRACTICE

Edited by **Yohei Tanaka**

Photomedicine - Advances in Clinical Practice
http://dx.doi.org/10.5772/62699
Edited by Yohei Tanaka

Contributors

Carolina Constantin, Monica Neagu, Wei Liu, Weijie Gu, Hongmei Liu, Paola Savoia, Giorgio Delrosso, Yesim Oguz, Vladan Koncar, Cedric Cochrane, Serge Mordon, Abdullah Al-Shenqiti, Nora Bloise, Paolo Minzoni, Marcello Imbriani, Livia Visai, Toshihiro Kushibiki, Hong Cai, Jang-Ming Lee, Ke-Cheng Chen, Priscila Jesus, Antonio Tedesco, Tomasz Kocki, Tomasz Goslinski, Beata Czarczynska-Goslinska, Katarzyna Kocka, Magdalena Stolarska, Sebastian Lijewski, Tomasz Koczorowski, Daria Wachowska, R. Glen Calderhead, Yohei Tanaka

Published by InTech

Janeza Trdine 9, 51000 Rijeka, Croatia

Publishing Process Manager Romina Skomersic
Technical Editor SPi Global
Cover InTech Design team

First published May, 2017
Printed in Croatia
Legal deposit, Croatia: National and University Library in Zagreb

Additional hard copies can be obtained from orders@intechopen.com

Photomedicine - Advances in Clinical Practice, Edited by Yohei Tanaka
p. cm.
Print ISBN 978-953-51-3155-7
Online ISBN 978-953-51-3156-4

For EU product safety concerns:
IN TECH d.o.o., Prolaz Marije Krucifikse Kozulić 3, 51000 Rijeka, Croatia,
info@intechopen.com or visit our website at intechopen.com.

Meet the editor

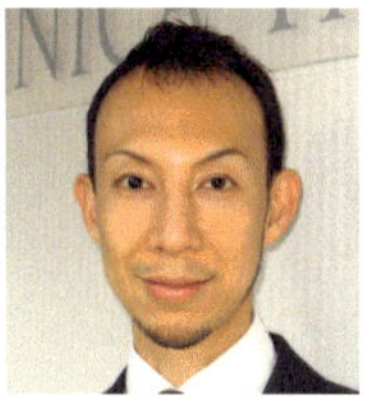

Dr. Tanaka is a board certified plastic surgeon who specializes in photobiology as well as an enthusiastic researcher. He received his MD degree from Shinshu University School of Medicine in 2000 and PhD degree from Shinshu University Graduate School of Medicine in 2010. As one of the leading plastic surgeons in Japan, Dr. Tanaka brings with him years of experience and a wealth of knowledge in the fields of plastic and reconstructive surgery, dermatology, antiaging, and photobiology. As well as being the founder of Clinica Tanaka Plastic, Reconstructive Surgery and Anti-aging Center and a visiting professor of Niigata University of Pharmacy and Applied Life Sciences, he is also a member of many Japanese and international institutions and societies. Dr. Tanaka has published over 40 peer-reviewed papers in English in a number of prestigious international journals and has edited 2 international open access books regarding melanoma and photomedicine.

Contents

Preface

In the beginning, there was—Nothing. "And God said, 'Let there be light!' and there was ... LIGHT" (Old Testament, Genesis 1:3). I have always harbored a particular fondness for light. Of course, we all need it, because without light, life will wither and fade, so light is intrinsically bound to life—the circadian cycle (light and life). We all instinctively lean toward light, positive phototaxis, because we know we need it. How elegant it is, therefore, to harness the natural phenomenon of photon energy to heal—the art of photomedicine.

Photomedicine is one of the most inspiring and interdisciplinary fields in medicine that involves the research and application of photobiology with respect to health and disease. Over the past few decades, an explosion of technological advances for phototherapies and diagnostic methods occurred with the general public's demand for safe, effective, and innovative phototherapies including anticancer therapy, photorejuvenation, and so on.

Photomedicine has contributed to the clinical practice of a variety of medical fields, including dermatology, surgery, radiology, diagnostics, cardiology, and anticancer therapy. Furthermore, expansion of its scope and contribution can be expected.

This book delivers basic and clinical findings and procedures to improve the knowledge and application of these techniques in medical science. It covers mechanistic studies and clinical applications of photomedicine. A wide range of aspects and issues related to photomedicine brings together researchers from many countries. The book consists of 12 chapters written by over 30 authors.

The first three chapters describe the basic science of photodynamic therapy and clinical applications in skin cancers, pleural photodynamic therapy in lung cancer, and photodynamic therapy for other skin diseases. The subsequent four chapters describe the use of photodynamic therapy in other medical specialties, including antimicrobial photodynamic therapy, nanotechnology, photoregeneration for wound healing and antiaging, light-emitting fabric for photodynamic therapy, and interdisciplinary team in photodynamic therapy. The last five chapters discuss photochemotherapy (PUVA) for dermatological diseases, laser therapy for musculoskeletal pain, intense pulsed light therapy for photorejuvenation, biological function of low-level laser therapy (LLLT), and photobiology for skin rejuvenation.

I would like to express my sincere appreciation and gratitude to all authors who contributed to this book with their research and to the InTech team who accomplished their mission with professionalism and dedication.

I hope that this book will not only be beneficial for readers but will also contribute to scientists making breakthroughs in photomedicine.

Yohei Tanaka, MD, PhD
Clinica Tanaka Plastic, Reconstructive Surgery and Anti-aging Center
Japan

Section 1

Photodynamic Therapy

Chapter 1

Photosensitizers Imprinting Intracellular Signaling Pathways in Dermato-Oncology Therapy

Carolina Constantin and Monica Neagu

Additional information is available at the end of the chapter

http://dx.doi.org/10.5772/65979

Abstract

This chapter describes the main deregulated intracellular pathways at both genetic and proteomic levels that are found in three main skin cancers: basal cell carcinoma, squamous cell carcinoma and melanoma. In basal cell carcinoma, the main intracellular signaling pathways is the Sonic Hedgehog pathway, while in squamous cell carcinoma, it is the p53 pathway. However, in both nonmelanoma skin cancers, these major pathways trigger cross-activation with other important ones. In melanoma, mitogen-activated protein kinase pathway and PI3K/Akt pathways are deeply deregulated, and moreover due to the disease complexity, BRAF, RAS (N/H/K), NF1 and Triple-WT melanoma subtypes need additional molecular stratification. The stage in which photodynamic therapies' clinical application is in the treatment of these diseases is another subject tackled by the chapter. Thus, if basal cell carcinoma and squamous cell carcinoma possess in their therapeutical armamentarium photodynamic therapies approach, melanoma, with its particularities, still needs thorough molecular investigations to adapt this particular therapy. Based on the accumulated knowledge on pathological intracellular pathways, the chapter describes the molecular details that reside in applying photodynamic therapy. *In vivo* and *in vitro* models of cutaneous malignancy and photodynamic therapies' molecular events are further detailed.

Keywords: skin cancer, intracellular signaling, biology, photodynamic therapy, photosensitizer, proteomics

1. Introduction

Skin cancers, especially cutaneous melanoma, remain a complex therapeutic challenge owing to a multiangle problem such as the emergent incidence in white population, the inefficiency of classical therapies like surgery and owing to transition to the new wave treatments like targeted therapies, immunotherapy and alternative therapies like photodynamic therapy (PDT). Skin tumors are classified as melanoma and nonmelanoma type. Basal cell carcinoma (BCC) and squamous cell carcinoma (SCC) along with actinic keratosis (AK) are considered nonmelanoma skin cancers (NMSC), being the most frequent skin cancers in comparison with melanoma which is more rare (only 4%) but highly deadly [1]. Similarly, organ transplant recipients (OTR) record an extremely high risk of developing NMSC [2]. All these types of cancers are generated by complex molecular events that favor tumor proliferation and invasion. At the core of this diseases' pathology intracellular pathways deregulation dwell. Therapies that are developed in each cancer type should acknowledge the molecular events particularities. In the therapeutical armamentarium of skin cancer, PDT has already gained its place. As further presented, the intracellular molecular pattern triggered in each type of skin cancer by PDT has both common outlines and particularities.

2. Skin cancer, photodynamic therapy and signaling pathways

2.1. Biology of skin cancer in the light of new therapeutical era

Deepening the biology of skin cancer by unraveling the intracellular mechanisms that trigger the neoplastic transformation could lead to deciphering new therapy targets and new therapeutical approaches. Both cellular and molecular basis of a successful therapy still needs new explorations and additional biomedical technologies in order to manage this high morbidity and mortality group of diseases.

2.1.1. Basal cell carcinoma

As described in the early 1990 [3], basal cell carcinoma (BCC) is the most common malignancy in humans, and although rarely metastatic, accounts for about two-thirds of all skin cancers with a worldwide incidence steady increase [4]. The diversity in the phenotypic appearance of BCCs relies on the fact that the majority of BCCs represent monoclonal tumors and anatomically distinct BCCs may sometimes share the same cellular origin [5]. An extensive genetic study on BCC profiling was published in 2016 investigating around 300 tumor tissue that displayed the highest mutation rate in cancer (65 mutations per mega base). About 85% of all tumors have mutations in the Sonic Hedgehog (Hh) pathway. These genes are PTCH1, SMO, SUFU and TP53. Other mutations were found in MYCN, PPP6C, STK19, LATS1, ERBB2, PIK3CA and NRAS. Loss-of-function and deleterious missense mutations were found in PTPN14, RB1 and FBXW7 genes [6]. Moreover, 2016 studies have shown that genetic predisposition in familial BCC has the most commonly gene mutated, PTCH1, main player in the Hh pathway. Another gene associated with familial BCC is SUFU being involved in the same pathway. This gene is loosing its function and hence inducing BCC predisposition. Understanding the deregulated genes that trigger BCCs can lead to new targeted therapy trials [7]. In the last five years, studies on the biology of BCC have shown that Hh pathway is deeply involved in the initiation of this skin tumor. This pathway cross-talks with other main intracellular pathways involved in skin's homeostasis. Hence, Wnt pathway was found as having increased levels of beta-catenin, a critical mediator of Wnt signaling in BCCs [8, 9]. Another important pathway involved in BCC is EGFR/MEK/ERK that modulates GLI-dependent transcription in human keratinocytes and drives their oncogenic transformation [10, 11]. As epithelial-stromal interactions are creating a protumoral microenvironment, stromal cells isolated from BCCs, have high levels of gremlin 1. This protein antagonizes with the prodifferentiation factors BMP2 and BMP4, sustaining, therefore, tumor proliferation [12]. If Hh pathway is deregulated at gene and protein level, another deregulated pathway in BCC is the MEK-ERK pathway. Hence, acknowledging that IL-17 (IL-17A) sustains a chronic inflammatory microenvironment with protumoral consequences some important reports were published in 2015. IL-17 binding to its receptor activates the route IL-17R-Act1-TRAF4-MEKK3-ERK5 that directly stimulates keratinocyte proliferation and tumor formation. In the BCC context, this axis sustains the expression of Steap4-p63 through p63-mediated TRAF4 expression that directly enhances keratinocyte proliferation and further tumor formation [13].

2.1.2. *Squamous cell carcinoma*

Cutaneous squamous cell carcinoma (SCC) is the second most common human skin malignancy after BCC, and opposed to BCC, it can trigger metastasis. SCC originates the premalign lesions actinic keratosis (AK) and it develops from keratinocytes of the spinous layer. The progression of AK to malignancy relies on the sequential DNA mutations in oncogenes and tumor suppressor genes. This multistep process triggered by chronic UV irradiation leads to increased genomic instability and loss of cell cycle control, thus driving the malignant uncontrolled proliferation of keratinocytes. Details of the molecular pathogenesis of SCC are still a subject of intense research [14]. Intracellular signaling deregulated pathways in SCC pinpoint to p53 pathway as mutated p53 is the most common genetic abnormality found in SCC. AK lesions can harbor mutated p53, and remain as such through the malignization process toward SCC [15, 16]. Whole transcriptome analysis published in 2016 has shown in SCC cancer cells, in comparison to normal human epidermal keratinocytes, an overexpression of long intergenic non coding RNA (LINC00162). LINC00162 is upregulated by the inhibition of the p38α and p38δ mitogen-activated protein kinases. Knockdown of LINC00162 inhibited proliferation and migration of SCC cells *in vitro* and inhibited extracellular signal-regulated kinase 1/2 activity, up regulating dual specificity phosphatase 6 (DUSP6) [17]. Other, recently published molecules involved in the complex biology of SCC are Ets2 and Elk3 genes, required for malignant progression from AK lesions to SCC. ETS2-overactivation in epidermal cancer stem cells induces hyperproliferation and SCC superenhancer-associated genes Fos, Junb and Klf5 expression [18]. Epidermal cancer stem cells are characterized by alterations in keratinocyte stem cells (KSC) and survivin gene expression. Silencing survivin reduces the classical expression of stem cell markers (OCT4, NOTCH1, CD133 and β_1-integrin), and increases differentiation markers (K10 and involucrin). Recently published results indicate survivin as a key gene in SCC development [19]. Another recently published protein, involved in SCC, is S100A8, whose overexpression regulates SCC differentiation [20].

2.1.3. *Cutaneous melanoma*

Cutaneous melanoma is one of the solid tumors that bear the highest rate of mutations. In 2015, The Cancer Genome Atlas Network has proposed a new genomic classification of these tumors divided into genomic subtypes: BRAF, RAS (N/H/K), NF1 and Triple-WT [21]. These subtypes have significant intracellular pathways deregulations. A BRAF mutation is present in the majority of melanomas, and an NRAS isoform is present in 15–30% of melanomas [22]. The mitogen-activated protein kinase (MAPK) pathway (Ras/Raf/MEK/ERK pathway) has several mutated points so that uncontrolled cellular proliferation may occur [23, 24]. Alike to the MAPK pathway, the PI3K/Akt pathway can also be activated by Ras. Once this pathway is activated, cell proliferation and invasion are promoted. Although PI3K mutations are believed to be rare, downstream components of the PI3K/Akt pathway steadily increase during melanoma progression, and are altered in 50–60% of melanomas [25]. CDKN2A is another gene that encodes proteins involved in cell cycle regulation. Approximately 10% of all melanomas have a familial susceptibility linked to the CDKN2A gene. Somatic CDKN2A mutations have been reported in 30–70% of sporadic melanomas [25].

The pathophysiology of each skin cancer can have different gene/protein/intracellular signaling foundation or can share the same molecular pathways. **Figure 1** resumes the main intracellular pathways that trigger the three main skin cancers in humans.

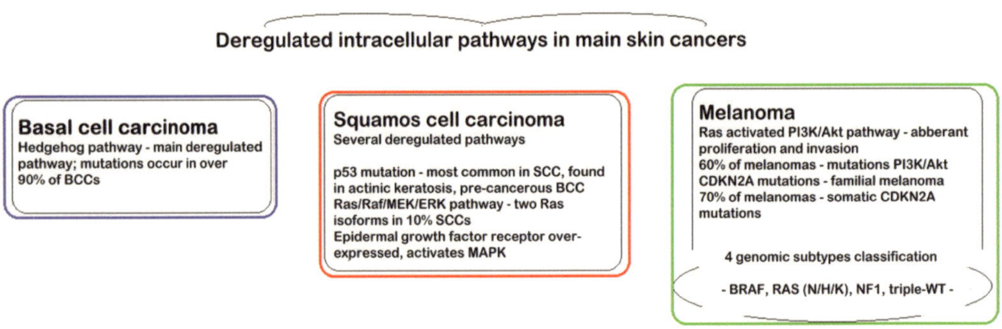

Figure 1. Intracellular signaling pathways that characterize the main skin cancer types: basal cell carcinoma (BCC), squamous cell carcinoma (SCC) and melanoma.

2.2. PDT in the clinical management of skin cancers

Owing to a constantly increasing incidence, malignant skin tumors need a multidisciplinary approach regarding their clinical management, comprising specialists and therapeutical lines, which could be personalized for every situation [26]. In this context, PDT is involved in the management of nonmelanoma skin cancers, primary superficial BCCs, low-risk nodular BCCs and superficial SCCs [27]. In recent years, even for melanoma, PDT starts to be considered as an alternative treatment option.

2.2.1. *PDT in BCC therapy*

Predominantly located in head and neck region, there are three types of BCC: nodular, superficial and morpheic with an increased heterogeneity [28, 29]. Due to this heterogeneity, there are several therapy lines and several ongoing clinical trials that are thoroughly resumed in Ref. [10]. Among all these therapies, PDT gains its place. Thus, topical PDT with methyl ester-based photosensitizer (PS) is currently accepted for superficial BCC. Accordingly, 16% methyl ester methyl aminolevulinate (MAL) is approved for topical PDT of BCC in Europe (Metvix®) while in the USA the corresponding approved drug is Levulan® (20% of 5-aminolevulinic acid in ethanol solution) [28]. The clinical response for PDT in BCC is not clear-cut. Thus evaluating more than 130 patients treated with MAL-PDT the best response was obtained for superficial BCC (82%) compared to nodular BCC (only 33%). Analyzing the subtypes some predictor factors emerged, nodular infiltrative histotypes, ulceration tumor thickness and localization on limbs were the negative ones [30]. Trying to improve the clinical outcome, two-fold illumination scheme for aminolevulinic acid-photodynamic therapy (ALA-PDT) was investigated and one-year post-treatment clinical evolution was assessed. For small BCC located outside the head and neck area, this activation scheme has proven good clinical outcome [31]. For a three-year follow-up in patients treated with MAL-PDT, fluorouracil and MAL-PDT have proven the same efficacy in the treatment of superficial BCCs [32].

2.2.2. *PDT in SCC therapy*

SCC and AK represent the same skin disease but in different stages of evolution, as AK is superficial, SCC involves also the dermis. Local PDT is suitable for AK and for *in situ* SCC [33]. Therapeutical protocols in SCC implies surgery (cryosurgery, electrosurgery and radiotherapy), topical treatments with 5-fluorouracil and imiquimod or PDT [34], successful ALA-PDT and blue light being reported several years ago [35]. In this type of cancer, although, surgical excision is the first therapeutical choice, PDT is a noninvasive approach and it can provide optimum cosmetic outcomes. As in SCC, resistant or recurrent tumors can appear, and PDT should be combined with other therapeutic modalities. Hence PDT can be combined with immunomodulatory (Imiquimod) and/or chemotherapeutic agents (5-fluorouracil, methotrexate, diclofenac or ingenol mebutate), and/or inhibitors of molecules involved in tumorigenesis, such as COX2 or MAPK [36].

2.2.3. *PDT in melanoma therapy*

There is an interesting link between melanoma patients and the subsequent appearance of BCC or SCC. In a study published in 2016, the associations between melanoma diagnosis and SCC were studied. The study showed a clear correlation between age, sex, skin characteristics, sun exposure and the existence of p.R163Q/p.D294H MC1R variants in melanoma patients, parameters that favor the risk of developing a SCC. This study has shown that melanoma patients with increased risk of developing another skin cancer should be further stratified [37].

Although in cutaneous melanoma targeted immune-therapies are the best clinical option, there is a therapeutical niche for PDT with second generation PS, especially as postsurgery adjuvant treatment or even as a preventive approach [38]. PDT exerts specific effects in melanoma cells both upon melanocytic antioxidant system and multidrug resistance cellular machinery decreasing these functions essential for melanoma survival. While successful in other skin cancers, PDT is not effective in pigmented melanoma due to photophysical properties of melanin from melanocyte-transformed cells, as melanin absorbs light over the entire wavelength region used by PS for PDT (400–750 nm). Amelanotic melanoma with low melanin pigment load has been more approached in PDT studies [38]. Still only few studies are reported in this topic, and clinically there are some promising results for PDT with chlorin e(6) in skin metastases [39] and ocular choroidal melanomas [40, 41]. PDT with verteporfin alone or in combination with bevacizumab may be useful as primary or preoperative procedure for ocular melanoma. There are also recent experimental studies involving amelanotic melanoma, the nonpigmented melanoma type owned to a poor differentiation of melanocytes, which produce less melanin, refractive to classic treatments and for which alternative therapies are taking into account [42]. Thus, in a mouse C57/BL6 model bearing B78H1 amelanotic melanoma, it was tested a novel PS assembly comprising a Zn(II)-phthalocyanine, a polyethylene glycol (PEG) derivative and gold nanoparticles. The deposition of PEG on the nanoparticle surface makes the conjugate hydrosoluble prolonging the retaining in serum, improving thus the PDT efficacy. The nanoparticle conjugates were significantly accumulated and retained in the tumor 3 h postinjection followed by PDT. The experimental approach lead to 40% survival of the treated mice, without tumor relapses. These types of PS functionalized with nanoparticles have good potential in PDT for difficult to treat cancers such as amelanotic melanoma [43]. Another strategy is to use natural compounds as PS in PDT of skin cancer; hence, positive results were obtained with hypericin in human melanoma cells, Where an inhibition of proliferation was registered [44]. In addition, natural compounds are "back in fashion" and hypericin was tested also in NMSC treatment approaches.

2.3. Specific intracellular networks triggered by PDT in skin tumor cells

PDT is an alternative therapy for some type of cancers and several nonmalignant diseases, involving application and preferentially accumulation of a PS in the target cell/tissue, followed by PS photoactivation with a light wavelength fitting the compound's absorption. The actual effect of PDT depends on many factors but the cell/tissue where the PS is accumulating triggers the main process (**Figure 2**).

Typically the structure of many PSs is based on the tetrapyrrole ring—porphyrins and phthalocyanines, including their derivatives (porphycenes)—or natural products such as hypericin, riboflavin or curcumin [45]. Several conditions should be attained by a potential PS, namely: chemical purity, stability, high solubility in water, preferentially loading in the target cell/tissue, low "dark" toxicity and high quantum yield of singlet oxygen ($^1O_2$) generated upon photoactivation [45]. This light activation causes the transition of PS first in a short-lived excited state then in a long-lived energetic state triggering reactive oxygen species (ROS) as main agents of tumor vasculature damage, immune response generation and further tumor eradication [46, 47]. Among relatively innovative approaches in skin tumors treatment, especially in NMSC, PDT could reveal new lines in terms of novel PSs embossing different insights in key intracellular pathways influenced by the PDT treatment. Elucidation of mechanisms in PDT has gained advance within the last decade, data regarding signaling pathways, transcription factors related to cell cycle control, inflammation and cellular death accumulated lately. Nevertheless in a living cell, all these processes are deeply overlapped so

http://dx.doi.org/10.5772/65979

minute understanding should be proceeded step by step [48]. Furthermore, survival mechanisms are activated in PDT-treated cells and some transcription factors have been identified to be involved in cell resistance following PDT, such as AP-1 transcription factor family members, NRF2, hypoxia-inducible factor-1 alpha (HIF-1), nuclear factor-kappa B (NF-κB), HSF1 and unfolded protein response (UPR) protein group [47]. Involvement of a certain signaling pathway could define the response of a treatment. For instance PDT with ALA as PS has been widely used to treat SCC. However, a segment of SCC patients does not respond well to this PDT therapy, the lack of efficacy being evoked at molecular level by the MAPK signaling pathway. *In vitro* studies on SCL-1 human squamous carcinoma cell line revealed that adding inhibitors of MAPK on ALA-treated SCL-1 cells could augment the cytotoxic effects of ALA-PDT. More specific, the addition of inhibitors for key components belonging MAPK, namely ERK1/2, p38 and JNK, induced a more dramatic decrease on cellular viability than induced with ALA-PDT alone [49].

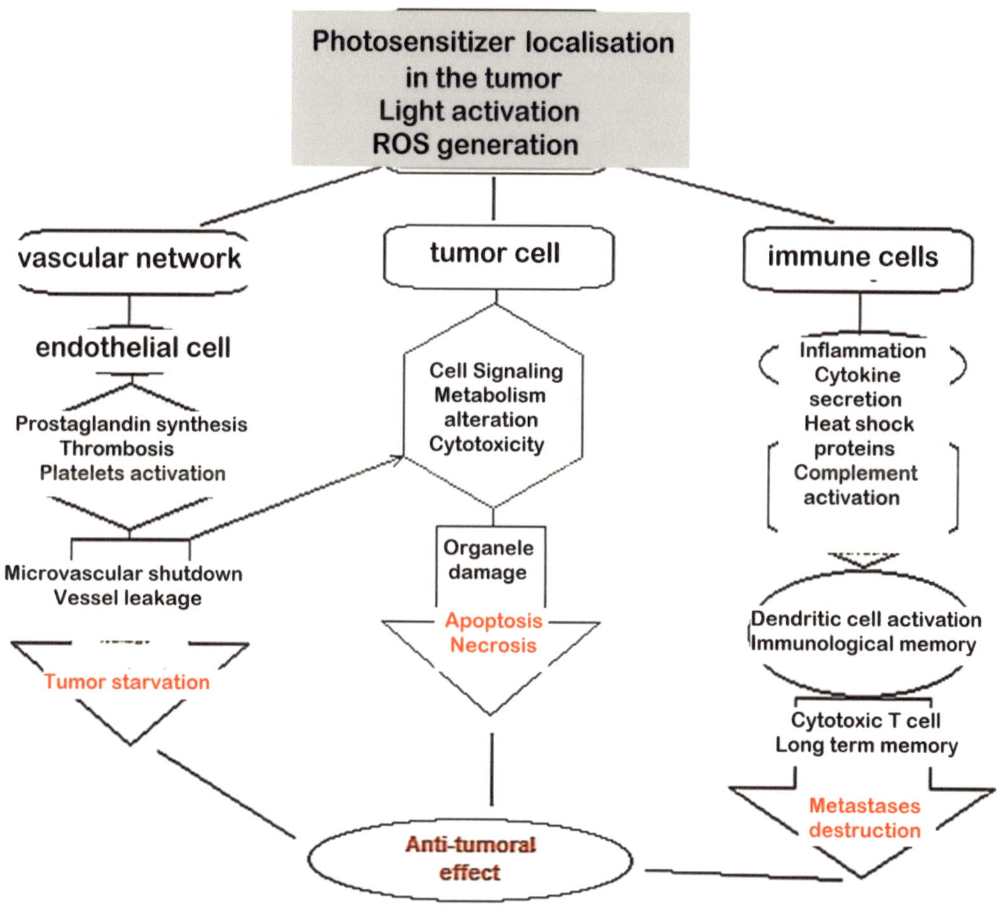

Figure 2. PDT effect inflicted upon localization in different cells and tissues. Regardless of the localization there is an overall antitumoral effect.

Figure 3 resumes intracellular events triggered by PDT in cells that were uptaking PS.

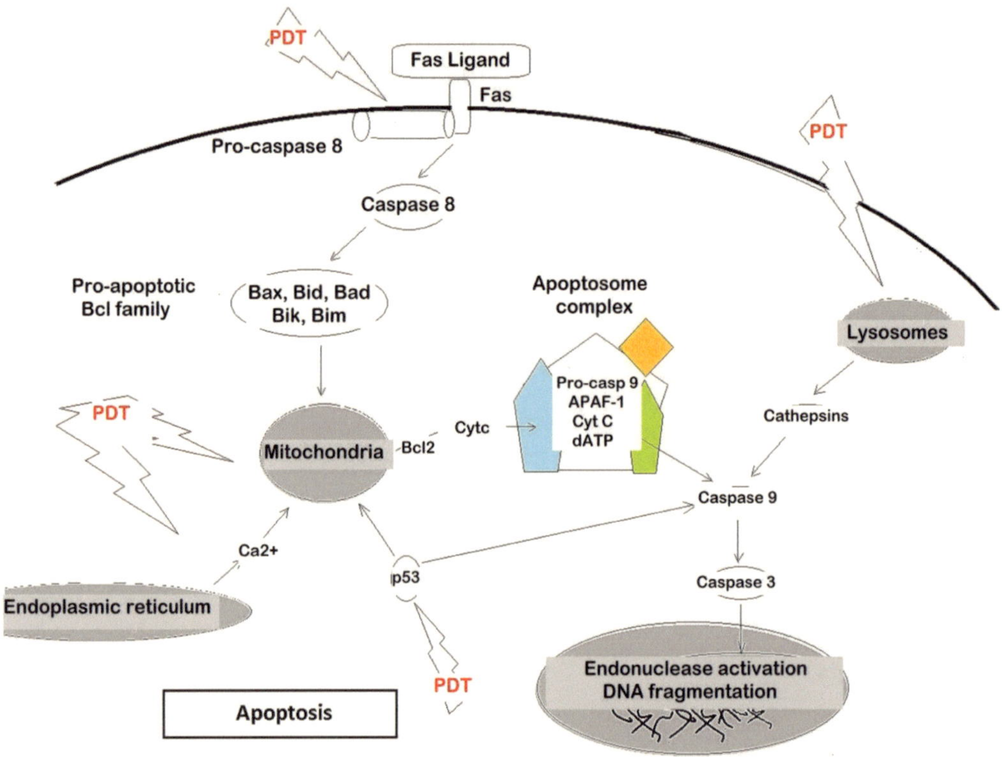

Figure 3. Intracellular events triggered by PDT in cells that were uptaking PS. PDT is inflicting upon cellular membrane an activation of procaspase 8 to caspase 8 that activates the proapoptotic Bcl family of proteins (Bax, Bid, Bad, Bik and Bim). PDT acting on mitochondria induces Bcl-2 that further induces cytochrome C (Cyt C) to form the apoptosome that comprises Procaspase 9, APAF-1, cytochrome C and dATP; the result is the formation of active caspase 9 that through caspase 3 activates intra-nuclear endonucleases and induces hence DNA fragmentation. When PDT acts on lysosomes the cathepsin activation induces activation of caspase 9 with the same fate of DNA fragmentation. When PDT acts on the endoplasmic reticulum it induces Ca^{2+} increase that acts upon the mitochondria to generate Bcl-2 family. PDT can activate directly p53 that will act upon mitochondria and upon caspase 9 activation. The overall effect is the cell death in PDT-treated cells by apoptotic mechanisms.

2.3.1. Pathways in intracellular events triggered by various photosensitizers used in PDT

As a general picture, in skin cancers, the PDT is a topic procedure, especially applied for NMSC while for melanoma could be an adjuvant postsurgery alternative. As PS used in dermatopathology, only two of them are known to be approved by FDA, namely 5-ALA and MAL, which are prodrugs becoming active upon intracellular metabolization [50], while other PS attempts are currently made with novel (bio) structures related to porphyrin skeleton such as porphycenes [51, 52]. Once activated in tumor cell, a PS triggers different pathways depending on intracellular localization of PS, PS's dose and type, light dose, cell genotype, affecting cell fate in terms of death and proliferation. PDT triggers the death of cellular target, occurred primarily by apoptosis, necrosis and, as recently shown, by autophagy [47]. The PS generations evolve continuously, hence from the first generation of PS, Photofrin, a partially purified form of hematoporphyrin derivative [53], the second generation was developed to overcome disadvantages of the first one, such as tetrapyrrole rings, substituted derivatives of porphyrin, chlorin and bacteriochlorin [54]. Recently the newer, third generation of PSs was put in scene in novel chemical compounds (e.g. fullerenes) or novel platforms such as PS coupled on different carriers [47]. Nowadays, a so called targeted PDT has emerged and in this type of therapy, antibodies, peptides, proteins, liposomes, cholesterol or other ligands are coupled to PS displaying an improved selective accumulation in the tumor [55].

An advanced generation of PS is always defined by longer wavelengths of light (as red as possible) which corroborates with a deeper penetration of target tissues and a decreased photosensitivity [56]. The antitumor PDT addresses two important issues: direct harmful effects on target cells and vascular injury that will limit blood and other nutrients supply to the affected region [57]. There are mainly two ways of cell fate following PDT: cellular death or cellular survival. The border between these two opposite processes is fine-lined by specific intracellular mechanisms development.

2.3.1.1. Cellular death induced by PDT

Once inside the target cell subjected to photoactivation, a variety of intracellular pathways are initiated by the PS. Although at first sight these biochemical pathways look complex, overlapped, multiple and hard to decipher, the target cell will act in one main direction, namely survival as a response to PDT-triggered aggression.

Generation of reactive oxygen species upon PDT: The first molecular steps in ROS generation are related to PSs' chemistry, depending on oxygen supply in the target tissue [58], and comprise the generation of ROS, as main tools for tumor/target cell destruction. Under the specific light action, the PS will absorb a photon moving from a low energetically short-lived singlet state to an excited long-lived triplet state able to react with molecular oxygen to produce superoxide anion $O_2^{\bullet -}$ (low reactivity, long lifetime—type I reaction) or singlet oxygen $^1O_2$ (high reactivity, short lifetime—type II reaction) [59].

What is the fate of ROS in photosensitized cells? Different types of ROS inflict different actions. Singlet oxygen being highly reactive but evanescent, will oxidize various many biomolecules (lipids, nucleic acids, proteins, etc.) at the level of their electron-dense regions [57, 60], while superoxide anion due to its low reactivity on direct biological target, will act mainly as a precursor for other reactive species (e.g. H_2O_2 or $^{\bullet}OH$) that will cause cellular fatal injuries triggering cell death through necrosis or apoptosis [61]. Also it is important to notice that since singlet oxygen is a short-lived species, will act immediately upon intracellular targets close to the site where PS was accumulated, influencing thus the type of response upon intracellular localization [57]. Regardless of ROS type, the outcome is tumor cell eradication by different mechanisms of cytotoxicity operated by PDT [46].

Cellular toxicity induced by reactive oxygen species: Three cytotoxicity modes are induced post-PDT: oxidative stress, hypoxia and antitumor immune response. Oxidative stress it's installed when generated ROS oxidize and irreversible damages nucleic acids (DNA and RNA) [62, 63], lipids [64] and proteins [65] with consequences upon the whole cellular physiology. Certain particular changes are related to cellular membrane where phospholipid peroxidation leads to alterations of membrane fluidity, permeability and the (photo)oxidation of cellular membrane contributing strongly to cell death [66, 67]. Oxidative stress is linked to locally induced hypoxia in the photosensitized tissue, which abort the ATP production by oxidative phosphorylation [68] thus leading to cellular death (namely necrosis, an ATP-independent process), and further to the antitumor immune response initiation which is the decisive piece for complete removal of photodamaged tissue [69]. Upon PDT-induced cellular death, namely apoptosis, necrosis, necroptosis [70] and/or autophagy [71]), intracellular damage-associated molecular patterns (DAMPs) [72] and tumor-associated antigens (TAAs) are released from the photosensitized cells and subsequently trigger an immune response aimed at removing the PDT-treated tumor [73].

2.3.1.2. Activation of intracellular survival pathways in photodynamic action

Although cellular death conducted by ROS is envisaged, tumor cells subjected to PDT could encounter this stress by triggering survival mechanisms when vascular shutdown was not completed following PDT action. This type of response is primarily mediated by several pathways raising in an interconnected manner where beside classical NF-kB-mediated proinflammatory and proangiogenic activity, is raising also a NRF2-mediated antioxidant response, a HIF-1-mediated hypoxia survival, a proteotoxic stress response interceded by certain transcription factors (HSF1, XBP1, ATF6 and ATF4) corroborated with an acute stress reply where factors from MAPK pathway are being involved. As PDT means an oxidative stress upon target cells, many studies related to signaling pathways were treated through the prism of oxidative stress and therefore extrapolated to PDT. Consequently, recent works refer to signaling pathways in PDT as to signaling pathways activated in cells subjected to oxidative stress [74].

NRF2 is the main transcription factor protecting against the oxidative stress by restoring the intracellular redox balance in a post-PDT–treated cell, promoting the transcription of the genes encoding for antioxidant enzymes, antioxidant proteins as well as for multidrug response proteins. Moreover, NRF2 is likely constitutively active in many cancer types potentially desensitizing these cells to PDT effects, mediated by ROS. Cells from various layers of the skin benefit from NRF2 protective actions, both in abnormal differentiation, wound healing and controlling inflammation. Thus in keratinocytes and melanocytes, NRF2 protects against mutation during keratinization and melanogenesis. Also, in fibroblasts, NRF2 protects against differentiation and fibrosis processes; therefore, NRF2 activity could be modulated in the context of skin diseases pharmacotherapy and in PDT in order to improve the PDT efficacy by impairing adaptation of target cells to oxidative stress. In addition, NRF2 could be a key biomolecule in the searching for new drugs for various skin disorders including vitiligo or even cutaneous melanoma [75].

NF-κB is a family of transcription factors with a crucial role in inflammation, apoptosis, innate immunity and also in cancer initiation. NF-kB interferes with an ample array of signaling pathways, including HIF-1, and certain biomolecules such as ROS [76]. The NF-κB activation following PDT could initiate the survival of tumor cells by inhibiting apoptosis and facilitating angiogenesis. Also, NF-κB pathway could display equally antitumor and protumor functions in different carcinogenesis processes, for instance in epidermal keratinocytes, NF-κB seems to exert mainly tumor growth inhibitory functions [77]. In melanoma, the NF-κB activity in tumorigenesis was demonstrated in a mouse model where HR as-mediated tumorigenesis onset relies on IKK2-mediated NF-κB activation [78].

HIF-1 is the central modulating pathway for hypoxic conditions in most tumor cells, as well as skin cancers, condition in which it is constitutively activated [79]. Thus, in a hypoxic or even anoxic milieu, HIF-1 becomes hyperactivate as a part of survival actions adopted post-PDT [80].

The ASK1 pathway directs the immediate early stress response, namely the rapid transcription of a set of genes encoding for stress adapting proteins. Classical ASK1 sends its signal *via* MAPKs proteins to the AP-1 transcription factors responsible for the rapid induction of immediate early gene transcription. Nevertheless, the direct ASK1 activation post-PDT is still difficult to demonstrate, so the actual involvement of ASK1 in PDT response can only be assumed from the effects on downstream kinases (MAPKs) and other transcription factors. This kind of indirect proof was reported in a model of PDT with murine PAM212 keratinocytes loaded with a benzoporphyrin derivative, where the activation of JNK and p38MAPK were associated with early stress response mediated by ASK1. In addition, the early survival response upon PDT means a transient JNK and p38MAPK activation triggered by AP-1 transcription factors phosphorylation from ASK-1 pathway. Thus, an approach for improving PDT efficacy could be the AP-1 pharmacological suppressing while preserving the JNK and p38MAPK functions [81].

The proteotoxic stress response arises as well as a survival mechanism in PDT stressed cells triggering certain transcriptional level responses known as the unfolded protein response (UPR), a form of endoplasmic reticulum (ER) stress. These resulted unfolded proteins activate further HSF transcription factors by which an adaptive response comprising chaperones upregulated and protein synthesis inhibition is raising, allowing protein refolding and degradation of those protein aggregates wrongly appeared during stress [82].

However, this UPR process should be analyzed in report with cell, type, PS nature, PS intracellular localization and PDT regimen. It is expected to launch an UPR response for those PS which accumulate preferentially in ER, such as hypericin. For instance, such ER-related oxidative stress was reported for a PDT model with sodium-porfimer photosensitizer, which conducts to protein polyubiquitination, carbonylation and ER lumen enlargement [65]. As a result, the UPR constitutively activated in tumors, as many other protection mechanisms [83], will protect tumor cells against anticancer therapies such as PDT [74].

2.3.2. Different effects triggered by in vitro PDT experimental models

Subtle changes triggered by photodynamic treatment are incompletely revealed, as signaling pathways regulate a myriad of cellular processes starting with genetic ones, such as transcription and translation, and ending with complex cellular behavior such as proliferation, apoptosis, differentiation, metabolism and overall cell survival upon a certain therapeutic regimen.

Such finest inquiries are needed to be explored with various techniques and experimental models that deliver data regarding the best way of PS delivery, the best PDT regimen, cellular and molecular characteristics imprinted by a certain PS, therapeutical outcome and so on. The "practical" history of experimental PDT begun in the mid-1970s when it was discovered that a hematoporphyrin derivative activated with red light "cured" a mammary tumor in a mouse model [84]. The studies are in continuous development as an arsenal of in vitro cellular models were settled for studying PDT effects on various cancers including skin cancers. Experimental *in vitro* models for PDT implying novel PS to be used in skin tumors, are related to cell types or types of cellular cultures (adherent, suspension, 2D or more recently 3D cellular cultures). For instance, three dimensional spheroid culture cells provide very convenient approaches for *in vitro* assessment of new PS and new PDT responses and, in addition, they could mimic many *in vivo* intercellular interactions. Their convenient growth characteristics and exploitable features in imagistic approaches allow *in vitro* PDT multiple parameters studies in an "all in one" manner [85].

2.3.2.1. *In vitro models for nonmelanoma skin cancer PDT therapy*

Among PS tested for NMSC, hypericin a natural quinone extracted from *Hypericum perforatum*, gain constant attention due to its good photosensitizing properties, an ideal candidate for PDT applied in skin tumors [86]. Hypericin as PS was currently investigated in a recent report where was tested in an *in vitro* system with human normal primary cells (keratinocytes, melanocytes and fibroblasts) mimicking thus the epidermis and dermis of human skin. Fibroblasts were the most susceptible to hypericin-PDT, followed by melanocytes and keratinocytes in terms of viability. The cellular morphologies were affected by PDT for all investigated cell types, keratinocytes being the most unaffected even at highest PS doses. Other results indicate a cytoplasmic localization of hypericin in all investigated skin cell types whereas the intracellular generated ROS were the most elevated in fibroblasts. This study describes the effects induced by *in vitro* PDT using hypericin on different human skin cells, gathering hence data on PS efficacy that could impacts *in vivo* application for NMSC [87].

2.3.2.2. *In vitro models for melanoma PDT therapy*

The main stream of the studies regarding PDT applied in melanoma encounter a major issue raised by this type of cancer: an evident resistance to this therapy owing to melanin that will compete with the PS for photons in the detriment of molecular oxygen, leading to an impaired phototoxicity upon target cell [47]. Therefore, the attempts regarding PDT in malignant melanoma have tried to combine PDT with a complementary procedure such as magneto-hyperthermia [88], or use an improved PS delivery system, namely a liposome formula including a second generation PS such as metallated phthalocyanines. This *in vitro* model with B16-F10 standard cell line was used for melanoma studies [89].

Although PDT seems not to be an option in melanoma, recent publication has shown that in a B16-melanoma cell line and also in a B16 ectopic tumor model, ALA-SDT had been more

http://dx.doi.org/10.5772/65979

efficacious when compared to ALA-PDT. SDT is sonodynamic therapy in which the activation of a nontoxic sensitizer drug is performed using low-intensity ultrasound to produce cytotoxic ROS. SDT can activate sensitizers at a greater depth within human tissue because of the low tissue attenuation of ultrasound. In PDT for melanoma the low efficacy was attributed to the dark pigmentation of the melanoma that filters the excitation light. In SDT, the sensitizer is activated by ultrasound and it is not hindered by pigmentation. These results suggest SDT as a better approach in comparison to PDT when treating highly pigmented cancerous skin lesions [90].

Nanocarriers for delivering one or even simultaneously two PSs [91] seem to be a good instrument to outcome the recognized melanoma resistance, and have been tested further in a mouse model of xenograft melanoma proving an increased efficacy of treatment and an enhanced accumulation in melanoma cell [92].

2.4. Proteomics technologies in intracellular signaling events triggered by PDT

The complex and intermingled intracellular mechanisms triggered by PDT claim high-throughput proteomic tools to thoroughly quest the signaling events occurred in cancer cell followed PS activation. The cellular signaling events are first triggered by the activation of plasma membrane events [93]. Recently emerged, the proteomics branch focusing on these events is plasma membrane proteomics. From antibody-based techniques to large-scale "precision proteomics" centered on mass spectrometry, posttranslational modifications, protein-protein interactions and changes in protein expression could be analyzed by large scale proteomics. Proteomics in this domain is important as it conveys accurate information concerning (patho) physiological changes in terms of qualitative and quantitative terms of thousands of proteins as response to a certain antitumor therapy.

Skin cancers alterations affect specific genes and thus specific protein mediators from different signaling pathways including the Sonic Hedgehog and NF-kB, targeting these proteins being the trigger for new approaches in skin cancers therapy [94].

Before tackling the proteomic involvement in PDT pattern, it must be underlined that genomic technologies' advancements paved the road to molecular insights in skin cancers and related signaling pathways. In skin tumors, advances in sequencing techniques were driven at the beginning of 2000s in receptor tyrosine kinases studies, and were the tools that identified and indicated the presence of BRAF mutations in 50% of skin melanomas [95]. This imprints a major impact in development of selective BRAF inhibitors (vemurafenib and dabrafenib) triggering impressive remissions in melanoma patients who benefit now from an improved treatment, leading to a new era in targeted therapy [96]. Starting from this crossing-point, it could be further underlined that proteomics is continuing to make major progresses in biological processes discoveries as well as in establishing an "universal" assay platform for measuring proteins status and levels in any biological system subjected to different physiological milieu. A strength of proteomic approach is that it can translate almost in "real-time" fundamental science achievements into clinical practice helping in outlining personalized medicine and precision medicine [97].

2.4.1. Proteomic technologies in skin cancers at a glance

Proteomics includes a number of methods that could be classified depending on several criteria, such as scope (for identification—quality *versus* measurement—quantity; discovery *versus* validation of biomarkers) and detection method (labeling *versus* label-free), and are broadly comprising spectrometry, electrophoresis and array methods. Regardless of classification criteria, for analyzing PDT events, all approaches could be used to obtain important data in comprehending the dynamic biology of malignant transformation, tumor cell behavior and therapy outcome [98].

It is not the chapters' intend to go in depth with proteomic techniques but one should keep in mind that there are several main stream approaches currently in use in different experimental sets in cancer research [97, 99] as resumed in **Table 1**.

Technology type	**Characteristics**
Two-dimensional gel electrophoresis (2-DE)	Quantitative method allowing extraction and separation in two dimensions (isoelectric point, molecular mass) of proteins from sample of interest
Mass spectroscopy (MS)	Generates peptide mass fingerprints for protein detected on 2-DE; MS has multiple variants—electrospray ionization-liquid chromatography tandem mass spectroscopy (ESI-LC-MS); matrix-assisted laser desorption ionization time of flight (MALDI-TOF); surface-enhanced laser desorption ionization time of flight (SELDI-TOF); MALDI MS imaging (MALDI-MSI); laser capture microdissection-MS (LCM-MS)—optimum for extracting cells from biological specimens preserving the morphologies of captured cells and the nearby tissues
Protein microarray (PM) technology	Proteins/antibodies/other biomolecules covalently attached to a solid support like glass are used to detect various interactions such as protein-protein, enzymatic targets, protein-small molecule (peptide, DNA, etc.), based on the antigen-antibody reaction; it has also many recent variants—cell arrays—it can analyze particular molecular targets expression triggered in in vivo experimental models; tissues array—it can analyze the molecular targets in situ across a panel of primary tissues in order to evaluate their clinical significance

Table 1. Main proteomic technologies applied for intracellular mechanisms investigation in skin cancer.

The future in the proteomic domain relies in multianalyte investigation with different congruent methods based on molecular characteristic evaluation such as 2-DE, MS and protein microarrays. As the proteomic approach is complex, so the future therapeutical approaches in skin cancer need the same multitargeted approach. In this aspect, photo-immune-theranostics reagents are the future compounds that will enter the PDT scene. This future to be therapeutical method combines molecular optical imaging, photodynamic therapy and immunotherapy using SNAP-tag technology which is a derivative of the O(6)-alkylguanine-DNA alkyltransferase (AGT) with the ability to efficiently conjugate to O(6)-benzylguanine (BG) molecules under physiological conditions depending on its folding pattern. An approach like this could simultaneously monitor and suppress the growth of skin squamous carcinoma and melanoma cells expressing EGFR [100].

2.4.2. *Proteomic data for skin cancers*

Data for cutaneous tumors were obtained from proteomic studies' involving MS. Referring strictly to cutaneous cancers, ESI-LC-MS was used for investigating in paraffin-embedded metastatic melanomas for comparative proteomic study [101]. This method quantifies peptide spectra that have been sequenced by the MS and can be used for biomarkers discovery through comparing the peak intensities derived from multiple LC-MS data set [102].

Biomarker identification in melanoma along with other type of cancers was also subjected of SELDI-TOF-MS analysis [103]. In SELDI, the protein sample mixture is spotted on a specific solid surface with chemical functionality such as binding affinity where some analytes in the samples would attach while the others will be washed off. The spotted samples on an SELDI surface are analyzed with TOF mass spectrometry [104].

Nevertheless, proteomic studies concerning PDT in skin tumor are still missing and are limited to *in vitro* approaches by assessing various cell lines. Thus a recent study published in 2016 involves the hexyl-aminolevulinate-mediated PDT in the human epidermoid carcinoma cell line A431 [105]. This analysis is another attempt to elucidate the exact trigger mechanisms for various death-pathways induced by PDT which are still unknown. One of the alteration induced by PDT *via* ROS is the reversible oxidation of cysteine thiols groups (–SH), as potential redox switch for protein activity and cellular signaling. Using MS as proteomic tool, the authors found that over 2000 proteins were reversibly oxidized post-PDT, of which 115 of the high confidence proteins were related to the apoptotic mechanisms and 257 have not been reported yet to be reversibly oxidized on –SH group. This study is considered the first complete mapping of reversibly oxidized proteins following PDT, among which ATM, p63, RSK1 p38, APE1/Ref-1 and three 14-3-3 family members represent potential signaling core in apoptosis death. This "core protein" furnished an apoptotic map that can subsequently identify potentially new redox-regulated triggers as well as potential targets for PDT efficacy improvement, demonstrating the benefit of proteomics in PDT [97, 105].

PM methodology is not yet a routine approach in PDT topic, although possess all strengths to become a robust tool in deciphering the protein-pattern of this domain. Many formats have been developed with whole proteomes, peptides, nucleic acids and lectins, although antibodies platforms remain the most popular PM surfaces. High-throughput tools in a miniaturized format, the arrays could perform parallel analysis, interactions and protein function on a large scale for benefit of both basic research and clinical applications [106].

Using antibody microarray, we have assessed the probable intracellular pathways by which PDT with aluminum-substituted disulfonated phthalocyanine trigger apoptosis in dysplastic oral keratinocytes cells (DOK cell line), leading to the tumoral cells eradication. Among the analyzed apoptotic factors, Bcl-2, P70S6K kinase, Raf-1 and Bad proteins were the biomolecules whose expression changes with the greatest amplitude. Until now, the intimate apoptotic mechanisms activated by PDT with metallated phthalocyanine in this type of keratinocytes are still to be deciphered as well as PDT-related signaling events per se [107]. This complex methodology is a versatile tool allowing investigation in detail of molecular events related to cellular death induced by PDT.

3. Conclusion

PDT procedures have several lines of improvement in skin cancers treatment. For example, BCC superficial lesions, preferentially located on the trunk, have the best therapeutic response when treated with PDT. In SCC, PDT should be combined with immune modulators and chemotherapeutic agents. For melanoma, there is still a huge array of improvement due to its particularities and probably with the prospect of advances in gene discovery and translation, multidisciplinary team has to solve all the emerging issues for introducing PDT in melanoma.

The therapeutic future relies in the homogeneous photo-immune-theranostics reagents combining molecular imaging, PDT and immunotherapy. Using "next generation" proteomic technologies (SNAP-tag) it would be possible to simultaneously monitor and suppress the growth of skin squamous carcinoma and melanoma cells expressing specific markers, like EGFR.

Concluding at a glance, large-scale proteomics-based signaling research will be one of the leaders in future photomedicine by enlarging the basic knowledge regarding (photo)therapy-targeted networks and molecules, and by deciphering new intracellular avenues for future precision medicine in skin tumors. A deeper knowledge regarding signaling mechanisms in PDT could furnish new molecular targets and increase its clinical efficacy.

Acknowledgements

This work was financed by national grants PNII-ID-PCE-2011-3-0918 and PNII-PT-PCCA-2013-4-1407.

Author details

Carolina Constantin[1*] and Monica Neagu[1,2]

*Address all correspondence to: caroconstantin@gmail.com

1 "Victor Babes" National Institute of Pathology, Bucharest, Romania

2 Faculty of Biology, University of Bucharest, Bucharest, Romania

References

[1] Neagu M. The immune system—a hidden treasure for biomarker discovery in cutaneous melanoma. Adv Clin Chem. 2012;58:89–140. DOI: 10.1016/B978-0-12-394383-5.00011-4

[2] Bouwes Bavinck JN, Euvrard S, Naldi L, Nindl I, Proby CM, Neale R, et al. Keratotic skin lesions and other risk factors are associated with skin cancer in organ-transplant recipients: a case-control study in The Netherlands, United Kingdom, Germany, France, and Italy. J Invest Dermatol. 2007;127(7):1647–1656. DOI: 10.1038/sj.jid.5700776

[3] Miller SJ. Biology of basal cell carcinoma (Part I). J Am Acad Dermatol. 1991;24(1):1–13002E

[4] Wu L, Jemal A, Siegel R eds. American Cancer Society. Cancer Facts and Figures. 2011. Atlanta, Georgia, USA: American Cancer Society, Inc.; 60 p.

[5] Shulman O, Laitman Y, Vilan A, Leviav A, Friedman E. Monoclonal origin of anatomically distinct basal cell carcinomas. J Invest Dermatol. 2006;126(3):676–679.

[6] Bonilla X, Parmentier L, King B, Bezrukov F, Kaya G, Zoete V, et al. Genomic analysis identifies new drivers and progression pathways in skin basal cell carcinoma. Nat Genet. 2016;48(4):398–406. DOI: 10.1038/ng.3525

[7] Shanley S, McCormack C. Diagnosis and management of hereditary basal cell skin cancer.Recent Results Cancer Res. 2016;205:191–212. DOI: 10.1007/978-3-319-29998-3_11

[8] Adolphe C, Hetherington R, Ellis T, Wainwright B. Patched1 functions as a gatekeeper by promoting cell cycle progression. Cancer Res. 2006;66(4):2081–2088. DOI: 10.1158/0008-5472.CAN-05-2146

[9] Yang SH, Andl T, Grachtchouk V, Wang A, Liu J, Syu LJ, et al. Pathological responses to oncogenic Hedgehog signaling in skin are dependent on canonical Wnt/beta3-catenin signaling. Nat Genet. 2008;40(9):1130–1135. DOI: 10.1038/ng.192

[10] Kasper M, Schnidar H, Neill GW, Hanneder M, Klingler S, Blaas L et al. Selective modulation of Hedgehog/GLI target gene expression by epidermal growth factor signaling in human keratinocytes. Mol Cell Biol. 2006;26(16):6283–6298. DOI: 10.1128/MCB.02317-05

[11] Schnidar H, Eberl M, Klingler S, Mangelberger D, Kasper M, Hauser-Kronberger C, et al. Epidermal growth factor receptor signaling synergizes with Hedgehog/GLI in oncogenic transformation via activation of the MEK/ERK/JUN pathway. Cancer Res. 2009;69(4):1284–1292. DOI: 10.1158/0008-5472.CAN-08-2331

[12] Sneddon JB, Zhen HH, Montgomery K, van de Rijn M, Tward AD, West R, et al. Bone morphogenetic protein antagonist gremlin 1 is widely expressed by cancer associated stromal cells and can promote tumor cell proliferation. Proc Natl Acad Sci USA. 2006; 103(40):14842–14847. DOI: 10.1073/pnas.0606857103

[13] Chen X, Zhao J, Martin B, Zepp JA, Ko JS, Gu C, et al.A novel IL-17 signaling pathway controlling keratinocyte proliferation and tumorigenesis via the TRAF4-ERK5 axis. J Exp Med. 2015;212(10):1571–1587. DOI: 10.1083/jcb.2106OIA178

[14] Missero C. The genetic evolution of skin squamous cell carcinoma: tumor suppressor identity matters. Exp Dermatol. 2016. DOI: 10.1111/exd.13075. [Epub ahead of print]

[15] Wood GS, Gunkel J, Stewart D, et al. Nonmelanoma skin cancers: basal cell and squamous cell carcinomas. In: Abeloff MD, Armitage JO, Niederhuber JE, Kastan MB, McKenna WG eds. Abeloff's Clinical Oncology. 4th ed. Philadelphia, PA: Churchill Livingston Elsevier; 2008:1253–1270.

[16] Shulstad RM, Proper S. Squamous cell carcinoma: a review of etiology, pathogenesis, treatment and variants. J Dermatol Nurse Assoc. 2010;2(1):12–16. DOI: 10.1097/JDN.0b013e3181cecc51

[17] Piipponen M, Nissinen L, Farshchian M, Riihilä P, Kivisaari A, Kallajoki M, et al. Long noncoding RNA PICSAR promotes growth of cutaneous squamous cell carcinoma by regulating ERK1/2 activity.J Invest Dermatol. 2016;136(8):1701–1710. DOI: 10.1016/j.jid.2016.03.028. Epub 2016 Apr 2.

[18] Yang H, Schramek D, Adam RC, Keyes BE, Wang P, Zheng D, et al. ETS family transcriptional regulators drive chromatin dynamics and malignancy in squamous cell carcinomas. Elife. 2015;4:e10870. DOI: 10.7554/eLife.10870

[19] Lotti R, Palazzo E, Petrachi T, Dallaglio K, Saltari A, Truzzi F, et al. Survivin modulates squamous cell carcinoma-derived stem-like cell proliferation, viability and tumor formation in vivo. Int J Mol Sci. 2016;17(1). pii: E89. DOI: 10.3390/ijms17010089

[20] Shin JM, Chang IK, Lee YH, Yeo MK, Kim JM, Sohn KC, et al. Potential role of S100A8 in cutaneous squamous cell carcinoma differentiation. Ann Dermatol. 2016;28(2):179–185. DOI: 10.5021/ad.2016.28.2.179

[21] Cancer Genome Atlas Network. Genomic classification of cutaneous melanoma. Cell. 2015;161(7):1681–1696. DOI: 10.1016/j.cell.2015.05.044

[22] Ancuceanu R, Neagu M. Immune based therapy for melanoma. Indian Journal of Medical Research. 2016; 143(2):135–144. DOI: 10.4103/0971-5916.180197

[23] Huang PH, Marais R. Melanoma troops massed. Nature. 2009;459(21):336–337. DOI: 10.1038/459336a

[24] Russo AE, Torrisi E, Bevelacqua Y, Perrotta R, Libra M, McCubrey JA et al. Melanoma: molecular pathogenesis and emerging target therapies. Int J Oncol. 2009;34(6):1481–1489. DOI: 10.3892/ijo_00000277

[25] Hocker TL, Singh MK, Tsao H. Melanoma genetics and therapeutic approaches in the 21st century: moving from the benchside to the bedside. J Invest Dermatol. 2008;128(11): 2575–2595. DOI: 10.1038/jid.2008.226

[26] Chummun S, McLean NR. The management of malignant skin cancers. Surgery. 2014; 32(9):484–490. DOI: 10.1016/j.mpsur.2014.06.008

[27] Neville Julie A, Welch E, Leffell David J. Management of nonmelanoma skin cancer in 2007. Nat Clin Pract Oncol. 2007;4:462e9. DOI: 10.1038/ncponc0883

[28] Ericson MB, Wennberg A-M, Larkö O. Review of photodynamic therapy in actinic keratosis and basal cell carcinoma. Ther Clin Risk Manag. 2008;4(1):1–9. PMCID: PMC2503644

[29] Kasper M, Jaks V, Hohl D, Toftgård R. Basal cell carcinoma—molecular biology and potential new therapies. J Clin Invest. 2012;122(2):455–463. DOI: 10.1172/JCI58779

[30] Fantini F, Greco A, Del Giovane C, Cesinaro AM, Venturini M, Zane C, et al. Photodynamic therapy for basal cell carcinoma: clinical and pathological determinants of response. J Eur Acad Dermatol Venereol. 2011;25:896–901. DOI: 10.1111/j.1468-3083.2010.03877.x

[31] Kessels J, Hendriks J, Nelemans P, Mosterd K, Kelleners-Smeets N. Two-fold illumination in topical 5-aminolevulinic acid (ALA)-mediated photodynamic therapy (PDT) for superficial basal cell carcinoma (sBCC): a retrospective case series and cohort study. J Am Acad Dermatol. 2016;74(5):899–906. DOI: 10.1016/j.jaad.2015.12.009

[32] Roozeboom MH, Arits AH, Mosterd K, Sommer A, Essers BA, de Rooij MJ, et al.Three-year follow-up results of photodynamic therapy vs. imiquimod vs. fluorouracil for treatment of superficial basal cell carcinoma: a single-blind, non inferiority, randomized controlled trial. J Invest Dermatol. 2016;136(8):1568–1574. DOI: 10.1016/j.jid.2016.03.043

[33] Sidoroff A, Thaler P. Taking treatment decisions in non-melanoma skin cancer—the place for topical photodynamic therapy (PDT). Photodiagnosis Photodyn Ther. 2010;7(1):24–32. DOI: 10.1016/j.pdpdt.2009.12.004

[34] Ferrándiz C, Fonseca-Capdevila E, García-Diez A, Guillén-Barona C, Belinchón-Romero I, Redondo-Bellón P, et al. Spanish adaptation of the European guidelines for the evaluation and treatment of actinic keratosis. Actas Dermosifiliogr. 2014;105:378–393. DOI: 10.1016/j.adengl.2013.11.004

[35] Zelickson B, Counters J, Coles C, Selim M. Light patch: preliminary report of a novel form of blue light delivery for the treatment of actinic keratosis. Dermatol Surg. 2005;31(3):375–378

[36] Lucena SR, Salazar N, Gracia-Cazaña T, Zamarrón A, González S, Juarranz Á, et al. Combined treatments with photodynamic therapy for non-melanoma skin cancer. Int J Mol Sci. 2015;16(10):25912–25933. DOI: 10.3390/ijms161025912

[37] Espinosa P, Pfeiffer RM, García-Casado Z, Requena C, Landi MT, Kumar R, et al. Risk factors for keratinocyte skin cancer in patients diagnosed with melanoma, a large retrospective study. Eur J Cancer. 2016;53:115–124. DOI: 10.1016/j.ejca.2015.10.058

[38] Choromańska A, Kulbacka J, Chwiłkowska A, Skołucka N, Gamian A and Saczko J. Can photodynamic therapy be an alternative method in melanoma treatment? In: Ms.

Morton R, editor. Treatment of Metastatic Melanoma. InTech; 2011. p. 271–294. DOI: 10.5772/20168

[39] Sheleg SV, Zhavrid EA, Khodina TV, Kochubeev GA, Istomin YP, Chalov VN, et al. Photodynamic therapy with chlorin e(6) for skin metastases of melanoma. Photodermatol Photoimmunol Photomed. 2004;20(1):21–26.

[40] Donaldson MJ, Lim L, Harper CA, Mackenzie J, Campbell GW. Primary treatment of choroidal amelanotic melanoma with photodynamic therapy. Clin Experiment Ophthalmol. 2005;33(5):548–549.DOI: 10.1111/j.1442-9071.2005.01083.x

[41] Canal-Fontcuberta I, Salomão DR, Robertson D, Cantrill HL, Koozekanani D, Rath PP, et al. Clinical and histopathologic findings after photodynamic therapy of choroidal melanoma. Retina. 2012;32(5):942–948. DOI: 10.1097/IAE.0b013e31825097c1

[42] Huang YY, Vecchio D, Avci P, Yin R, Garcia-Diaz M, Hamblin MR. Melanoma resistance to photodynamic therapy: new insights. Biol Chem. 2013;394(2):239–250. DOI: 10.1515/hsz-2012-0228

[43] Camerin M, Moreno M, Marín MJ, Schofield CL, Chambrier I, Cook MJ, et al. Delivery of a hydrophobic phthalocyanine photosensitizer using PEGylated gold nanoparticle conjugates for the in vivo photodynamic therapy of amelanotic melanoma. Photochem Photobiol Sci. 2016;15(5):618–625. DOI: 10.1039/c5pp00463b

[44] Menichini G, Alfano C, Marrelli M, Toniolo C, Provenzano E, Statti GA, et al. *Hypericum perforatum* L. subsp. perforatum induces inhibition of free radicals and enhanced phototoxicity in human melanoma cells under ultraviolet light. Cell Prolif. 2013; 46:193–202. DOI: 10.1111/cpr.12020.

[45] Abrahamse H, Hamblin MR. New photosensitizers for photodynamic therapy. Biochem J. 2016;473(4):347–364. DOI: 10.1042/BJ20150942.

[46] Dolmans DE, Fukumura D, Jain RK. Photodynamic therapy for cancer. Nat Rev Cancer. 2003;3(5):380–387. DOI: 10.1038/nrc1071

[47] Piette J. Signalling pathway activation by photodynamic therapy: NF-κB at the crossroad between oncology and immunology. Photochem Photobiol Sci. 2015; 14:1510–1517. DOI: 10.1039/c4pp00465e

[48] Castano AP, Demidova TN, Hamblin MR. Mechanisms in photodynamic therapy: part two-cellular signaling, cell metabolism and modes of cell death. Photodiagnosis Photodyn Ther. 2005;2(1):1–23. DOI: 10.1016/S1572-1000(05)00030-X

[49] Ge X, Liu J, Shi Z, Jing L, Yu N, Zhang X, et al. Inhibition of MAPK signaling pathways enhances cell death induced by 5-Aminolevulinic acid-photodynamic therapy in skin squamous carcinoma cells. Eur J Dermatol. 2016; 26(2):164–172. DOI: 10.1684/ejd.2015.2725

[50] Wan MT, Lin JY. Current evidence and applications of photodynamic therapy in dermatology. Clin Cosmet Investig Dermatol. 2014;7:145–163. DOI: 10.2147/CCID.S35334

[51] Stockert JC, Cañete M, Juarranz A, Villanueva A, Horobin RW, Borrell JI, et al. Porphycenes: facts and prospects in photodynamic therapy of cancer. Curr Med Chem. 2007;14(9):997–1026. DOI: 10.2174/092986707780362934

[52] Davids LM, Kleemann B. The menace of melanoma: a photodynamic approach to adjunctive cancer therapy. In: Guy Huynh Thien Duc, editor. Melanoma-from early detection to treatment. InTech; 2013. p. 583–628. DOI: 10.5772/53676

[53] Ormond AB, Freeman HS. Dye sensitizers for photodynamic therapy. Materials. 2013;6:817–840. DOI: 10.3390/ma6030817

[54] Il Y, Jia Zhu L, Young Key S. Advance in photosensitizers and light delivery for photodynamic therapy. Clin Endosc. 2013;46(1):7–23. DOI: 10.5946/ce.2013.46.1.7

[55] Allison RR, Sibata CH. Oncologic photodynamic therapy photosensitizers: a clinical review. Photodiagnosis Photodyn Ther. 2010;7:61–75. DOI: 10.1016/j.pdpdt.2010.02.001

[56] Anand S, Ortel BJ, Pereira SP, Hasan T, Maytin EV. Biomodulatory approaches to photodynamic therapy for solid tumors. Cancer Lett. 2012; 326(1):8–16. DOI: 10.1016/j.canlet.2012.07.026

[57] Almeida RD, Manadas BJ, Carvalho AP, Duarte CB. Intracellular signaling mechanisms in photodynamic therapy. Biochimicaet Biophysica Acta. 2004;1704(2):59–86. DOI: 10.1016/j.bbcan.2004.05.003

[58] Gołab J, Olszewska D, Mróz P, Kozar K, Kamiński R, Jalili A, et al. Erythropoietin restores the antitumor effectiveness of photodynamic therapy in mice with chemotherapy-induced anemia. Clin Cancer Res. 2002;8:1265–1270.

[59] Mroz P, Yaroslavsky A, Kharkwal GB, Hamblin MR. Cell death pathways in photodynamic therapy of cancer. Cancer. 2011;3:2516–2539. DOI: 10.3390/cancers3022516

[60] O'Connor AE, Gallagher WM, Byrne AT. Porphyrin and nonporphyrin photosensitizers in oncology: preclinical and clinical advances in photodynamic therapy. Photochem Photobiol. 2009;85:1053–1074. DOI: 10.1111/j.1751-1097.2009.00585.x

[61] Debele TA, Peng S, Tsai HC. Drug carrier for photodynamic cancer therapy. Int J Mol Sci. 2015;16(9):22094–22136. DOI: 10.3390/ijms160922094

[62] Cadet J, Douki T, Ravanat JL. Oxidatively generated damage to the guanine moiety of DNA: mechanisticaspects and formation in cells. Acc Chem Res. 2008;41(8):1075–1083. DOI: 10.1021/ar700245e

[63] Shan X, Chang Y, Lin CG. Messenger RNA oxidation is an early event preceding cell death and causes reduced protein expression. FASEB J. 2007;21:2753–2764. DOI: 10.1096/fj.07-8200com

[64] Sakharov DV, Elstak EDR, Chernyak B,Wirtz KWA. Prolonged lipid oxidation after photodynamic treatment. Study with oxidation-sensitive probe C11-BODIPY581/591. FEBS Lett. 2005;579:1255–1260. DOI: 10.1016/j.febslet.2005.01.024

[65] Szokalska A, Makowski M, Nowis D, Wilczynski GM, Kujawa M, Wójcik C, et al. Proteasome inhibition potentiates antitumor effects ofphotodynamic therapy in mice through induction of endoplasmic reticulum stress and unfolded protein response. Cancer Res. 2009;69:4235–4243. DOI: 10.1158/0008-5472.CAN-08-3439

[66] Catalá A. Lipid peroxidation of membrane phospholipids generates hydroxy-alkenals and oxidized phospholipids active in physiological and/or pathological conditions. Chem Phys Lipids. 2009;157:1–11. DOI: 10.1016/j.chemphyslip.2008.09.004

[67] Yukawa O, Nagatsuka S, Nakazawa T. Reconstitution studies on the involvement of radiation-induced lipid peroxidation in damage to membrane enzymes. Int J Radiat Biol Relat Stud Phys Chem Med. 1983;43(4):391–398. DOI: 10.1080/09553008314550451

[68] Hilf R. Mitochondria are targets of photodynamic therapy. J Bioenerg Biomembr. 2007;39(1):85–89. DOI: 10.1007/s10863-006-9064-8

[69] Wachowska M, Muchowicz A, Demkow U.Immunological aspects of antitumor photodynamic therapy outcome. Cent Eur J Immunol. 2015;40(4): 481–485. DOI: 10.5114/ceji.2015.56974

[70] Coupienne I, Fettweis G, Rubio N, Agostinis P, Piette J. 5-ALA-PDT induces RIP3-dependent necrosis in glioblastoma. Photochem Photobiol Sci. 2011;10(12):1868–1878. DOI: 10.1039/c1pp05213f

[71] Reiners JJ, Agostinis P, Berg K, Oleinick NL,Kessel DH. Assessing autophagy in the context of photodynamic therapy. Autophagy. 2010;6(1):7–18.

[72] Garg AD, Krysko DV, Vandenabeele P, Agostinis P. DAMPs and PDT-mediated photo-oxidative stress: exploring the unknown. Photochem Photobiol Sci. 2011;10(5):670–680. DOI: 10.1039/c0pp00294a.

[73] Mroz P, Hashmi JT, Huang YY, Lange N, Hamblin MR.Stimulation of anti-tumor immunity by photodynamic therapy. Expert Rev Clin Immunol. 2011;7(1):75–91. DOI: 10.1586/eci.10.81.

[74] Broekgaarden M, Weijer R, van Gulik TM, Hamblin MR, Heger M. Tumor cell survival pathways activated by photodynamictherapy: a molecular basis for pharmacologicalinhibition strategies. Cancer Metastasis Rev 2015;34:643–690. DOI: 10.1007/s10555-015-9588-7

[75] Gęgotek A, Skrzydlewska E. The role of transcription factor Nrf2 in skin cells metabolism. Arch Dermatol Res. 2015;307(5):385–396. DOI: 10.1007/s00403-015-1554-2

[76] Hoesel B, Schmid JA. The complexity of NF-κB signaling in inflammation and cancer. Mol Cancer. 2013;12:86. DOI: 10.1186/1476-4598-12-86

[77] Kim C, Pasparakis M. Epidermal p65/NF-κB signalling is essential for skin carcinogenesis. EMBO Mol Med. 2014; 6(7):970–983. DOI: 10.15252/emmm.201303541

[78] Yang J, Splittgerber R, Yull FE, Kantrow S, Ayers GD, Karin M, et al. Conditional ablation of Ikkb inhibits melanoma tumor development in mice. J Clin Invest. 2010;120:2563–2574. DOI: 10.1172/JCI42358.

[79] Singh M, Suman S, Shukla Y. New enlightenment of skin cancer chemoprevention through phytochemicals: in vitro and in vivo studies and the underlying mechanisms. Biomed Res Int. 2014;2014:243452. DOI: 10.1155/2014/243452

[80] Mitra S, Cassar SE, Niles DJ, Puskas JA, Frelinger JG, et al. Photodynamic therapy mediates the oxygen-independent activation of hypoxia-inducible factor 1α. Mol Cancer Ther. 2006;5:3268–3274. DOI: 10.1158/1535-7163.MCT-06-0421

[81] Tao JS, Sanghera JS, Pelech SL, Wong G, Levy JG. Stimulation of stress-activated protein kinase and p38HOG1 kinase in murine keratinocytes following photodynamic therapy with benzoporphyrin derivative. J Biol Chem. 1996;271(43):27107–27115.

[82] Hetz C. The unfolded protein response: controlling cell fate decisions under ER stress and beyond. Nat Rev Mol Cell Biol. 2012; 13(2):89–102. DOI: 10.1038/nrm3270

[83] Koumenis C. ER stress, hypoxia tolerance and tumor progression. Curr Mol Med. 2006;6:55–69.

[84] Dougherty TJ, Grindey GB, Fiel R, Weishaupt KR, Boyle DG. Photoradiation therapy. II. Cure of animal tumors with hematoporphyrin and light. J Natl Cancer Inst. 1975;55(1):115–121.

[85] Evans CL. Three-dimensional in vitro cancer spheroid models for photodynamic therapy: strengths and opportunities. Front Phys. 2015;3:15. DOI: 10.3389/fphy.2015.00015

[86] Chinembiri TN, du Plessis LH, Gerber M, Hamman JH, du Plessis J. Review of natural compounds for potential skin cancer treatment. Molecules. 2014;19:11679–11721. DOI: 10.3390/molecules190811679

[87] Popovic A, Wiggins T, Davids LM. Differential susceptibility of primary cultured human skin cells to hypericin PDT in an in vitro model. J Photochem Photobiol B. 2015;1(49):249–256. DOI: 10.1016/j.jphotobiol.2015.06.009

[88] Park SI, Hwang YH, Lim JH, Kim JH, Yun HI, Kim CO. Biological and thermic effects of magnetic fluids for photodynamic therapy and hyperthermia. J Magn Magn Mater. 2006; 304:e403–e405. DOI: 10.1016/j.jmmm.2006.01.204

[89] Bolfarini GC, Siqueira-Moura MP, Demets GJF, Morais PC, Tedesco AC. *In vitro* evaluation of combined hyperthermia and photodynamic effects using magnetoliposomes loaded with cucurbit [7]uril zinc phthalocyanine complex on melanoma. J Photochem Photobiol B. 2012;115:1–4. DOI: 10.1016/j.jphotobiol.2012.05.009

[90] McEwan C, Nesbitt H, Nicholas D, Kavanagh ON, McKenna K, Loan P, et al. Comparing the efficacy of photodynamic and sonodynamic therapy in non-melanoma and melanoma skin cancer. Bioorg Med Chem. 2016;24(13):3023–3028. DOI: 10.1016/j.bmc.2016.05.015

[91] Idris NM, Gnanasammandhan MK, Zhang J, Ho PC, Mahendran R, Zhang Y. In vivo photodynamic therapy using up conversion nanoparticles as remote-controlled nanotransducers. Nat Med. 2012;18(10):1580–1585. DOI: 10.1038/nm.2933

[92] Chen J, Shao R, Zhang XD, Chen C. Applications of nanotechnology for melanoma treatment, diagnosis, and theranostics. Int J Nanomedicine. 2013;8:2677–2688. DOI: 10.2147/IJN.S45429

[93] Cordwell SJ, Thingholm TE. Technologies for plasma membrane proteomics. Proteomics. 2010;10:611–627. DOI: 10.1002/pmic.200900521

[94] Franssen ME, Zeeuwen PL, Vierwinden G, Van De Kerkhof PC, Schalkwijk J, Van Erp PE. Phenotypical and functional differences in germinative subpopulations derived from normal and psoriatic epidermis. J Invest Dermatol. 2005;124(2):373–383. DOI: 10.1111/j.0022-202X.2004.23612.x

[95] Davies H, Bignell GR, Cox C, Stephens P, Edkins S, Clegg S, et al. Mutations of the BRAF gene in human cancer. Nature. 2002;417(6892):949–954. DOI: 10.1038/nature00766

[96] Medina T, Amaria MN, Jimeno A. Dabrafenib in the treatment of advanced melanoma. Drugs Today (Barc). 2013;49(6):377–385. DOI: 10.1358/dot.2013.49.6.1968669

[97] Mesri M. Advances in proteomic technologies and its contribution to the field of cancer. Adv Med. 2014;2014:238045. DOI: 10.1155/2014/238045

[98] Boja E, Hiltke T, Rivers R, Kinsinger C, Rahbar A, Mesri M, et al. Evolution of clinical proteomics and its role in medicine. J Proteome Res. 2011;10(1):66–84. DOI: 10.1021/pr100532g

[99] Roy P, Shukla Y. Applications of proteomic techniques in cancer research. Cancer Ther. 2008;6:841–856.

[100] von Felbert V, Bauerschlag D, Maass N, Bräutigam K, Meinhold-Heerlein I, Woitok M, et al. A specific photoimmunotheranostics agent to detect and eliminate skin cancer cells expressing EGFR. J Cancer Res Clin Oncol. 2016;142(5):1003–1011. DOI: 10.1007/s00432-016-2122-7

[101] Huang SK, Darfler MM, Nicholl MB, You J, Bemis KG, Tegeler TJ, et al. LC/MS-based quantitative proteomic analysis of paraffin-embedded archival melanomas reveals potential proteomic biomarkers associated with metastasis. PLoS One. 2009;4(2):e4430. DOI: 10.1371/journal.pone.0004430

[102] Griffin NM, Yu J, Long F, Oh P, Shore S, Li Y, et al. Label-free, normalized quantification of complex mass spectrometry data for proteomic analysis. Nat Biotechnol. 2010;28(1):83–89. DOI: 10.1038/nbt.1592

[103] Wilson LL, Tran L, Morton DL, Hoon DS. Detection of differentially expressed proteins in early-stage melanoma patients using SELDI-TOF mass spectrometry. Ann N Y Acad Sci. 2004;1022:317–322. DOI: 10.1196/annals.1318.047

[104] Zhou M, Veenstra TD. Mass spectrometry: m/z 1983–2008. Biotechniques. 2008;44(5):667–668, 670. DOI: 10.2144/000112791

[105] Helander L, Sharma A, Krokan HE, Plaetzer K, Krammer B, Tortik N, et al. Photodynamic treatment with hexyl-aminolevulinate mediates reversible thiol oxidation in core oxidative stress signaling proteins. Mol Biosyst. 2016;12(3):796–805. DOI: 10.1039/c5mb00744e

[106] Tu S, Jiang HW, Liu CX, Zhou SM, Tao SC. Protein microarrays for studies of drug mechanisms and biomarker discovery in the era of systems biology. Curr Pharm Des. 2014;20(1):49–55.

[107] Matei C, Tampa M, Caruntu C, Ion RM, Georgescu SR, Dumitrascu GR, et al. Protein microarray for complex apoptosis monitoring of dysplastic oral keratinocytes in experimental photodynamic therapy. Biol Res. 2014;47:33. DOI: 10.1186/0717-6287-47-33

Chapter 2

Pleural Photodynamic Therapy and Surgery in Thoracic Cancer Patients with Pleural Spread

Ke-Cheng Chen and Jang-Ming Lee

Additional information is available at the end of the chapter

http://dx.doi.org/10.5772/intechopen.68722

Abstract

Pleural spread from non-small cell lung cancer is a difficult situation. The average survival in the situation is about 6–9 months. We investigate the current management of this challenging condition. Although, there is no much evidence found in the literature, we do see the pleural photodynamic therapy giving some promising light in the dark night. However, the patients still require complete neoadjuvant and adjuvant therapies, as well as radical tumor resection. Pleural PDT is one of the multi-modality treatments, which combined can achieve satisfactory oncological results. The long-term survival can be achieved in more than half the patients. However, the side effects of pleural PDT include skin hypersensitivity, trachea and esophageal perforation, and ARDS, which we should keep in mind.

Keywords: PDT, lung cancer, thymic cancer, pleural spread

1. Introduction

Photodynamic therapy (PDT) is one of the established treatment modality for non-small cell lung cancer (NSCLC). Early-stage lung cancer and superficial endobronchial lesions less than 1 cm in thickness can be effectively treated with external light sources. Thicker lesions and peripheral lesions may be amenable to interstitial PDT, where the light is delivered intratumorally. The primary adverse event, phototoxicity, is expected to be minimized with the introduction of new photosensitizers that have shown promising results in phase I and II clinical studies. Moreover, the addition of PDT to standard-of-care surgery and chemotherapy (or target therapy) can improve survival and outcomes in patients with pleural dissemination. Therefore, intra-operative PDT has shown promise in the treatment of non-small cell lung cancer with pleural spread.

The presence of pleural spread in non-small cell lung cancer (NSCLC) without distant metastases was classified as stage III b in the previous International System for Staging Lung Cancer [1]. The seventh edition of the TNM classification of lung cancer was published in 2009, and the changes to the sixth edition of this document were according to proposals from the International Association for the Study of Lung Cancer (IASLC). The IASLC lung cancer staging project committee suggested that pleural disseminations (pleural nodules or malignant pleural effusions) be reclassified to M1a from T4. In patients with pleural carcinomatosis, the reported median survival time ranged from 6 to 9 months [2–8]. Currently, the management options for pleural spread include chemotherapy, surgery with pleurectomy, and photodynamic therapy. Thymomas are neoplasms arising from epithelial thymic cells. They rarely metastasize to distant sites; on the contrary, they more often show pleural implantation at diagnosis or during follow-up. Thymoma with pleural spread is also a difficult clinical situation to manage, and the treatment is controversial [9–11].

Photodynamic therapy (PDT) is an anticancer treatment combining photosensitizer, oxygen, and visible light. PDT anticancer effect occurs when the photosensitizer captures light energy and transfers that energy to oxygen. The excited oxygen species are responsible for the effect and can directly kill tumor cells, damage the tumor blood supply, or both [10]. Porfimer sodium (Photofrin; Axcan Pharma Inc, Birmingham, AL, USA), a first-generation photosensitizer that is a mixture of porphyrin monomers and oligomers, is used most often. They are activated by 630 nm red light. Successful treatment of malignant mesothelioma by photodynamic therapy has been reported as a new approach for pleural malignancy dissemination [12]. Moreover, as with malignant pleural mesothelioma, PDT may be utilized as part of a multi-modality management strategy for non-small cell lung cancer with pleural spread. A phase II trial enrolling 22 patients with pleural spread and clinical T4 NSCLC was conducted in which patients underwent surgery with complete or partial tumor debulking, followed by hemithoracic pleural PDT or PDT alone. The median overall survival was 21.7 months, compared with 6–9 months for similar patients based on historical controls [13].

2. Operative procedures

Thoracotomy was performed for either multiple wedge resection or lobectomy. The particular pulmonary resection was chosen by the same criteria as those used for performing resections with curative intent in patients with early lung cancer. Anatomic resections (pneumonectomy, lobectomy, or segmentectomy) were performed only in patients in whom it was possible to resect all gross disease. After finishing lung resection, total parietal pleurectomy was performed subsequently. The parietal pleura were stripped from the bony hemithorax as radical parietal pleurectomy. The mediastinum was debulked of all gross tumor. For thymoma patients, the radical thymothymectomy was performed concurrent with radical pleural pleurectomy. The goal was to have no visible or palpable tumor left in the affected hemithorax at the end of the operation [14].

We sewed flat photodiodes into seven regions of the pleural space, which include the apex, anterior chest wall, posterior chest wall, posterior costophrenic sulcus, anterior costophrenic sulcus, posterior mediastinum, and pericardium. Moreover, we handle it with a dosimetry system. The dosimetry system provided both the real-time luminescence and the cumulative

http://dx.doi.org/10.5772/intechopen.68722

light dose for the seven regions. The cavity was filled with diluted intralipid solution (0.01%) to act as scattering agent, giving a more homogeneous light delivery. The light was delivered with an optical fiber sheathed within a modified endotracheal tube. This delivery system was moved around the chest cavity until a measured dose of 40 J/cm^2 of 630 nm light was recorded at all seven regions (**Figures 1** and **2**). During the light delivery of PDT, the chest retractors were removed to avoid shielding. We use 20 L of intralipid solution to maintain a clear intrathoracic area and to minimize light absorption affected by hemoglobin. Sterile photodiodes were removed from the pleural cavity after completion of light administration. The overall time of the light delivery portion of PDT was about 1 h. Then, the operation is completed after wound closure and setting two 28 fr chest tubes.

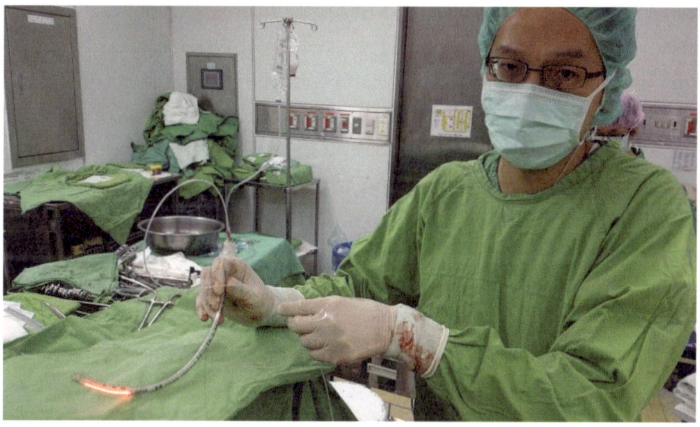

Figure 1. The operator and the 630 nm light source. The operator is hoding the laser light source which can activate the photosensitizer in tumor cells. The laser probe is within the endotracheal tube which enhance the convenience of irradiation in the pleural space.

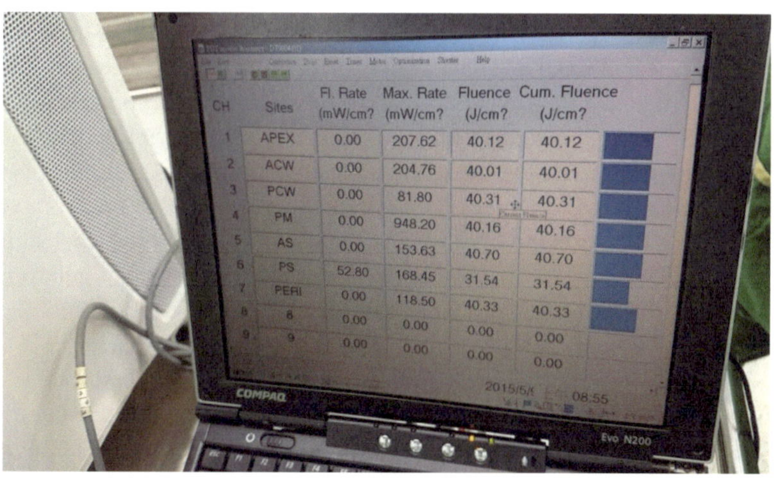

Figure 2. The dosimetry system. The dosimetry system provided both the real-time luminescence and the cumulative light dose for the seven regions.

3. Comments

The pleural spread of thoracic malignancy is difficult to manage. The standard care of the condition is non-operative worldwide. Currently, surgery is not considered part of the treatment for these patients. It is usually treated with palliative chemotherapy but is barely cured. Surgery alone has been ineffective in treating cancer with pleural dissemination because residual microscopic disease remains in the chest cavity, even after what appears to be a "complete" resection [2–8]. Photodynamic therapy offers several potential advantages for treating disseminating surface cancer. First, preclinical studies demonstrate a greater retention of photosensitizers in tumor compared with normal tissues [15]. Second, the PDT penetrates several millimeters into tissue. It results in surface cell killing, while sparing the underlying tissues. Therefore, PDT is suitable for the treatment of cancers that have spread to organ surfaces, including pleura or peritoneum [16, 17]. Moreover, PDT is a localized therapy that can be performed intraoperatively. Intraoperative pleural PDT was used as one of the multimodal approaches for treating patients with pleural carcinomatosis. The hypothesis was that, upon complete resection of all gross disease, immediate intraoperative PDT might be effective in treating the residual microscopic disease. For lung cancer, the phase II trial at the University of Pennsylvania proved our point of view. It showed 73.3% of 6-month localized disease control for the cohort and a median overall survival of 21.7 months, compared with 6–9 months survival for similar patients treated with the non-operative standard of care and based upon historical controls [13]. Compared with surgery without PDT for patients of lung cancer with pleural spread in literature, the outcome of patients receiving surgery plus PDT is better [18, 19]. The best median overall survival of the lung cancer patients was 39.0 months, conducted by our group (**Figure 3**) [20]. The comparison of these results is listed in **Table 1**. Therefore, we found that the result was good, and the morbidity was acceptable. However, the PDT is only one of the multi-modality treatments, so the adjuvant or neoadjuvant therapy is important, too. Our group conducted another experiment about the significance of the Epidermal Growth Factor Receptor (EGFR) profile to the PDT-sensitive cancer cells [21]. Because tyrosine kinase inhibitor (TKI) was popularly used in the advanced lung cancer, we investigated the roles of this two common therapies combined. Although photodynamic therapy (PDT) has been demonstrated to be an effective minimally invasive treatment modality for thoracic cancer, the molecular action in thoracic cancer during PDT is hardly known. EGFR has been known to downregulate in various cancer cells during PDT. In the study, we investigated the effects of Photofrin-mediated PDT on cell death and expression of EGFR in CE48T/VGH (CE48T) squamous carcinoma cells. We found that the photosensitizer Photofrin in the absence of light exposure can downregulate the expression of EGFR at both transcription and translation levels. Higher concentrations of Photofrin result in cytotoxicity, whereas lower doses of Photofrin inhibit EGFR expression under dark control without inducing significant cell death. This Photofrin-associated inhibition of EGFR was repeated in lung cancer, cervical cancer, and glioblastoma cells. Another squamous cell carcinoma cell line CE81T/VGH (CE81T) was found to be resistant to Photofrin-induced inhibition of EGFR as well as to Photofrin-mediated dark toxicity compared with CE48T. The resistance to the cytotoxicity in CE81T cells became insignificant when the Photofrin-treated cells were further irradiated by red light (Photofrin-PDT). We suggest Photofrin modulates the expression of EGFR in cancer cells. However, efficient cell death still requires the combination of Photofrin and light irradiation in squamous cell carcinoma cells.

http://dx.doi.org/10.5772/intechopen.68722

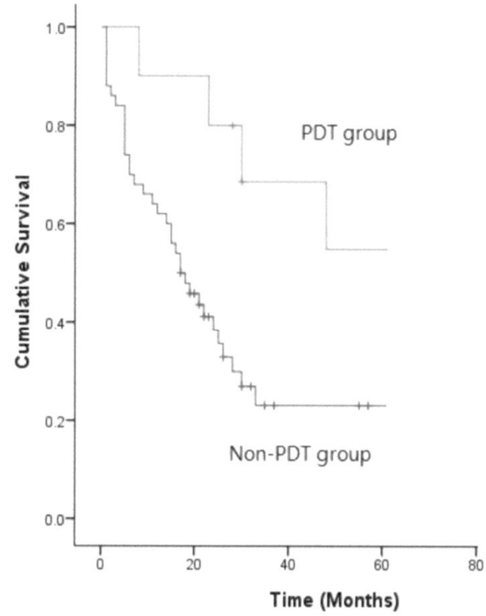

Figure 3. Kaplan-Meier survival analysis of the patients undergoing PDT vs. non-PDT for pleural spread (P = 0.047).

Studies	Year	Country	Mean age ± SD (years)	No. of patients	5-year survival rate (%)
Wang et al.	2011	Taiwan	62.3 ± 11.2	90	21.7
Mordant et al.	2011	France	59.0 ± 8.8	32	16.0
Chen et al.	2013	Taiwan	51.9 ± 11.9	10	56.3

Table 1. Comparison with other series for lung cancer patients.

4. Conclusion

Photodynamic therapy is a promising treatment modality for thoracic malignancy. With proper patient selection, intrapleural photodynamic therapy for pleural spread in patients with lung cancer or thymoma is feasible and may provide a survival benefit.

Author details

Ke-Cheng Chen and Jang-Ming Lee*

*Address all correspondence to: jangminglee@gmail.com

Department of Surgery, National Taiwan University Hospital, Taipei, Taiwan

References

[1] Mountain CF. Revisions in the international system for staging lung cancer. Chest. 1997;**111**(6):1710–1717

[2] Werner-Wasik M, Scott C, Cox JD, Sause WT, Byhardt RW, et al. Recursive partitioning analysis of 1999 Radiation Therapy Oncology Group (RTOG) patients with locally advanced non-small-cell lung cancer (LANSCLC): Identification of five groups with different survival. International Journal of Radiation Oncology Biology Physics. 2000;**48**(5): 1475–1482

[3] Martini N, Bains MS, Beattie EJ Jr. Indications for pleurectomy in malignant effusion. Cancer. 1975;**35**(3):734–738

[4] Reyes L, Parvez Z, Regal AM, Takita H. Neoadjuvant chemotherapy and operations in the treatment of lung cancer with pleural effusion. The Journal of Thoracic and Cardiovascular Surgery. 1991;**101**(5):946–947

[5] Mott FE, Sharma N, Ashley P. Malignant pleural effusion in non-small cell lung cancer--time for a stage revision? Chest. 2001;**119**(1):317–318

[6] Rami-Porta R, Ball D, Crowley J, Giroux DJ, Jett J, et al. The IASLC Lung Cancer Staging Project: Proposals for the revision of the T descriptors in the forthcoming (seventh) edition of the TNM classification for lung cancer. Journal of Thoracic Oncology. 2007;**2**(7):593–602

[7] Postmus PE, Brambilla E, Chansky K, Crowley J, Goldstraw P, et al. The IASLC Lung Cancer Staging Project: Proposals for revision of the M descriptors in the forthcoming (seventh) edition of the TNM classification of lung cancer. Journal of Thoracic Oncology. 2007;**2**(8):686–693

[8] Goldstraw P, Crowley J, Chansky K, Giroux DJ, Groome PA, et al. The IASLC Lung Cancer Staging Project: Proposals for the revision of the TNM stage groupings in the forthcoming (seventh) edition of the TNM Classification of malignant tumours. Journal of Thoracic Oncology. 2007;**2**(8):706–714

[9] Lucchi M, Davini F, Ricciardi R, Duranti L, Boldrini L, et al. Management of pleural recurrence after curative resection of thymoma. The Journal of Thoracic and Cardiovascular Surgery. 2009;**137**(5):1185–1189

[10] Yu L, Jing Y, Ma S, Li F, Zhang YF. Cytoreductive surgery combined with hyperthermic intrapleural chemotherapy to treat thymoma or thymic carcinoma with pleural dissemination. OncoTargets and Therapy. 2013;**6**:517–521

[11] Ishikawa Y, Matsuguma H, Nakahara R, Suzuki H, Ui A, et al. Multimodality therapy for patients with invasive thymoma disseminated into the pleural cavity: The potential role of extrapleural pneumonectomy. The Annals of Thoracic Surgery. 2009;**88**(3):952–957

[12] Friedberg JS, Culligan MJ, Mick R, Stevenson J, Hahn SM, et al. Radical pleurectomy and intraoperative photodynamic therapy for malignant pleural mesothelioma. The Annals of Thoracic Surgery. 2012;**93**(5):1658–1665

[13] Friedberg JS, Mick R, Stevenson JP, Zhu T, Busch TM, et al. Phase II trial of pleural photodynamic therapy and surgery for patients with non-small-cell lung cancer with pleural spread. Journal of Clinical Oncology. 2004;**22**(11):2192–2201

[14] Liu TJ, Lin MW, Hsieh MS, Kao MW, Chen KC, et al. Video-assisted thoracoscopic surgical thymectomy to treat early thymoma: A comparison with the conventional transsternal approach. Annals of Surgical Oncology. 2014;**21**(1):322–328

[15] Gomer CJ, Dougherty TJ. Determination of [3H]- and [14C]hematoporphyrin derivative distribution in malignant and normal tissue. Cancer Research. 1979;**39**(1):146–151

[16] Dougherty TJ, Gomer CJ, Henderson BW, Jori G, Kessel D, et al. Photodynamic therapy. Journal of the National Cancer Institute. 1998;**90**(12):889–905

[17] Hahn S, Glatstein E. The emergence of photodynamic therapy as a major modality in cancer treatment. Reviews in Contemporary Pharmacotherapy. 1999;**10**:69–74

[18] Wang BY, Wu YC, Hung JJ, Hsu PK, Hsieh CC, et al. Prognosis of non-small-cell lung cancer with unexpected pleural spread at thoracotomy. Journal of Surgical Research. 2011;**169**(1):e1–e5

[19] Mordant P, Arame A, Foucault C, Dujon A, Le Pimpec Barthes F, et al. Surgery for metastatic pleural extension of non-small-cell lung cancer. European Journal of Cardio-Thoracic Surgery. 2011;**40**(6):1444–1449

[20] Chen KC, Hsieh YS, Tseng YF, Shieh MJ, Chen JS, Lai HS, Lee JM. Pleural photodynamic therapy and surgery in lung cancer. Plos One. 2015;**10**(7):e0133230. DOI: 10.1371/journal.pone.0133230. eCollection 2015

[21] Yang P-W, Hung M-C, Hsieh C-Y, Tung E-C, Wang Y-H, Tsai J-C, Lee J-W. The effects of Photofrin-mediated photodynamic therapy on the modulation of EGFR in esophageal squamous cell carcinoma cells. Lasers in Medical Science. 2013;**28**(2):605–614. DOI: 10.1007/s10103-012-1119-y. Epub 2012 May 15

Chapter 3

Photodynamic Therapy

Wei Liu and Hong Cai

Additional information is available at the end of the chapter

http://dx.doi.org/10.5772/66420

Abstract

Photodynamic therapy (PDT) employs light activation of tissue-localized photosensitizer in an oxygen-dependent process which initiates oxidative stress, inflammation, and cell death. Photodynamic therapy (PDT) involves the activation of a previously administered photosensitizing agent by visible light to induce tumor necrosis. Photosensitizers are topically applied in the treatment of skin tumors to avoid systemic side effects. The main dermatology indications for topical PDT are superficial nonmelanoma skin cancer and dysplasia, notably superficial basal carcinoma (BCC), Bowen's disease (BD), and actinic keratosis (AK). In this chapter, we evaluated the feasibility and efficacy of aminolevulinic acid (ALA) as a photosensitizer (ALA-PDT) in combination with CO_2 laser in the treatment of dermatological disease from basics to clinic research.

Keywords: photodynamic therapy, photosensitizer, Bowen's disease, actinic keratosis, aminolevulinic acid

1. Photodynamic therapy for actinic keratoses

Skin aging is often divided into natural aging and photoaging. Photoaging is caused by excessive exposure to the ultraviolet (UV) irradiation. The skin becomes thick and rough, with coarse wrinkles, mottled pigmentation, and precancerous lesions, including actinic keratoses (AK). Actinic keratosis (AK) is a growth of dysplastic cells within the epidermis that presents clinically with a scaly localized macule or papule on chronically sun-exposed skin [1]. Over the last few years, the relationship between AK and SCC has been a topic for much debate in the literature, as AK is believed not to be a separate entity but an SCC *in situ*.

Some researchers also consider actinic keratoses equivalent to squamous cell carcinoma (SCC). Yet, SCC is capable of metastasis [2, 3]. So it can be life threatening. AK is a precancerous lesion, therefore should be treated early. There are a lot of methods for AK, while not all treatments are appropriate for all patients or lesions, especially cosmetic outcome may be generally less than optimal [4, 5]. The ideal treatment for AKs should be effective, well tolerated, and have an excellent cosmetic outcome, particularly in cosmetic-sensitive areas such as the face.

Photodynamic therapy (PDT) has been under development for the treatment of various tumors by the end of the 1970s. Topical ALA-PDT was originally used for superficial non-melanoma skin cancers and their precursors. However, other benign diseases, such as acne vulgaris, sebaceous gland hyperplasia, and hidradenitis suppurativa, have been shown to improve with this treatment. Photodynamic therapy (PDT) is an alternative, minimally invasive treatment. Oxygen, photosensitizer, and light are the three principal elements of PDT. When illuminated by a light source with an appropriate wavelength, the photosensitizer is activated and will react with oxygen to produce singlet oxygen and reactive oxygen species (ROS) to cause the selective destruction of target tissues [6]. As a metabolic precursor of endogenous porphyrins in heme biosynthesis, the absorption of 5-ALA induces the production and accumulation of protoporphyrin IX (Pp IX), a fluorescent substance that is as effective as a light sensitive agent (408, 506, 532, 580, and 635 nm).

An ideal treatment for AK would only affect lesional skin, leaving normal surrounding skin unharmed. In the 1990s, Kennedy et al. using topic 5-aminolaevulinic acid (5-ALA) that has restricted the phototoxicity at the application site. Since AK lesions are capable of selectively accumulating PPIX, they are excellent targets for PDT.

Forty-two patients with a total of 56 AK lesions on the face were enrolled in our study. The 5-ALA (Zhangjiang, China) was prepared at a concentration of 20% in physiological saline. A thick layer of the formulation was applied to cover the AK lesions for 5 h. Then the lesions were illuminated by laser (λ = 630 nm, light dose 100 mW/cm^2) for 30 minutes All patients were reviewed in at least 2-week intervals. The response to the PDT was evaluated 1 month after the therapy, and treatment is repeated if necessary [7].

Initially, AKs lesions were detected among the patients (**Figure 1**). The treated skin lesions were evaluated macroscopically at several time points following the treatment. Immediately after ALA-PDT, it showed limited edema and erythema in the treated area. Conversely, the lesions were covered with necrotic tissue after 1 day. A red granulation tissue developed after 4–7 days and gradually atrophic flatten (**Figure 2**). Afterwards, a pink-red contracted atrophic scar could be observed that progressively healed after 3 weeks. All the 56 lesions from 42 patients showed a complete response by histologic examination (remission rate, 85.71%) 1 month after PDT treatment. The epidermis of the photodamaged skin became thinner and more even. Clinically, there was no significant scarring or pigmentary changes after treatment (**Figure 3**).

There were six patients with persistent lesions, the six patients with eight lesions received one or two additional PDT treatments; the AKs in the follow-up biopsy resolved, and the lesions were all cleared in the end.

Before treatment, histopathological analysis of the lesions showed the presence of atypical keratinocytes characteristic for AK (**Figure 4**). After treatment, the epidermis of the

http://dx.doi.org/10.5772/66420

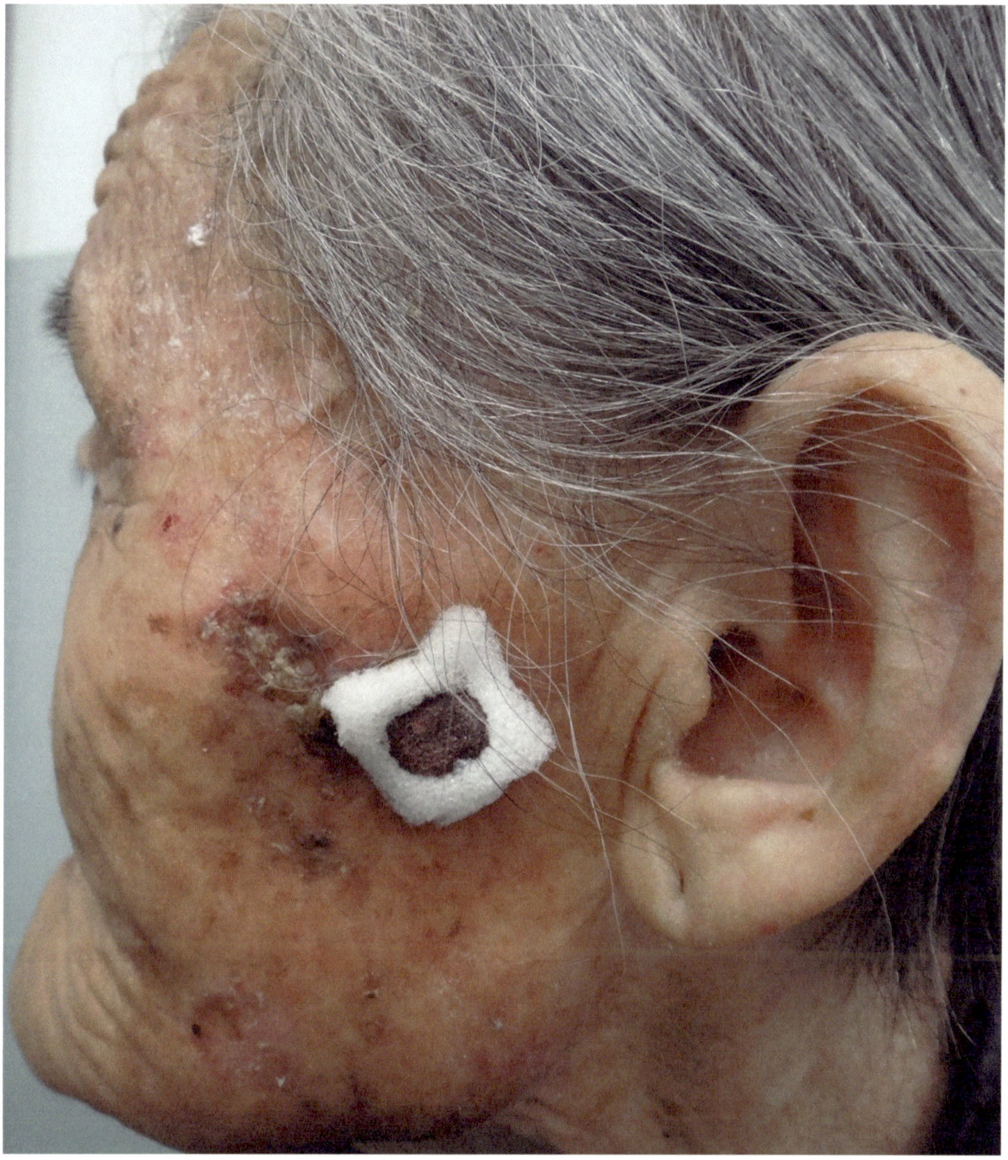

Figure 1. After biopsy.

photodamaged skin became thinner and more even, and the skin structure in responsive lesions had returned to normal and the atypical cells of AK were replaced by normal keratinocytes (**Figure 5**). The epidermis was fully regenerated by day 30 following PDT.

The facial lesions' mean epidermal thickness significantly decreased from 155.22 ± 70.45 to 74.35 ± 18.65 μm after treatment ($P < 0.05$) (**Figure 6**). We can observe a large number of infiltrating cells in the dermis before the treatment, and those were significantly reduced after treatment. In 5 h of 5-ALA occlusive treatment, there were no reports of irritation, local or

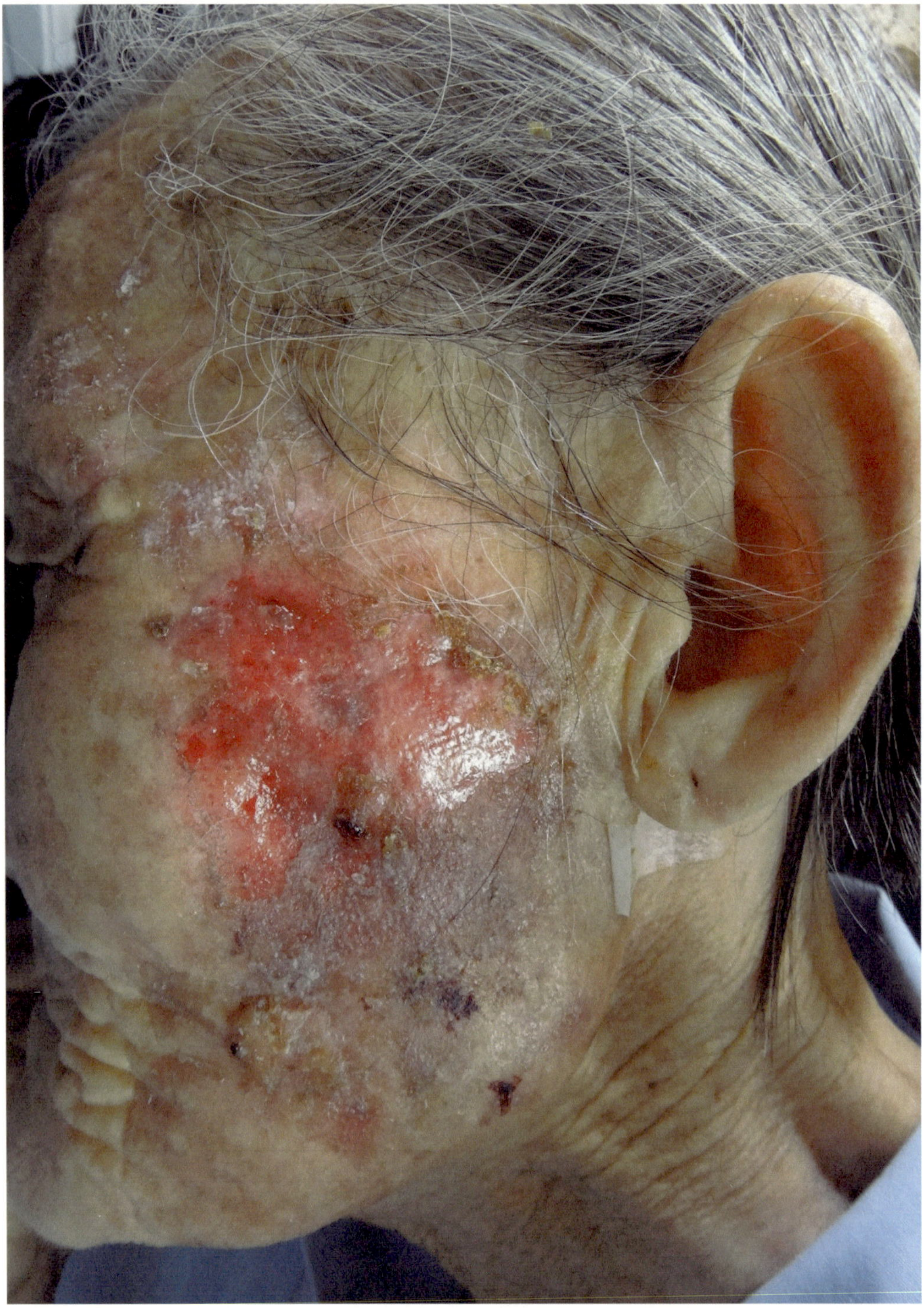

Figure 2. 1 week after PDT.

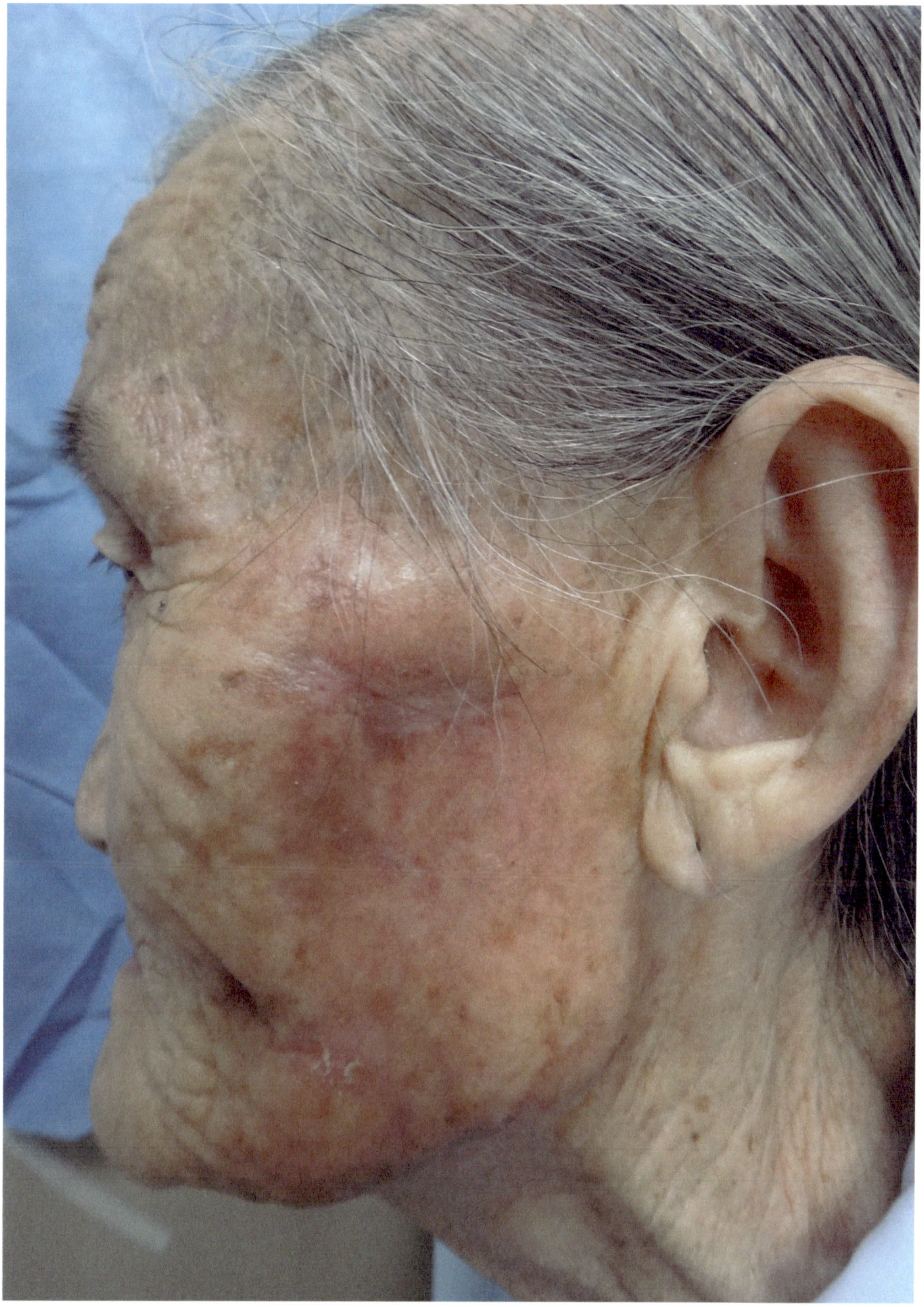

Figure 3. 1 month after PDT.

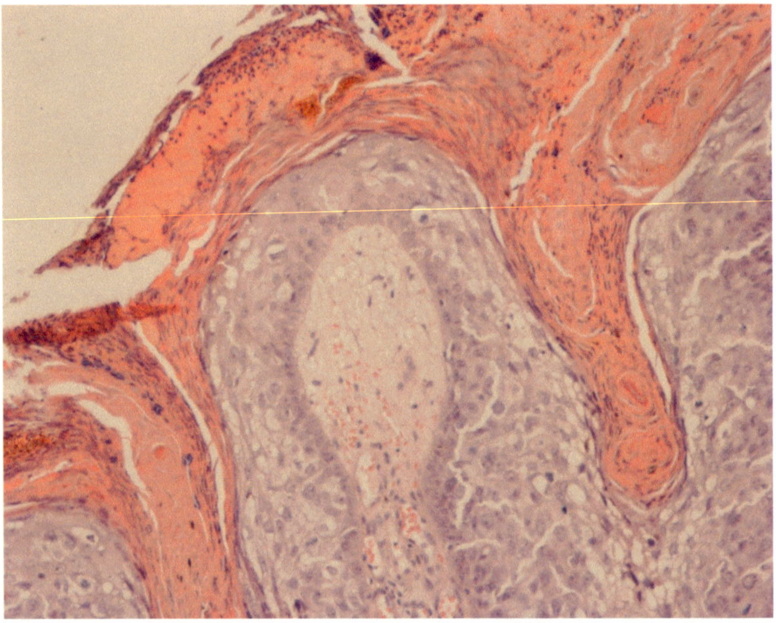

Figure 4. Before PDT.

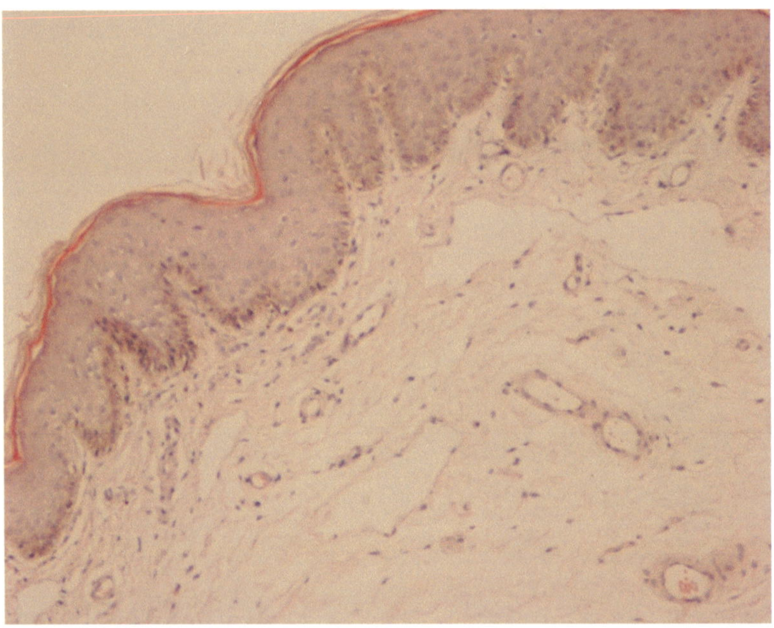

Figure 5. After PDT.

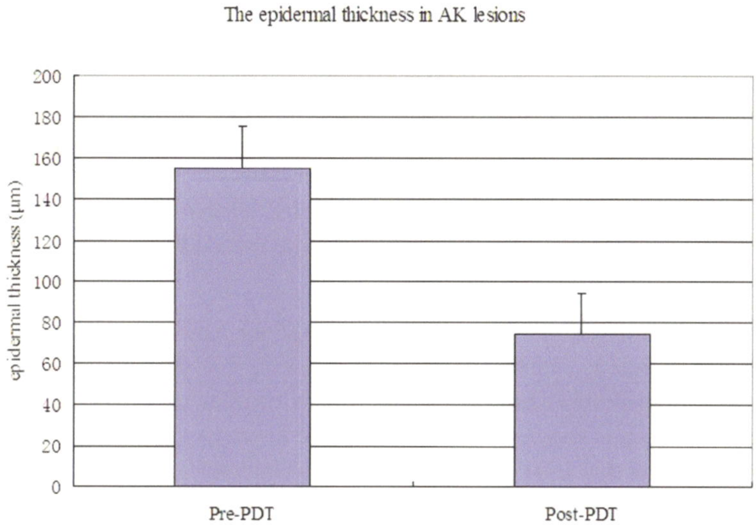

Figure 6. Epidermal thickness.

systemic light sensitization reaction. During the exposure to the light source all patients complained about a burning sensation, ranging from light to intense. During the treatment, variable degrees of erythema, blistering and edema occurred, all of these events were of short duration and completely reversible. During the treatment, it was possible to see progressive and evident edema and erythema on the application site. Despite the pain, none of the patients asked or interrupted the light exposition treatment.

The cosmetic outcome in all cured AKs was excellent, except for one patient; after additional sun exposure, postinflammatory hyperpigmentation developed. The method of topical application of ALA is a minimally invasive treatment. Photosensitizer's metabolic cycle is very quick, the period of photosenisitization is short, and can give good cosmetic effect.

The investigations of the action of light on living organisms began in the nineteenth century. Since Dougherty [8] in the 1970s began clinical trials for photodynamic destruction of cutaneous and subcutaneous malignancies, PDT has been used to treat esophageal [9], laryngeal, endobronchial, gastrointestinal, genitourinary, nervous, head and neck [10], oral leucoplakia, and skin malignancies [11].

Photodynamic therapy (PDT) is an oxygen-dependent process involving the use of a photosensitizing drug which accumulates in diseased tissue. The main topical agents used in dermatology are 20% 5-aminolaevulinic acid (ALA). It produced porphyrins via the heme biosynthetic pathway. It is an endogenous chemical, which participates in heme biosynthesis in the body. As a precursor of the hemoglobin content, its production has strong photosensitive function after the activation of ALA anhydrase and a series of enzymes. Porphyrin IX (protoporphyrin IX, Pp IX) is the last step of heme biosynthesis intermediate [12]. Under normal circumstances, heme biosynthesis pathway by regulating the body negative feedback mechanism, the synthesis of ALA is regulated by the hemoglobin content in the cell, so there will not be too much ALA accumulation in the body. When given overdoses of exogenous ALA, it can increase the intracellular concentration of Pp IX to therapeutically useful concentrations. Photoactivation by visible light results in cell damage of targeted abnormal cells while preserving normal structures. This effect of PDT is connected with direct photochemical reactions mediated by singlet oxygen and other reactive species. The cooperation of photosensitizing substances with light leads to the release of cytotoxic substances. It has been described that tumor destruction of PDT is connected with indirect effects of PDT: blood vessel occlusion within vascularized tumors. These effects demonstrated [9] that PDT induces apoptosis and vascular endothelial damage [13, 14]. It has also been mediated by the release of prostaglandin E2 (PGE2) and cytokines (IL-2, IL- 1, TNF).

In this study, we observed pre- and post- ALA-PDT specimens for AK and determined whether ALA-PDT induced histologic changes reversing the destructive connective tissue events. Normally, we selected 1 month after the PDT as the point time to evaluate the histologic changes for lots of results showing this time point of the assessment might be an important consideration. The fact that 1–20% of AKs progress to squamous cell carcinoma and approximately 60% of all squamous cell carcinomas develop from AKs underscores the importance of early treatment of AKs [3]. Our findings showed approximately 85% of AKs are already cured after a single PDT exposure. As a result, the majority of patients need only one treatment, and we only performed one PDT session followed by clinical examinations at 1 and 3 months after PDT. Only those lesions that showed an incomplete response need further treatment.

- The results of this study provide histologic evidence supporting the beneficial effects of ALA-PDT for photodamaged skin. PDT appears to be a more feasible alternative to conventional therapy of skin malignancies. Our results showed that the thickness of epidermis decreased significantly after ALA-PDT. We could see hyperkeratosis, stratum spinosum hypertrophy before the treatment. And the acanthocyte arranged in disorder. There are atypical keratinocytes in the central of the epidermis. We evaluated the histologic changes 1 month after the PDT, suggesting that the point in time of the assessment might be an important consideration. The epidermis was fully regenerated by day 30 following PDT. After treatment, the epidermis of the photodamaged skin became thinner and more even, and the skin structure in responsive lesions had returned to normal and the atypical cells of epidermis were replaced by normal keratinocyte [7]. Although the light source itself might affect the histologic changes in AKs, we still consider that ALA-PDT is the most important reason leading to the histologic changes in the present study where the light energy is very low.

Topically applied photosensitizers are preferred for dermatological PDT because of the reduced risk for prolonged skin photosensitivity. As we all know, topical application of ALA is a minimally invasive treatment. It has a short photosenisitization period, can treat multiple lesions at the same time, and can give good cosmetic effect. Studies have shown that the depth of penetration for most tissues using 630 nm light is about 1 cm [15, 16]. This percutaneous penetration is the most important factor influencing response rates for topical ALA PDT. Photodynamic therapy is associated with epidermal necrosis and dermal inflammation, which in turn gives a series of side effects in dermatology, including pain, ecchymosis, ulceration, and blistering [17].

Selective photodynamic destruction of treated premalignant and malignant areas without injury of normal tissue, ability to repeat PDT without loss of normal tissue proves PDT to be a more acceptable option than surgical resection. At the same time, laser-induced PDT almost left no obvious scar in our study. Patients treated with PDT may also benefit from minimal invasiveness, low recurrence, as well as excellent cosmetic effects in premalignant and malignant lesions of the skin.

The present study is limited by the follow-up time. In our study at 1 and 3 months after PDT, previous reports are in good agreement with the overall CR rates of 85.71 and 100% that were found, respectively. However, there are still existed residual malignant cells in the epidermis but not apparent by visual inspection. It will lead to clinical recurrence of the AKs at a later examination if the malignant cells continue to proliferate. That is the important reason why we need to observe the clearance rate after PDT for a long follow-up time.

In conclusion, the results of this study provide histologic evidence supporting the beneficial effects of PDT for AK. PDT using topical ALA was a safe and effective treatment for actinic keratoses with an excellent cosmetic outcome. It is a promising treatment that could benefit from further study. Topical PDT for AKs is now a well-established treatment modality that showed easy handling of 5-ALA administration with excellent efficacy and safety results.

2. Photodynamic therapy for the treatment of Bowen's disease

Bowen's disease (BD), or squamous cell carcinoma *in situ*, usually presents as a well-defined erythematous plaque on photoexposed sites [18]. Although any body part can be involved, BD lesions are common on the head and neck and lower limbs. The diagnosis is often delayed because of the symptoms are often untypical. The early skin changes may often appear to be eczema, tinea corporis, and psoriasis. Therefore, pathological diagnosis might be necessary when clinical differentiation between these diseases is difficult [3].

BD is a more aggressive form of intraepidermal (*in situ*) squamous cell carcinoma. Risk factors for BD include fair skin, protracted sunlight damage, radiation exposure, immune compromise and human papillomavirus infection [19]. Most BD lesions are found in the elderly patients commonly at high risk for surgery.

Several equally efficacious treatment options are available for the treatment of BD including conventional surgery, Mohs' surgery, cryosurgery, and CO_2 laser. However, it is not indicated for patients with numerous or large lesions such as those located in face. Alternative treatments are needed to treat superficial malignancies on nose, ear, and other sites. CO_2 laser vaporizes lesional tissues by thermal effects and causes minimal injuries, but it often fails to entirely remove lesions, especially those invisible or infiltrating into adjacent tissues, resulting in disease persistence and recurrence.

Topical 5-aminolevulinic acid-mediated photodynamic therapy (ALA-PDT) is a minimally invasive procedure, represents a relatively new treatment modality, and, with some unique features, it is especially suitable for the local treatment of superficial epithelial disorders. It causes less damage to normal tissues than surgical treatment, radiation therapy, or chemotherapy. In addition, since PDT does not produce cumulative effect and systemic phototoxicity, it allows repetitive treatments for new, partially responding or recurrent lesions. In this study, ALA-PDT treatment was performed following local pretreatment with CO_2 laser. By the pretreatment, we could enhance photosensitizer absorption, reduce the thickness of the BD lesion, and even increase the penetration depth of the irradiation, to achieve a multiplier effect [20].

Twenty-two lesions from 18 patients were randomized into two groups [21]; 11 lesions were treated with CO_2 laser alone, serving as control group. The remaining 11 lesions were treated with topical ALA-PDT (180 J/cm^2 at 100 mW/cm^2) + CO_2 laser for 1–3 sessions.

Biopsies were taken from BD lesions prior to treatment. BD is histopathologically characterized by the presence of atypical keratinocytes (**Figure 7**). Skin biopsies from the erythematous plaque exhibited proliferation of atypical squamous cells across the entire thickness of the epidermis and the BD diagnosis was based on the finding. The initial evaluation was undertaken 1 month after treatment and biopsies were harvested for histological evaluation. The epidermis fully regenerated in the point of 30 days after ALA-PDT + CO_2 laser treatment. The epidermis of the BD lesion became thinner and more even following the treatment. Moreover, the atypical BD cells were replaced by normal keratinocytes and the skin structure in responsive lesions returned to normal (**Figure 8**). All patients were reviewed at ≤1-week intervals. Patients who did not respond to the three sessions of treatment were referred to surgical treatment [21].

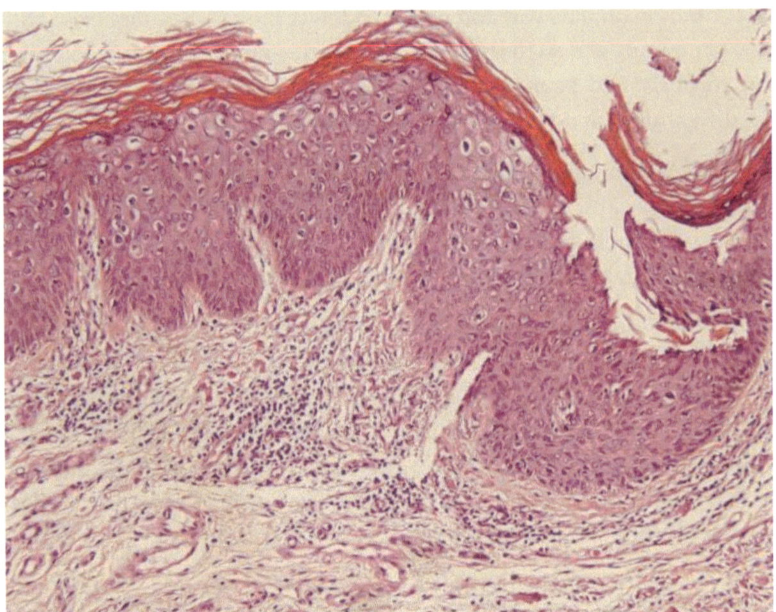

Figure 7. Before PDT (×20).

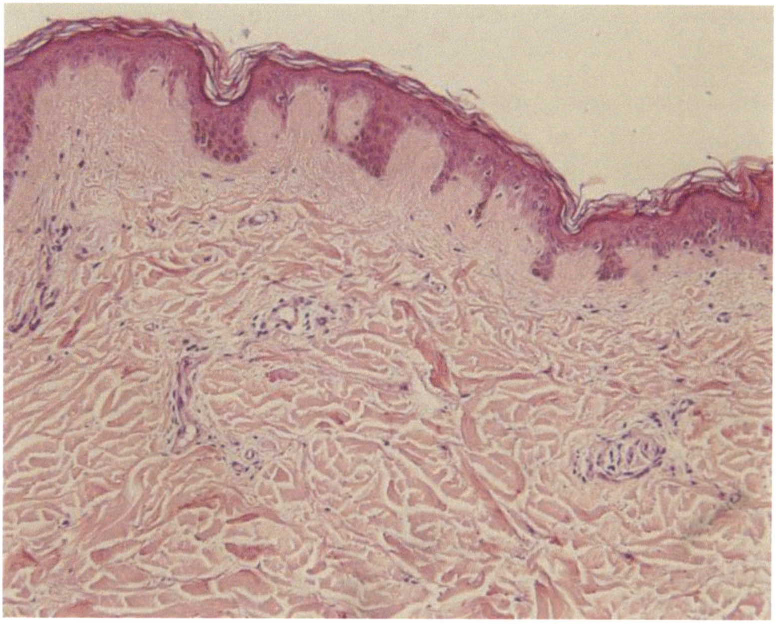

Figure 8. After PDT (×20).

In the CO_2 laser group, eight patients who underwent 1–3 sessions of laser treatment alone showed response to the therapy. Seven lesions (63.63%) achieved complete recovery, three (27.27%) showed partial response but another five lesions (45.45%) relapsed within 6 months during follow-up. Five out of eight (62.5%) patients were satisfied with the therapeutic results of CO_2 laser therapy.

In the ALA-PDT + CO_2 laser group, complete response was achieved in 72.73% of the lesions after 1–3 treatment sessions. Three lesions (27.27%) showed partial response during the treatment. ALA-PDT + CO_2 laser was repeated in the cases of partial response after a single session. Out of eight lesions that initially responded completely, 1 month later one relapsed. The recurrence rate was 9.1% (1/11) and the overall clearance was 90.9% (10/11). Eight out of 10 (80%) patients were satisfied with their therapeutic outcome after ALA-PDT + CO_2 laser treatment, which is much higher than control group [21].

BD lesions are commonly seen on the head, neck, and lower limbs, although any site can be involved. The combination treatment of ALA-PDT and CO_2 laser could achieve a much better cosmetic outcome. Compared with CO_2 laser alone, histopathological examination of the BD lesions confirmed that the response to the combination therapy was more uniform after ALA-PDT + CO_2 laser. PDT appears to be a more feasible alternative to conventional therapy for skin malignancies. BD lesions predominantly consisted of atypical keratinocytes before the treatment. We can see the large number of atypical cells in the epidermis and superficial layers of the dermis, a few lymphocytes and dilated capillaries. Following ALA-PDT + CO_2 laser treatment, the epidermis was found to have fully regenerated 30 days. Furthermore, the stratum spinosum become thinner after treatment, the atypical BD cells were replaced by normal keratinocytes and the photodamaged skin architecture in responsive lesions returned to normal.

Our study also showed that local ALA-PDT after CO_2 laser was highly effective for BD lesions and could be used as an ideal alternative for large and multiple BD lesions, or for other modalities of treatment (surgical or nonsurgical) are inappropriate or have failed. There was no difference in the complete remission rate between the two groups ($P > 0.05$). However, recurrence of BD at the treated site is common. The recurrence rate was substantially higher in the control group than in the ALA-PDT + CO_2 laser group ($P < 0.05$). While the overall clearance was higher in the ALA-PDT + CO_2 laser group than in the control group ($P < 0.05$). A complete response was seen in 72.73% of lesions after 1–3 treatment sessions. Only one lesion developed recurrence 6 month after ALA-PDT + CO_2 laser treatment. The post-treatment recurrence rate was 45.45% (5/11) in CO_2 laser alone group, and five lesions relapsed within 6 months during follow-up. In general, we consider incomplete clearance after four or more times of PDT treatments to be a PDT failure. In terms of our experience, the vast majority of patients were cured within two or three treatment cycles. We would advise patients select alternative treatments in this failure situation. Recurrent disease can be retreated by PDT. This is another advantage of PDT and particularly applied for large or multiple areas and field change. **Figure 9** showed a 55-year-old male hepatitis B patient who has 6-month history of genital BD lesions. He underwent three sessions of ALA-PDT + CO_2 laser treatments, and he completely recovered from BD. He revealed no recurrence during the 6-month follow-up after treatment (**Figure 10**).

In most cases, PDT plus superficial laser vaporization was usually given as a single outpatient treatment that gave good therapeutic results. Most treatments are not suitable for BD lesions involving large and multiple lesions, but we used PDT for BD lesions in some sites such as peri-genital areas, and succeed in the end. The efficacy of local ALA-PDT after CO_2 laser for Bowen's disease lesions reaches almost 80–90%. Compared with the efficacy of PDT with laser in the treatment of Bowen's disease demonstrated that PDT was better than laser alone [14, 22]. Compared with other treatments, PDT causes the low incidences of ulceration and absence of infections.

BD may be a prototype of a non-melanoma skin cancer, and clinically PDT should be seen as a first-line therapy, especially for elderly patients who find the need for hospital attendance limiting [23]. Many BD lesions require immediate surgical intervention in order to avoid the risk of malignant change. With local ALA and light illumination combined with CO_2 laser, good results can be accomplished usually with a single outpatient treatment session without causing serious side effects except a few patients had transient pain, erythema, and scabby.

The most common side effect experienced with PDT is pain, with up to 20% of patients describing pain as being "severe". This can sometimes persist for a few hours after treatment, and it tends to be severest during the early period of irradiation. Postinflammatory hyper or hypopigmentation can also occur. Persistent erythema is often seen at 3 months but does not necessarily indicate residual disease [24, 25].

http://dx.doi.org/10.5772/66420

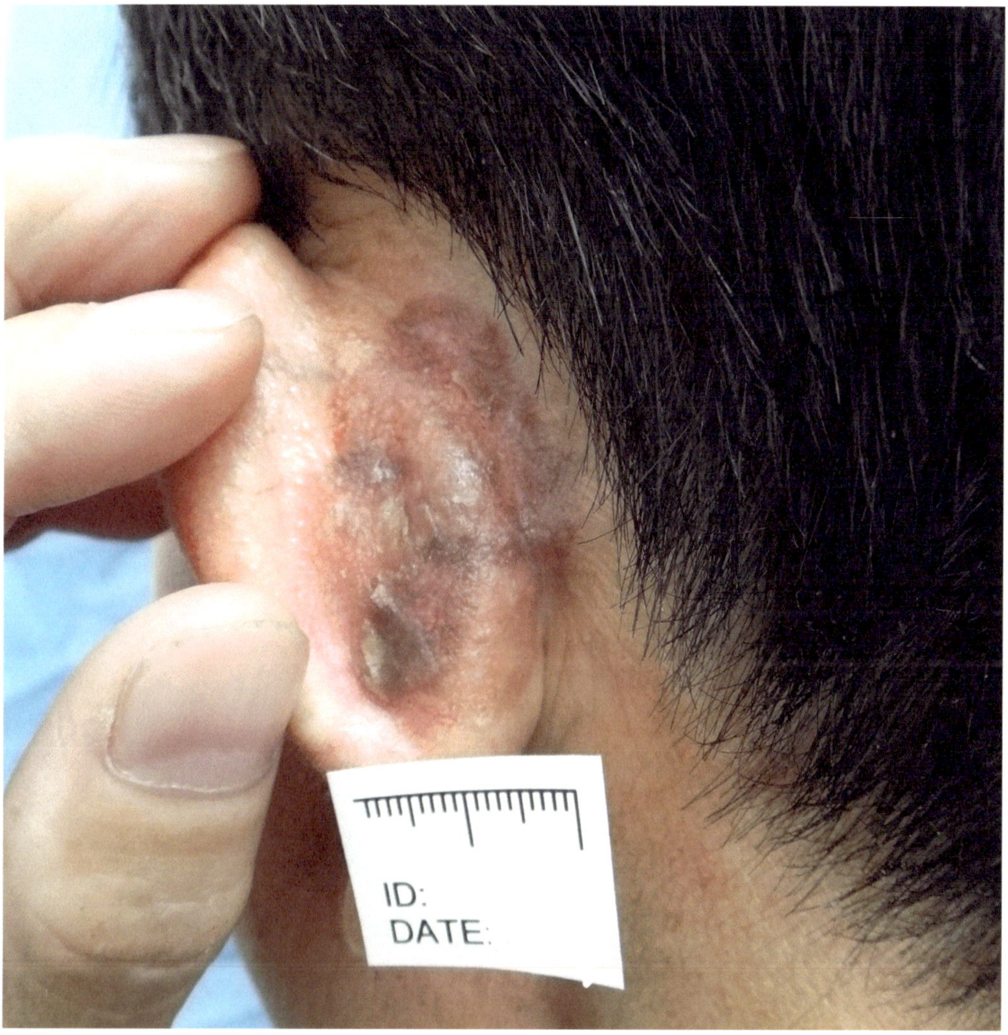

Figure 9. Before PDT.

This study explored the feasibility of using topical ALA-PDT combined with CO_2 laser for BD. Our preliminary results proved that the ALA-PDT after CO_2 laser is safe and effective and is associated with a low recurrence rate. The main limiting factors for PDT at the moment are pain and the inconvenience of hospital attendance. However, this study provided histological evidence that supports the beneficial effects of ALA-PDT + CO_2 laser for the treatment of BD. PDT is quite promising and could be the potential alternative, especially for large and multiple lesions; or for patients where other modalities of treatment (surgical or non-surgical) are inappropriate or have failed.

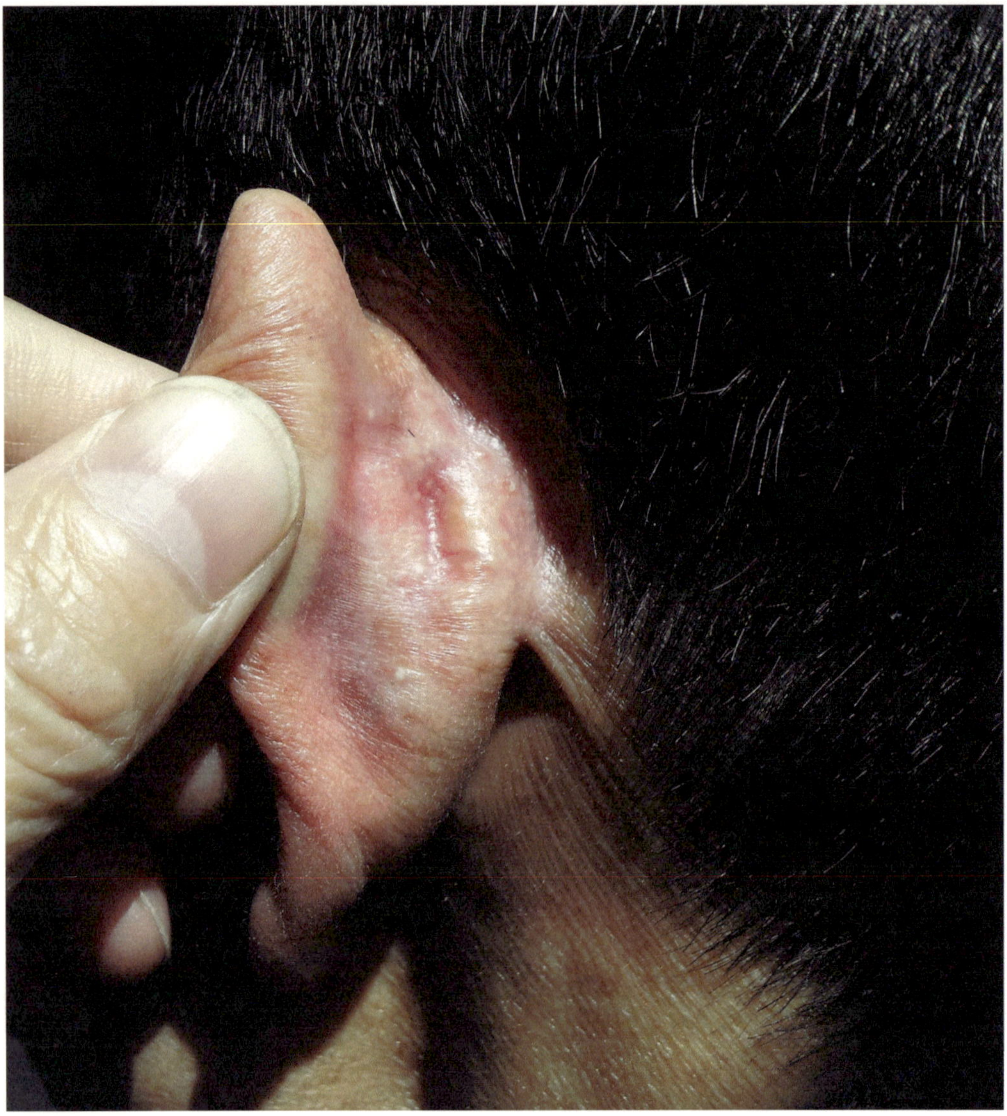

Figure 10. After PDT.

3. Photodynamic therapy for the treatment of port wine stains

Port-wine stain (PWS) is congenital vascular malformation characterized by ectatic capillaries in the papillary layer of the dermis. PWS occurs in an estimated 0.3% of births, affecting males and females and all racial groups equally. It may be located anywhere on the body, but more often on the face. PWS are permanent, do not disappear spontaneously. They usually appear at birth and tend to become darker and thicker with age [26, 27], deepening in color from faint pink to deep red or purple or developing nodularity. It is usually isolated but may be associated with other vascular malformations or occurs as a component of a variety of congenital syndromes.

Because persistent PWS lesions can cause serious psychological problems, therapy for PWS is considered a medical necessity. Many therapeutic methods have been used to treat PWS, including surgical excision, cryosurgery, dermabrasion, tattooing, and cosmetic camouflage makeup [28]. These methods are no longer used because of ineffectiveness and scarring.

PDT is a relatively new therapeutic modality for skin disease. The vascular effects of PDT on tumors leads to endothelial injury, vasoconstriction, thrombus formation, and blood flow stasis. These results suggest that PDT is a potential treatment for certain vascular diseases, including PWS. The advantage of PDT is its dual selectivity: precise direction of laser light to the specific target area and selective uptake of photosensitizer to target tissues. PWS have a histologic characteristic of dilated capillary vessels, the target of PDT. *In vivo* 23–26 and *in vitro* 25 studies have shown that photosensitizer accumulation occurs rapidly in vascular endothelial cells after intravenous administration.

Recently, the General Hospital of the Peoples' Liberation Army in China reported their decade-long experience of PWS with PDT. Gu et al. [29, 30] reported that among 1942 PWS lesions in 1385 patients treated by either PSD-007 or HMME from April 1991 to May 2003 showed that, after one PDT treatment session, total clearance was achieved in 128 lesions (6.6%), achieved excellent results, 746 (38.3%) good results, 923 (47.4%) fair results, 145 (7.4%) results, and seven (0.3%) with no visible change. Their data showed that PDT was an effective treatment in all patients with PWS, especially for dark-skinned patients or patients with papules or nodules.

Acknowledgements

The authors are grateful to Ying Gu academician (Department of Laser Medicine, Chinese PLA General Hospital) for constructive suggestions and the members of the department of dermatology of the Air Force General Hospital for their technical support. This work was supported by the National Natural Science Foundation of China (No. 81301386) and the China Postdoctoral Science Foundation (no. 2013M532225 and no. 2014T71009).

Author details

Wei Liu* and Hong Cai

*Address all correspondence to: lwei5811@126.com

Department of Dermatology, Air Force General Hospital, PLA, Beijing, P. R. China

References

[1] Zalaudek I, Giacomel J, Schmid K, et al. Dermatoscopy of facial actinic keratosis, intraepidermal carcinoma, and invasive squamous cell carcinoma: a progression model. J Am Acad Dermatol. 2012; 66(4):589–597.

[2] Feldman SR, Fleischer AB Jr. Progression of actinic keratosis to squamous cell carcinoma revisited: clinical and treatment implications. Cutis. 2011; 87(4):201–207.

[3] Butani AK, Arbesfeld DM, Schwartz RA. Premalignant and early squamous cell carcinoma. Clin Plast Surg. 2005; 32(2):223–235.

[4] Borgonjen RJ, van Everdingen JJ, Bik CM, et al. Prospective comparison of three guideline development methods for treatment of actinic keratosis. BMJ Qual Saf. 2011; 20(10):832–841.

[5] Demetriou C. Reversing precancerous actinic damage by mixing wavelengths (1064 nm, 532 nm). J Cosmet Laser Ther. 2011; 13(3):113–119.

[6] Inada NM, Costa MM, Guimarães OC, et al. Photodiagnosis and treatment of condyloma acuminatum using 5-aminolevulinic acid and homemade devices. Photodiagnosis Photodyn Ther. 2012; 9(1):60–68.

[7] Cai H, Wang YX, Sun P, et al. Photodynamic therapy for facial actinic keratosis: a clinical and histological study in Chinese patients. Photodiagnosis Photodyn Ther. 2013; 10(3):260–265.

[8] Dougherty TJ. Introduction. Methods Mol Biol. 2010; 635:1–6.

[9] Nava HR, Allamaneni SS, Dougherty TJ, et al. Photodynamic therapy (PDT) using HPPH for the treatment of precancerous lesions associated with barrett's esophagus. Lasers Surg Med. 2011; 43(7):705–712.

[10] Biel MA. Photodynamic therapy of head and neck cancers. Methods Mol Biol. 2010; 635:281–293.

[11] Guyon L, Ascencio M, Collinet P, et al. Photodiagnosis and photodynamic therapy of peritoneal metastasis of ovarian cancer. Photodiagnosis Photodyn Ther. 2012; 9(1):16–31.

[12] Mitra S, Cassar SE, Niles DJ, et al. Photodynamic therapy mediates the oxygen-independent activation of hypoxia-inducible factor 1 alpha. Mol Cancer Ther. 2006; 5(12):3268–3274.

[13] Ferrario A, Gomer CJ. Targeting the tumor microenvironment using photodynamic therapy combined with inhibitors of cyclooxygenase-2 or vascular endothelial growth factor. Methods Mol Biol. 2010; 635:121–132.

[14] Sailer R, Strauss WS, Wagner M, et al. Relation between intracellular location and photodynamic efficacy of 5-aminolevulinic acid-induced protoporphyrin IX in vitro. Comparison between human glioblastoma cells and other cancer cell lines. Photochem Photobiol Sci. 2007; 6(2):145–151.

[15] Camp WL, Turnham JW, Athar M, et al. New agents for prevention of ultraviolet-induced nonmelanoma skin cancer. Semin Cutan Med Surg. 2011; 30(1):6–13.

[16] Lee Y, Baron ED. Photodynamic therapy: current evidence and applications in dermatology. Semin Cutan Med Surg. 2011; 30(4):199–209.

[17] Apalla Z, Sotiriou E, Panagiotidou D, et al. The impact of different fluence rates on pain and clinical outcome in patients with actinic keratoses treated with photodynamic therapy. Photodermatol Photoimmunol Photomed. 2011; 27(4):181–185.

[18] Wang X-L, Wang H-W, Yuan K-H, Li F-L, and Huang Z. Combination of photodynamic therapy and immunomodulation for skin diseases—update of clinical aspects. Photochem. Photobiol. Sci. 2011; 10(2):704–711.

[19] Kaushal S, Merideth M, Kopparthy P, Pulanic TK, Stratton P. Treatment of multifocal Bowen's disease in immunocompromised women with surgery and topical imiquimod. Obstet Gynecol. 2012; 119(2):442–444.

[20] Young LC, Tuxen AJ, Goodman G. Mohs' micrographic surgery as treatment for squamous dysplasia of the nail unit. Australas J Dermatol. 2012; 53(2):123–127.

[21] Cai H, Wang YX, Zheng JC, et al. Photodynamic therapy in combination with CO_2 laser for the treatment of Bowen's disease. Lasers Med Sci. 2015; 30(5):1505–1510.

[22] Hasegawa T, Suga Y, Mizuno Y, Haruna K, Ogawa H, Ikeda S. Efficacy of photodynamic therapy with topical 5-aminolevulinic acid using intense pulsed light for Bowen's disease. J Dermatol. 2010; 37(7):623–628.

[23] Sidoroff A, Thaler P. Taking treatment decisions in non-melanoma skin cancer - the place for topical photodynamic therapy (PDT). Photodiagnosis Photodyn Ther. 2010; 7(1):24–32.

[24] Steinbauer JM, Schreml S, Babilas P, Zeman F, Karrer S, Landthaler M, Szeimies R-M. Topical photodynamic therapy with porphyrin precursors—assessment of treatment-associated pain in a retrospective study. Photochem Photobiol Sci. 2009; 8(8):1111–1116.

[25] Arits AH, van de Weert MM, Nelemans PJ, Kelleners-Smeets NW. Pain during topical photodynamic therapy: uncomfortable and unpredictable. J Eur Acad Dermatol Venereol. 2010; 24(12):1452–1357.

[26] Zhao Y, Tu P, Zhou G, et al. Hemoporfin photodynamic therapy for port-wine stain: a randomized controlled trial. PLoS One. 2016; 11(5):e0156219.

[27] Huang Z. Photodynamic therapy in China: 25 years of unique history – Part one: history and domestic photosensitizers. Photodiagnosis Photodyn Ther. 2006; 3(2):3–10.

[28] Huang NY. What is the optimal PDT protocol for treating port wine stains (PWS)? Photodiagnosis Photodyn Ther. 2007; 4(2):145–146.

[29] Gu Y, Huang NY, Liang J, Pan YM, Liu FG. Clinical study of 1949 cases of port wine stains treated with vascular photodynamic therapy (Gu's PDT). Ann Dermatol Venereol. 2007; 134(3):241–244.

[30] Qiu H, Gu Y, Wang Y, et al. Twenty years of clinical experience with a new modality of vascular-targeted photodynamic therapy for port wine stains. Dermatol Surg. 2011; 37(11):1603–1610.

Chapter 4

Can Nanotechnology Shine a New Light on Antimicrobial Photodynamic Therapies?

Nora Bloise, Paolo Minzioni, Marcello Imbriani and Livia Visai

Additional information is available at the end of the chapter

http://dx.doi.org/10.5772/65974

Abstract

Recent developments in light-controlled therapies (e.g., photodynamic and photothermal therapies) provide promising strategies to prevent and suppress bacterial infections, which are a leading cause of morbidity and mortality. Antibacterial photodynamic therapy (aPDT) has drawn increasing attention from the scientific society for its potential to kill multidrug-resistant pathogenic bacteria and for its low tendency to induce drug resistance. In this chapter, we summarize the mechanism of action of aPDT, the photosensitizers, as well the current developments in terms of treating Gram-positive and Gram-negative bacteria. The chapter also describes the recent progress relating to photomedicine for preventing bacterial infections and biofilm formation. We focus on the laser device used in aPDT and on the light-treatment parameters that may have a strong impact on the results of aPDT experiments. In the last part of this chapter, we survey on the various nanoparticles delivering photoactive molecules, and photoactive-nanoparticles that can potentially enhance the antimicrobial action of aPDT.

Keywords: bacterial infections, biofilm, antimicrobial photodynamic therapy, laser, nanotechnology

1. Introduction

"It is not difficult to make microbes resistant to penicillin in the laboratory by exposing them to concentrations not sufficient to kill them, and the same thing has occasionally happened in the body" Alexander Fleming, 1945.

In the 1940s, the introduction of the *penicillin*, discovered in the 1926 by Fleming, opened the era of the antibiotics, recognized as one of the greatest advances in the therapeutic medicine.

However, the appearance of resistance phenomena came very quickly: by 1944, half of all clinical *Staphylococci spp.* isolates failed to respond to the so-called "miracle-drug" [1]. The World Health Organization (WHO) has recently recognized the multidrug-resistance (MDR) as one of the most important problems facing human health all over the world [2]. The need to overcome this rising problem has stimulated research into alternative antimicrobial approaches with less potential of developing resistances in microorganisms toward controlling the growing incidence of infectious diseases. An innovative light-based approach to achieve this goal is antimicrobial photodynamic therapy (aPDT). The aPDT involves harmless visible light in combination with nontoxic and light-sensitive dye, the so-called "photosensitizer (PS)," and oxygen that can selectively control bacterial infections [3]. Nanotechnology is an emerging technology that may change the face of PDT by new photoactive molecules, with numerous advantages to gain a successful bacterial infections eradication.

1.1. Photodynamic therapy as antimicrobial strategy: how it works

The photodynamic therapy has gained considerable attention as an emerging treatment modality for many forms of neoplastic diseases [4]. However, the PDT was originally discovered over 100 years ago when Oscar Raab observed that *Paramecium spp.* protozoans could be killed by particular combinations of dyes (acridine orange) and bright light [5]. For many years the potential of this finding was forgotten because of the discovery of antibiotics since the relentless increase in antibiotic resistance worldwide has spurred a migration of PDT research effort to its origin in microbiology. Numerous findings strongly support the hypothesis that PDT can represent a viable alternative since the mode of action of photodynamic sensitizers on microbial cells is markedly different from that typical of most antibiotic drugs [6]. aPDT has been successfully applied *in vivo* and *ex vivo* tissue or in biological materials for blood sterilization, in animal models of localized infections as surface wounds, burns, oral sites, abscesses, and in the middle ear. aPDT is being clinically studied for several dermatological infections, such as leishmaniosis and mycobacteria [7]. As mentioned before, PDT combines the action of three components: the PS, visible light, and molecular oxygen. The absorption of the light by the PS leads to a transition from its initial ground state (PS_0) to an energetically excited state ($^1PS^*$) that can relax to the more long-lived triplet state ($^3PS^*$). This triplet state can interact with molecular oxygen by two mechanism of reaction, letting the PS regain its ground state. Type I photoreactions occurs by an electron and/or proton transfer, where the PS interacts directly with the cellular substrate (i.e., lipids, proteins, nucleic acids, etc.). The generated radicals react with molecular oxygen, yielding several different oxygen intermediates collectively called reactive oxygen species (ROS), such as for instance the superoxide anion (O_2^-), the hydroxyl radical (OH), and hydrogen peroxide (H_2O_2). Alternatively, Type II photoreactions proceed by energy (not electron) transfer, while the oxygen is the primary acceptor. The interaction of molecular oxygen in its ground triplet state ($^3O_2$) with $^3PS^*$ generates a more reactive form of oxygen, i.e., singlet oxygen ($^1O_2$). This nonradical species is highly reactive toward electron-rich substrates such as aromatic rings, amines, and thioesters [8]. The contribution of both Type I and Type II reactions to cell death depends on several factors including, among others, the PS itself, the subcellular localization, the substrate, and molecular oxygen concentration within the target cells. Although the detailed mechanism of

http://dx.doi.org/10.5772/65974

PDT and the concomitant processes are not yet fully understood, it is generally accepted that Type I and Type II reactions both produce ROS that cause oxidation of biomolecules (lipids, proteins, and nucleic acids) in the cell. For a reason not entirely understood, hyper proliferating cells selectively uptake PS [9]. This, together with the fact that cell death is spatially limited to regions where light of the appropriate wavelength is applied, makes PDT a highly selective and useful modality. Because microbial cell possess very fast growth rate, it was suggested that PDT could be effective against microbial cells (**Figure 1**). In most instances, aPDT predominantly proceeds via Type II processes. However, by comparing PSs that tend to undergo either Type I or Type II mechanism, Huang et al. reported that Gram-negative species are more susceptible to •OH than $^1O_2$ [10]. A Type I reaction is therefore favored when targeting Gram-negative species.

1.2. Antimicrobial efficacy of PDT: the photosensitizers

The photosensitizer plays a crucial role in determining the therapeutic outcome. Accumulating selectively in diseased tissue and, via generation of cytotoxic species, PS provokes the desired biological effect, without causing excessive damage to the host tissue. In general, a PS used for antimicrobial PDT should be endowed with the following properties [11]: (i) high triplet-state quantum yields ($\Phi\tau \geq 0.5$), triplet-state with lifetimes long enough (τ microsecond range), and sufficiently energetic ($\geq$94 kJ/mol) to produce $^1O_2$ ($\Phi\Delta \geq 0.5$); (ii) high-binding affinity for microorganism (positively charged PS for good adherence to negatively charged bacterial cell wall) and low-binding affinity for mammalian cells; (iii) broad spectrum of action, since one photosensitizer can act on bacteria, fungi, yeasts, and parasitic protozoa; (iv) minimum dark toxicity and negligible cytotoxicity in the absence of light; (v) not yield toxic and mutagenic

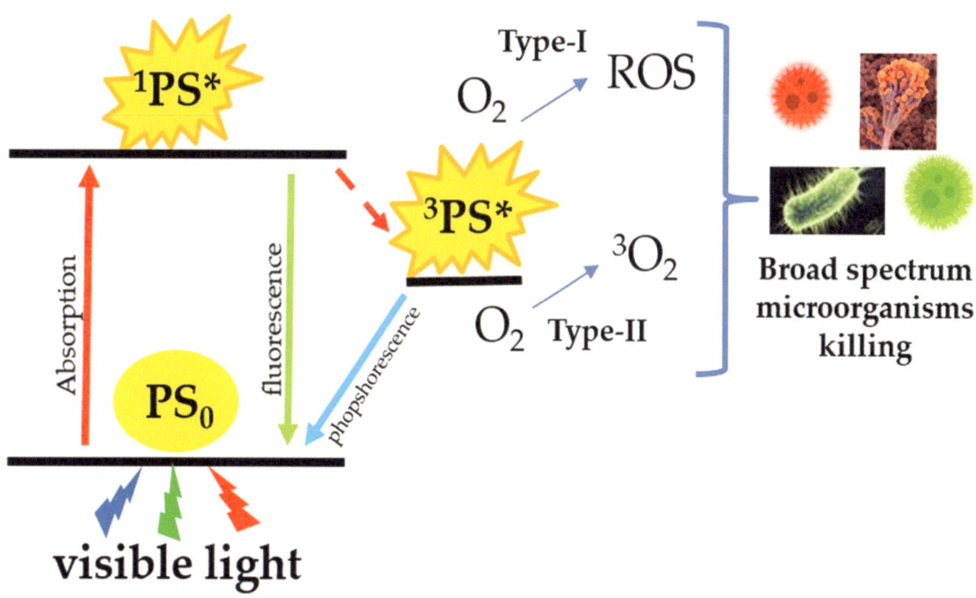

Figure 1. Schematic illustration of photodynamic action.

metabolites; (vi) greater retention in target tissue/cells over healthy ones, and (vii) high molar extinction coefficients, with high absorbance, particularly in the red and near-infrared UV-vis spectral regions (600–800 nm range), for a maximum light penetration and minimum light scattering within the "*therapeutic window.*" PSs are usually organic aromatic molecules with a high degree of electron delocalization. They contain a central chromophore with auxiliary branches (auxochromes) which add further electron delocalization to the PS and thus alter the absorption spectra of the PS [12]. As reviewed in [13], different classes of natural and synthetic molecules have demonstrated antimicrobial efficacy against a broad spectrum of antibiotic-resistant microorganisms upon illumination. These include porphyrins, chlorins, bacteriochlorins, phthalocyanines, as well dyes with different molecular framework such as halogenated xanthenes (e.g., Rose Bengal (RB)), perylenequinones (e.g., hypericin), phenothiazinium salts (e.g., toluidine blue oral (TBO), and methylene blue (MB)), and merocianine and cationic fullerenes (e.g., derivatives of C60). PS binding to the bacterial cell and uptake are dependent on the microbial species. In general, aPDT has been more effective against Gram-positive and fungal cells than Gram-negative, especially when neutral or anionic PS was used. Gram-negative bacterial cells are relatively resistant to these compounds [14]. The high susceptibility of Gram-positive bacteria and fungi was explained by their physiology as a relatively porous layer of peptidoglycan and lipoteichoic acid, or beta-glucan and chitin, respectively, surrounds their cytoplasmic membrane and both these structures allow non-cationic PSs to cross [14, 15]. Gram-negative bacteria are less prone to take up exogenous compounds due to the extra outer membrane and the permeability barrier imparted by lipopolysaccharides [16]. This outer membrane provides also an effective permeability barrier and limits the binding and penetration of anionic and lipophilic PS. These critical characteristics guided the research efforts toward approaches that would allow PDI of Gram-negative species [14]. A method adopted by numerous groups is to use a PS molecule with an intrinsic positive charge [17–19]. An increase of the PDI efficacy has been addressed recently both in bacteria using the polycationic biopolymer chitosan [20]. Another method includes the using of metal chelators (ethylenediaminetetraacetic acid (EDTA)) or polypeptide polymixin B [21]. These agents destabilize the lipopolysaccharides coating by removing the Ca^{2+} and Mg^{2+} ions, thereby increasing permeability of the Gram-negative outer membrane and allowing PSs, that are normally excluded from the cell, to penetrate to a location where the reactive oxygen species (ROS) generated on illumination that can execute fatal damage [21]. At present, there is a consensus that aPDT can be effective to kill all known classes of microorganism, including methicillin-resistant *Staphylococcus aureus* (MRSA), multidrug-resistant (MDR) and pandrug-resistant (PDR) fungi, protozoa, viruses, etc., whether *in vitro* or *in vivo* [13].

1.3. PDT for inactivate biofilm formation

Most important in the chronic infections is the formation of a thick, multilayered biofilm [22]. A biofilm is defined as a microbially derived sessile community surrounded by a self-producing extracellular polymer matrix. The biofilm matrix, a homoglycan composed of β-1,6-linked N-acetylglucosamine residues, is involved in intercellular adhesion and is referred to as polysaccharide intercellular adhesion (PIA) [23]. Biofilm formation includes several sequential steps in which planktonic bacteria initially attach to a solid surface, that may be either unmodified or coated with host plasma proteins, followed by cell proliferation, cell-cell interaction, and production of an extracellular polymeric matrix, where bacteria accumulate in multilayered clusters (**Figure 2**).

Biofilms generally do not restrict penetration of antibiotics [24], but they do form a barrier to the larger components of the immune system [25]. As a consequence, biofilm-associated infections can only be resolved by removal of the infected device, determining high-threat care costs. PDT is a possible alternative to inactivate biofilms and may represent a different treatment for several recalcitrant infections. There is a wealth of literature that focuses on PDT-based antibiofilm strategies against a variety of microbial species [26–28]. On the contrary, the effects of PDT on phenotypic biofilm elements (e.g., adhesions and extracellular polysaccharide) are poorly investigated [29, 30]. Staphylococci are one of the most important human pathogens and a major cause of morbidity and mortality worldwide. In particular, *S. epidermidis* and *S. aureus* are emerging as the most important agents of persistent infections, especially in implanted medical devices [31, 32]. The use of tri-meso (N-methyl-pyridyl) and meso (N-tetradecyl-pyridyl) porphine (C14) for inactivation of two structurally distinct *S. epidermidis* biofilms grown on Ti6Al4V alloy has been observed and its photosensitizing efficiency with that of the parent molecule, tetra-substituted N-methylpyridyl-porphine (C1), was compared [26]. In another work, the antimicrobial activity of merocyanine 540, a photosensitizing dye used for purging malignant cells from autologous bone marrow grafts, has been evaluated against *Staphylococcus epidermidis* biofilms. Merocyanine 540-mediated PDT showed a significant inactivation effect on the viability and structure of biofilms of two *Staphylococcus epidermidis* strains, RP62A and 1457, respectively [27]. Moreover, it was found that erythrosine-induced PDT was also more potent than MB, RB, and TBO against *Aggregatibacter actinomycetemcomitans* biofilm

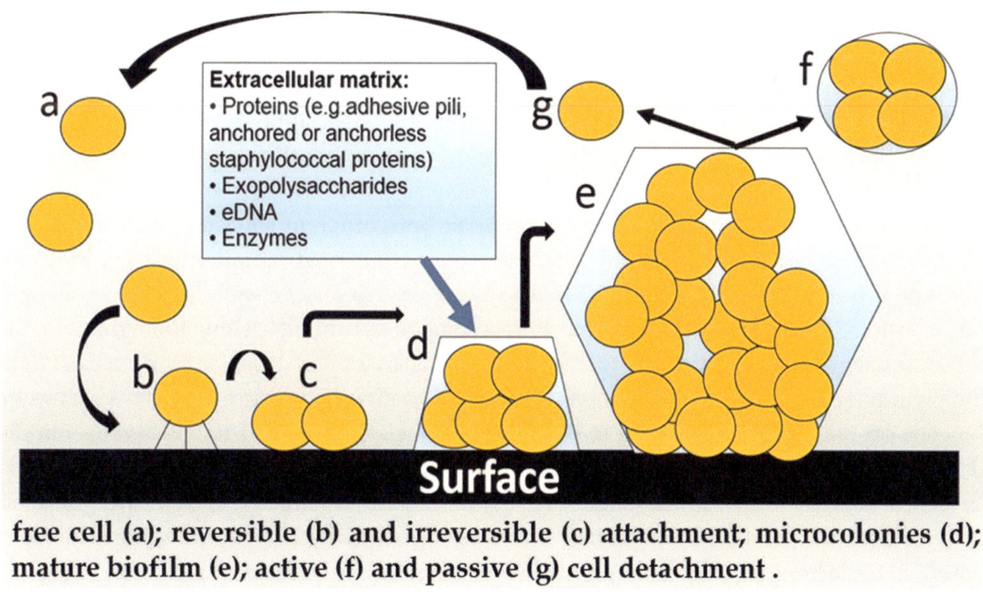

Figure 2. Biofilm development.

[33–35]. A recent paper described the photokilling propensity of the curcumin (a yellow pigment derived from the root of the *Curcuma longa* plant) in *S. epidermidis* biofilm and suspended cells in two *in vitro* models [28]. Finally, although in many systems the PDT seem promising it yields inconsistent results mainly due to the lack of standard reproducible models for assessing PDT efficacy against biofilms, as well as the lack of robustness of the majority of methodologies used in the majority of published studies.

2. Laser source and parameters for PDT in microbial infections

Given the always present variability in biological experiments, and the need to allow for experimental results comparison, we give in this section a guide that will help the reader to understand the properties of laser sources, the physical phenomena occurring in the treated samples, the parameters to be defined in order to set a reproducible experiment, and also the technical aspects regarding the instruments required for a proper optical beam characterization. In order to understand why lasers are generally used to carry out PDT experiments, it is helpful to recall the main differences between the radiation emitted by a lamp and that emitted by a laser. As everybody knows the most "visible" differences between lamps and lasers are the directionality of laser light, and the fact that it is generally "colored" and not white. The directionality aspect of laser light is of fundamental importance when a selective illumination is required, as it allows illuminating certain portions of the sample/tissue, or a specific position of a multiwell plate without irradiating the neighboring area. The laser light directionality thus enables comparing the biological effect in treated versus untreated areas on the same substrate and makes it possible to exploit relatively simple components (lenses and mirrors) in order to control the optical beam properties, as direction and diameter. In particular, the possibility to properly control the beam properties is of great importance in some recently investigated techniques, as two-photons PDT [36] where the PDT is activated only in the focal region of the optical beam, thus making possible to induce PDT in "deep regions" without affecting all the biological material irradiated. From the physical point of view, the fact that the laser light is characterized by a specific "color" means that the emitted electromagnetic radiation has a very specific wavelength. On the contrary, the "white light" emitted by a lamp is given by the simultaneous presence of radiations with different wavelengths, covering the whole spectrum of visible light and generally comprising even radiation in the ultraviolet (UV) and infrared (IR) range. Even if it is always possible to select a well-defined wavelength (i.e., a "color") from a white light source by inserting an optical filter along the light path, the obtained beam characteristics are still quite different, mainly because of two reasons: light "line-width" and the achievable "power." It is worth noticing that the exact line-width value depends on many parameters and in certain cases, it can be reduced to reach values in the kHz range, but an in-depth discussion of the parameters affecting laser line-width is beyond the aim of this section [37]. The origin of these laser beams characteristics is strictly related to the structure of a laser source, which is thus briefly described in the following. The word "laser" is the acronym of light amplification by stimulated emission of radiation [38], thus immediately suggesting that what we call "laser light" is the result of an amplification mechanism, and that a "light amplifier" should be used in order to produce laser light. The laser source is composed by two main components: the "active medium," which is the element amplifying the light beam thanks to the stimulated emission process [39], and the "cavity," used to provide the feedback required to transform the amplifier in an oscillator. The "active medium" obviously requires some form of power supply, as otherwise no amplification could occur because of the general energy conservation principle, and the way that power is transmitted to the active medium is generally called "pumping method" (or scheme) (**Figure 3**). As the material used as active medium determines the frequency of the emitted laser light, laser sources are generally identified by describing the active medium; this is the reason why lasers are generally classified as either "solid state," "gas," "fiber," or "semiconductor" lasers. The role of the cavity is that of creating the "selection" of the light components to be emitted. This selection is both a "frequency (or wavelength) selection," and a "direction selection": only those wavelengths that are exact dividers of the cavity length can be in fact emitted by a laser source (the so-called "cavity autofrequencies") and only those rays propagating sufficiently aligned to the cavity axis, so that they can be reflected several times before transmission, are actually selected by the cavity feedback.

The most suitable laser for PDT experiments and applications is probably that of the so-called semiconductor lasers. The first demonstration of the possibility to produce laser light from a semiconductor dates back to 1962 [40, 41], just two years after the first ever demonstration of a laser source. The main advantage of semiconductor lasers with respect to the other laser types (gas, solid, and fiber lasers) is the possibility to electrically pump the active medium, without requiring the use of additional light sources, thus significantly increasing the system efficiency. Because of the combination of high efficiency (and thus small power supply requirements) and small size (generally <1 mm^3), semiconductor lasers are the ideal choice to realize portable, and maybe even battery-operated, hand-held laser devices. Regarding the optical wavelengths that can be emitted by semiconductor lasers, these are related to the so-called "energy-gap" of the semiconductor, which in turns depends on the semiconductor lattice composition. As an example, considering an $Ga_xAl_{1-x}As$ semiconductor it is thus possible in principle to tune the emission wavelength between 570 and 850 nm by changing the value

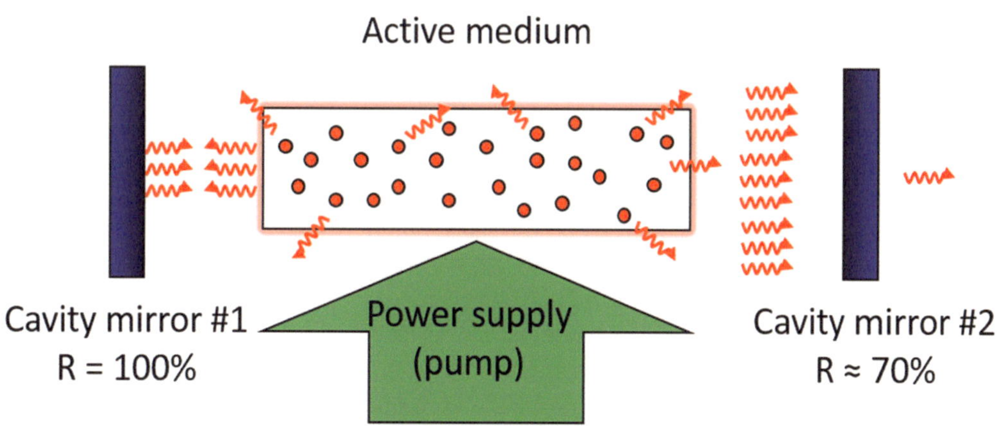

Figure 3. Example of the generation of laser beam into a cavity.

of the x parameter (while keeping it between 0 and 1) in the composition formula. From the practical point of view, commercial products, because of fabrication issues, cover not all the theoretically available wavelengths. The "unpleasant side" of semiconductor lasers is related to the properties of the optical beam. The small cross-section of the active medium makes the optical beam to be extremely small directly at the laser output, and in general with an elliptical shape. The very small size induces the beam diffraction phenomenon, making the beam profile broader and broader during propagation.

2.1. Laser wavelengths and irradiation system setup

A fundamental point in the preparation of the PDT experiments is the wavelength of the laser used in the system. In particular, it is useful to recall that the absorption spectrum of the photosensitizer (PS) is not the only parameter to be considered, but other elements, such as the light absorption due to the culture medium or the depth at which the target cells are located (when performing *in vivo* experiments), may impose significant constraints to the choice of the wavelength to be used, and hence on the laser choice. As a first step for the wavelength determination, it is necessary to measure the absorption spectrum of the PS, paying attention to the fact that slight modifications of the PS absorption curve may be observed when changing the medium where the PS is dispersed. After having determined the PS absorption peak, it is important to check if the corresponding wavelength may induce local medium/sample heating, generally checking if the absorption peak lies within the "biological window" (a wavelength range roughly going from 650 to 1300 nm) [42]. If the PS absorption peaks is within the biological window it is possible to assume a good penetration (>1 cm) of the light beam in a standard sample; conversely, if the absorption peak is out of the window a more detailed analysis is required, in order to understand which are the components that could cause light absorption, and the consequences of their presence in terms of heat production, light scattering, and penetration. When the desired wavelength has been selected, it is then necessary to find a suitable laser source. Limiting the discussion to semiconductor lasers, the most used in PDT, it is interesting to notice that even if several different sources are available inside the "biological window" they do not uniformly cover the required biological range and some "dark ranges" are present. This implies that even if a small (generally <1%) tuning of the emission wavelength is possible thanks to temperature tuning of the semiconductor chip, some "dark" wavelength range still exist, and thus custom solutions may be required. Additionally, from what has been reported it is probably now obvious that when multi-PS studies are considered it would be ideally required to have different laser sources, whose emission wavelengths correspond to the PS absorption peaks. As an alternative, if the absorption spectra of the tested PS all have a common "absorption region," it is possible to use a single laser, by fine-tuning the optical power to balance for the different absorption coefficient. As an additional possibility, if the laser system offers this possibility, the emission wavelength can be slightly changed (e.g., by controlling the source temperature in semiconductors lasers) to match the PS absorption peak. In order to realize a suitable irradiation system for PDT experiments, it is important to notice that the availability of the laser source is required but definitely not sufficient. We thus give a short list and description of the elements required for a proper setup preparation. The semiconductors lasers are generally sold as a "component," implying the use of a suitable mounting and right drivers for controlling both the current injected to the semiconductor (to tune the emitted-beam power) and the temperature. It is thus important, when planning a PDT experiment to: (i) acquire the right drivers, which can be relatively expensive, even if they can be often reused in future experiments simply changing the semiconductor sources; (ii) consider the set of lenses/mirrors to control and steer the optical beam, and the corresponding mechanical mounts, allowing to keep the optical elements in a stable and well-defined position. Moreover, for an accurate characterization three elements are required: (i) an optical spectrum analyzer, for guarantee the stability of the wavelength emitted by the laser source over time (as it may drift in case of nonaccurate thermal control); (ii) a power meter to verify that the laser operating conditions remain stable even after months of usage [43], and (iii) a properly calibrated camera to acquire the spatial intensity distribution and to analyze the obtained images so as to guarantee that the beam uniformity requirements are met on the whole surface.

2.2. The "light-treatment" plan

Finally, it is helpful to highlight which are the light-treatment parameters that may have a strong impact on the results of PDT experiments. While the idea of "light-dose" (measured in J/cm^2) is generally accepted and used in the scientific literature in this field, careful analysis must be performed before comparing results of experiments using the same light-dose on identical samples. A first parameter is the beam wavelength: even very small beam wavelength variations (e.g., <1 nm) can have a strong impact on the ability of the beam to excite the PS, especially if the considered beam wavelength is close to the absorption edge and not exactly in the middle of the absorption spectrum. A second parameter, which is often overlooked, is the beam intensity (i.e., the ratio of the optical power over the irradiated surface) impinging on the sample and measured in W/cm^2. As an example, a 1 W laser beam and a 10 MW beam impinging on the same surface may be used to apply the same "light-dose" by simply scaling (by a factor of 100) the irradiation times between the two beams. Nevertheless, in the first case the beam intensity will be two orders of magnitude higher, leading to a significantly different interaction between the light beam and the biological sample. As a consequence, this means that in order to properly define a suitable light-irradiation plan, it is not sufficient to keep the laser intensity at a fixed level and to investigate the role of different doses, but it is instead necessary to vary both the light intensity and the exposure-time parameter, so as to create a "data-grid" allowing to optimize both parameters (**Figure 4**).

Additionally, the role played by localized thermal heating, due to absorption, may become relevant in PDT experiments, with two consequences: it is necessary to properly evaluate the produced temperature increase, and if the heating is nonnegligible, it is important to model the thermal situation of the experiment. Furthermore, when very high intensities are considered (for example, by using pulsed lasers), several other aspects must be considered, such as the possibility to induce photoablation and two-photons light absorption (i.e., the light beam is absorbed even if the medium absorption at the beam wavelength is very low).

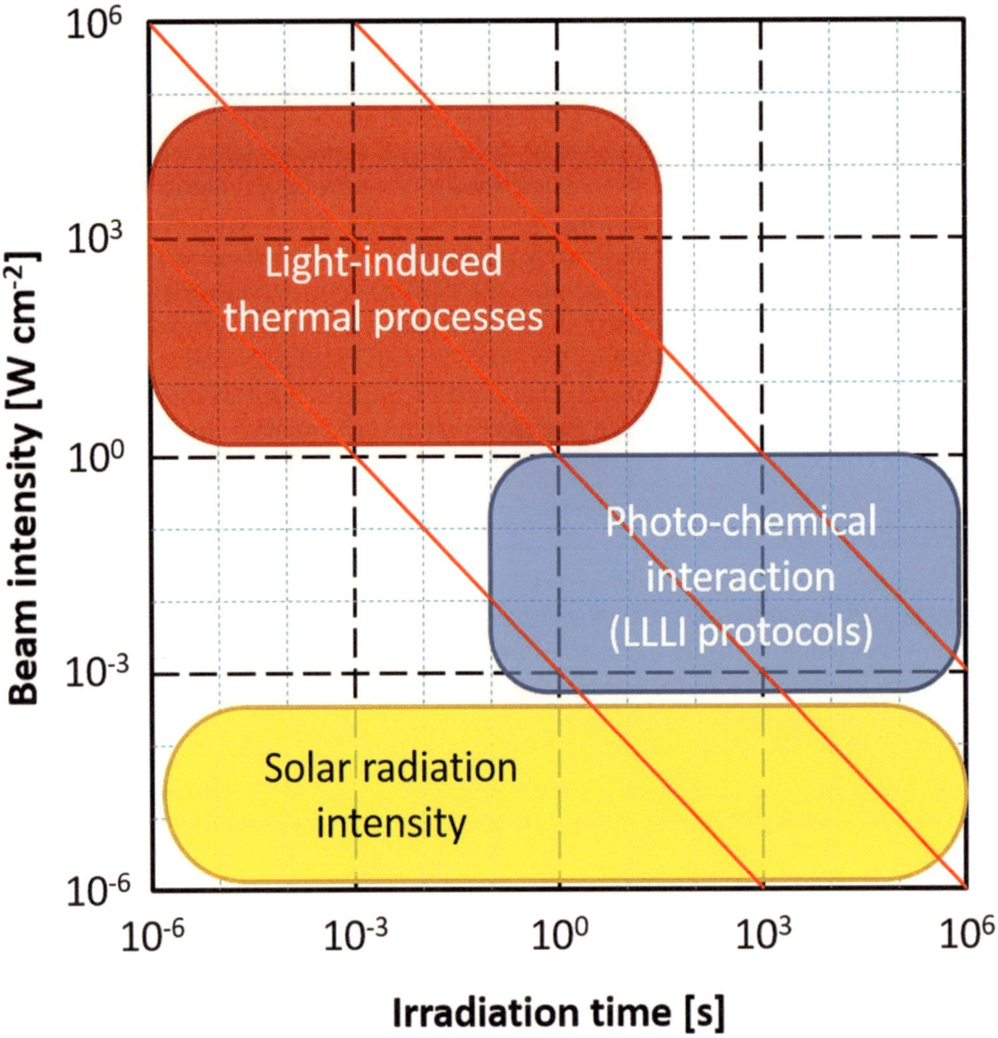

Figure 4. Log-log chart describing the interactions produced as a function of the beam intensity and of the irradiation time.

3. Nanotechnology shines a new light in antimicrobial PDT

Although the efficacy of PDT has been recognized, inefficient PS uptake by bacteria could result in insufficient therapeutic index. It is now clear that a nanotechnology-driven approach using nanoparticles can overcome this problem, increasing the efficiency and efficacy of aPDT. Several types of nanoparticle (NP) systems have been studied to potentiate antimicrobial PDT with the aim of improving photosensitizer solubility, photochemistry, photophysics, and targeting [44]. There are two different ways to combine nanoparticles and PDT for antimicrobial applications: (i) the noncovalent encapsulation or incorporation of PS in nanosystems, and (ii) the covalent binding of the PS to the surfaces of the nanoparticles. Furthermore, the nanomaterial itself can take part in the optics, physics, and chemistry of the photodynamic process, capable of photodynamically inactivate microorganisms. As reviewed in [44], compared to free the encapsulation of PS in nanoparticles show several advantages: (i) transport a larger concentrations of PS for the production of lethal reactive oxygen species; (ii) enhance the solubility of nonsoluble water PS; (iii) a controlled release of PS, concentrating the PS in inflammatory and infectious locations by virtue of their enhanced permeability and preservation; (iv) increase the targeting to specific cells and tissues and reduced ability of the target cell to pump out the PS, hence reducing the possibility of multidrug resistance; (v) stopping the PS from dimerizing and trimerizing as it occurs in the free state, forms that are ineffective; and (vi) a selectivity of treatment achieved through either passive targeting or by active targeting (charging of the nanoparticle surface). We will give some examples of nanostructures that have been investigated as PS-delivery systems. As the main application of aPDT is likely to be in the medical (wound and surfaces sterilization) and environmental fields (food industry and water purification), particular interest has been placed on biocompatible and biodegradables nanomatrix, such as polymeric nanoparticles [45], micelles [46], and liposomes [47]. The use of biodegradable polymeric nanoparticles as PS-delivery nanoparticles has been recently reported. Polylacticglycolic acid (PLGA), polyacrylamide (PAA), and calcium phosphate have been used as PS polymeric carriers. For example, see in [48], it has been demonstrated how preparation of poly(lactic-co-glycolic acid) nanoparticles loaded with the PS methylene blue (MB) is effectively not only against biofilm formation, but is also able to kill cells already formed in the biofilm. Moreover, calcium phosphate nanoparticles can be used as efficient carriers for MB and porphyrin, against *S. aureus* and *Pseudomonas aeruginosa* bacteria [45]. Hypericin (a natural potent photosensitizer) can be embedded in amphiphilic block copolymers to form Hypericin-NPs, that when light activated demonstrated better inhibition of biofilm cells compared with planktonic cells [49]. Therefore, the encapsulation of PS in nanoparticles opens a new door for the treatment of infections with minimal side effects. Recently, Chlorine 6 (Ce6), a potent PS used in cancer therapy, has been encapsulated in charge-conversion polymeric nanoparticles (NPs) for efficiently targeting and killing pathogenic bacteria in a weak acidic urinary tract infection environment [50]. Additionally, naturally occurring polymers, such as chitosan and cellulose can be used as novel starting material for the preparation of nontoxic nanoparticles with photobactericidal action [51]. Liposomes nanoparticles are also employed as antimicrobial drug delivery vehicles because their lipid bilayer structure imitates the cell membrane and can readily fuse with infectious microbes. The hydrophobic center of these bilayers can accommodate hydrophobic drugs or PS, while the hydrophilic central region or core can accommodate water-soluble drugs or PS [52]. Liposomes exert their antimicrobial activity through different mechanisms: (i) the fusion with the cell membrane and the release of PS into the cytosol; (ii) the increase in solubility and stability of PS; or (iii) the engulfment of these liposomes in phagocytic cells and their disintegration inside the endosomes or lysosomes, thereby releasing the active PS into the cell [51]. However, the properties of liposome influence mostly the action of liposomes to alter PS distribution. For example, their zeta potential is a determinant parameter influencing their aggregation. It has been showed that values close to zero induce their aggregation, thereby reducing the antimicrobial activity [53], on the contrary if these values are too high (>40 Mv), dark toxicity is present [54], whereas negative potentials result in repulsion between bacterial cells and nanoparticles. An important parameter is the surface charge of liposomes [55]. In particular, cationic liposomes are more effective than neutral or anionic ones in aPDT because of the establishment of electrostatic attraction with the negatively charged cell wall, which facilitate the interaction of liposome to microbial wall, and then the delivery of the PS into the microbial cells. Cationic liposomes for aPDT have been formed from different lipids including the lipid *N*-[1-(2, 3-dioleoyloxy)propyl]-*N,N,N*-trimethylammonium methylsulfate (DOTAP), the DL-a-dipalmitoyl-phosphatidyl-choline (DPPC), and the L-a-dimyristoyl-phosphatidyl-choline (DMPC) [55, 56]. As mentioned before, nanoparticles can also improve the efficacy of aPDT either increasing the $^1O_2$ yield of the PS and by covalently binding the PS to the surface of the nanoparticles. In this design, the PS appears to remain on the surface of the NP, but the NP itself still dictates pharmacokinetics [57]. Theoretically, the singlet oxygen would be more available when generated from the surface than from diffusing with a NP [58]. Rose Bengal is one of the most frequently used PS due to its availability, high water solubility, high singlet oxygen quantum yield, and low rate of photodegradation, and has been linked to polystyrene for inactivating *E. coli* and to silica nanoparticles to inactivate Gram-positive bacteria, including methicillin-resistant *Staphylococcus aureus* [59]. In another study, *S. aureus* has been inactivated with porphyrin bound to carbon nanotubes [60], while the toluidine blue oral (TBO) has been bound to the surface of Au nanoparticles and have been shown to be effective against *S. epidermidis* [61]. What promises to be even more exciting, are those applications where the nanomaterial can acts as PS. The carbon nanomaterials (fullerenes, nanotubes, and graphene) are being discovered to be photoactive in their own right, exhibiting intriguing photo-induced electron transfer properties. Such molecules are particularly attractive due to their long wavelength of absorption, the high quantum yield, and lack of acute toxicity, except in rare cases, in the absence of light. Fullerenes (C60) are the third type of carbon structure; they consist of 60 carbon atoms arranged in a spherical structure that can absorb light and be active PS [62], they generate different ROS according to the solvent, and in polar solvents they produce superoxide and hydroxyl radicals, while in nonpolar solvents they predominantly generate singlet oxygen. As shown from recent studies, their functionalization (with multiple attached cationic groups) make them more soluble in water or other biological fluids and more active for targeting and killing different bacterial species [63]. Titanium oxide (TiO_2) has been more widely studied as a PS among metal oxide nanoparticles in a process termed "photocatalysis," which has been proposed as an antimicrobial strategy for disinfection of surfaces, air, and water [64, 65]. Photocatalysis is the acceleration of a light-mediated reaction in the presence of a catalyst (usually an inorganic semiconductor) [64]. The advantage of photocatalysis is having sunlight or UV-radiation to trigger the disinfection process using a catalyst (TiO_2) [66, 67]. The process has been shown to be capable of killing a wide range of organisms including Gram-negative and Gram-positive bacteria, endospores, fungi, algae, protozoa, and viruses, and has also been shown to be capable of inactivating prions [68]. However, the use of UV-region is also the main obstacle to the use of TiO_2 nanoparticles for medical applications. As a consequence, the research efforts has been in shifting the absorbance spectrum of TiO_2 toward the visible region through doping the titanium surface with other elements, such as ytterbium (Yb^{3+}), erbium (Er^{3+}) [69], and argent [70] ions. Furthermore, the coating with argent and copper, both antimicrobial agents, can enhance the killing activity of TiO_2 [71, 72]. Metal nanoparticles usually are of very small size (i.e., ranging from one to a few nanometers)

http://dx.doi.org/10.5772/65974

and are characterized by a high monodispersity. Most applications of metallic NPs stem from the principle of their surface functionalization (unprotected metal NPS are highly sensitive to air), which allows loading them with large PS doses. Typical metals employed for this purpose include gold, silver, platinum, and palladium. Gold (Au) is not intrinsically antibacterial but gold nanoparticles possess two or more localized surface plasmon resonances (LSPR) that undergo thermal relaxation upon irradiation. This property has been employed to potentiate the photodynamic inactivation. Using different methods of preparation, Au-based nanomaterials such as Au nanospheres, Au nanostars, and Au nanorods can be obtained to inactive bacteria by a photothermic process [73]. Thus, Au-nanoparticles can be conjugated with specific antibody [74], PSs [75], and antibiotics [76], or have intrinsic antibacterial activity [77, 78]. Furthermore, it has been observed that the coating of glass materials with gold nanoparticles proved to be very efficient in photothermal biofilm laser treatment against *S. aureus* biofilms, suggesting the possibility of fabricating medical devices with the same coating: once internalized, they would not need to be removed if a biofilm is formed on their surface but may be treated *in situ*, i.e., through tissues, avoiding surgical removal (**Figure 5**) [79].

Finally, recent studies have proposed that rare earth mineral nanoparticles (the so-called upconversion nanoparticles, consisting of sodium yttrium fluoride ($NaYF_4$) codoped with ytterbium and erbium ions [80]) can be used to transduce near-infrared light into required short wavelength light for activate powerful photosensitizers and for a better penetration of PS into the tissues.

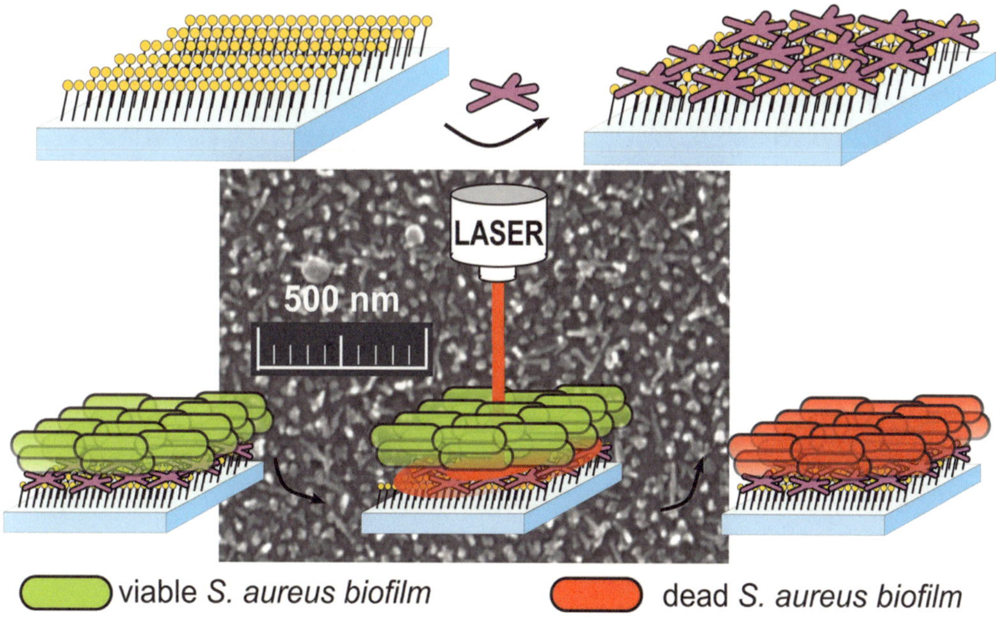

Figure 5. Monolayers of gold nanostars (GNS) grafted on mercaptopropyltrimethoxysilane-coated glass slides for aPDT application.

4. Conclusion

This chapter provides a state-of-the-art analysis about the use of phototherapy and nanotechnology to resist or counteract implant infections, together with a glimpse of the future possible applications and main trends occurring in the field. Progress in the field will correlate with a better understanding of photophysics, chemistry, materials science, biology, and clinical practice, which will allow a rational design of the whole investigation protocol, ranging from optimized formulations to the development of suitable tools for photosensitizers and light beams delivery. Nanotechnology is one of the most rapidly growing fields of translational medicine, and its potential impact on photodynamic therapies is extremely wide. The convergence of phototherapy and nanotechnology may provide new therapeutic modalities (e.g., new nanophotosensitizer formulations) that are easy to apply throughout the body in a targeted manner. In conclusion, exploring the current and possible future interactions between nanotechnology and PDT will offer new outlooks on their bactericidal potentiality.

Acknowledgements

Figure 2 is adapted from [31]. **Figure 5** is reproduced from [79] with permission from the Royal Society of Chemistry.

Author details

Nora Bloise*[1,4], Paolo Minzioni[2], Marcello Imbriani[3,4] and Livia Visai[1,4]

*Address all correspondence to: nora.bloise@unipv.it

1 Department of Molecular Medicine, Center for Health Technologies (CHT), INSTM UdR of Pavia, University of Pavia, Pavia, Italy

2 Department of Electrical, Computer, and Biomedical Engineering, University of Pavia, Pavia, Italy

3 Department of Public Health, Experimental Medicine, and Forensic, University of Pavia, Pavia, Italy

4 Department of Occupational Medicine, Toxicology and Environmental Risks, Istituti Clinici Scientifici Maugeri S.p.A, IRCCS, Pavia, Italy

References

[1] Livermore DM. Antibiotic resistance in staphylococci. Int J Antimicrob Agents. 2000; **16**(1):3–10. DOI: 10.1016/S0924-8579(00)00299-5.

[2] WHO. Antimicrobial resistance: global report on surveillance [Internet] 2014. Available from: http://www.who.int/drugresistance/documents/surveillancereport/en.

[3] Hamblin MR, Hasan T. Photodynamic therapy: a new antimicrobial approach to infectious disease? Photochem Photobiol Sci. 2004; **3**(5):436–450. DOI:10.1039/b311900a.

[4] Dolmans DEJGJ, Fukumura D, Jain RK. Photodynamic therapy for cancer. Nat Rev Cancer. 2003; **3**(5):380–387. DOI:10.1038/nrc1071.

[5] Raab O. The effect of fluorescent substances on infusoria. Zeit Bio. 1900;**39**:524–546.

[6] Wainwright M. Photodynamic antimicrobial chemotherapy (PACT). J Antimicrob Chemother. 1998; **42**(1):13–28. DOI: 10.1093/jac/42.1.13

[7] St Denis TG, Dai T, Izikson L, Astrakas C, Anderson RR, Hamblin MR, Tegos GP. All you need is light: antimicrobial photoinactivation as an evolving and emerging discovery strategy against infectious disease. Virulence. 2011; **2**(6):509–520. DOI:10.4161/viru.2.6.17889.

[8] Nava HR, Allamaneni SS, Dougherty TJ, Cooper MT, Tan W, Wilding G, Henderson BW. Photodynamic therapy (PDT) using HPPH for the treatment of precancerous lesions associated with Barrett's esophagus. Lasers Surg Med. 2011; **43**(7):705–712. DOI:10.1002/lsm.21112.

[9] Hunt DWC. Rostaporfin (Miravant Medical Technologies). IDrugs. 2002;5(2):180–186.

[10] Huang L, Xuan Y, Koide Y, Zhiyentayev T, Tanaka M, Hamblin MR. Type I and Type II mechanisms of antimicrobial photodynamic therapy: an in vitro study on gram-negative and gram-positive bacteria. Lasers Surg Med. 2012; **44**(6):490–499. DOI:10.1002/lsm.22045.

[11] Tim M. Strategies to optimize photosensitizers for photodynamic inactivation of bacteria. J Photochem Photobiol B. 2015; **150**:2–10. DOI:10.1016/j.jphotobiol.2015.05.010.

[12] Wainwright M, Byrne MN GM. Phenothiazinium-based photobactericidal materials. J Photochem Photobiol B. 2006; **84**(3):227–230. DOI:10.1016/j.jphotobiol.2006.03.002.

[13] Yin R, Dai T, Avci P, Serafim Jorge AE,de Melo W, Vecchio V, Huang YY, Gupta A, Hamblin MR. Light based anti-infectives: ultraviolet C irradiation, photodynamic therapy, blue light, and beyond. Curr Opin Pharmacol 2013; **13**:731–762. DOI: 10.1016/j.coph.2013.08.009.

[14] Malik Z, Ladan H, Nitzan Y. Photodynamic inactivation of Gram-negative bacteria: problems and possible solutions. J Photochem Photobiol B Biol. 1992; **14**(3):262–266. DOI :10.1016/1011-1344(92)85104-3.

[15] Malik Z, Hanania J, Nitzan Y. Bactericidal effects of photoactivated porphyrins—an alternative approach to antimicrobial drugs. J Photochem Photobiol B. 1990; **5**(3–4):281-–293.

[16] Jori G, Fabris C, Soncin MS, Coppellotti O, Dei D, et al. Photodynamic therapy in the treatment of microbial infections: basic principles and perspective applications. Lasers Surg Med. 2006; **38**(5):468–481. DOI:10.1002/lsm.20361.

[17] Nikaido H. Prevention of drug access to bacterial targets: permeability barriers and active efflux. Science. 1994; **264**(5157):382–388. DOI: 10.1126/science.8153625.

[18] Merchat M, Bertolini G, Giacomini P, Villaneuva A, Jori G. Meso-substituted cationic porphyrins as efficient photosensitizers of gram-positive and gram-negative bacteria. J Photochem Photobiol B Biol. 1996; **32**(3):153–157. DOI:10.1016/1011-1344(95)07147-4.

[19] Minnock A, Vernon DI, Schofield J, Griffiths J, Parish JH, Brown SB. Mechanism of uptake of a cationic water-soluble pyridinium zinc phthalocyanine across the outer membrane of Escherichia coli. Antimicrob Agents Chemother. 2000; **44**(3):522–527.

[20] Tsai T, Chien H-F, Wang T-H, Huang C-T, Ker Y-B, Chen C-T. Chitosan augments photodynamic inactivation of gram-positive and gram-negative bacteria. Antimicrob Agents Chemother. 2011; **55**(5):1883–1890. DOI:10.1128/AAC.00550-10.

[21] Valduga G, Bertoloni G, Reddi E, Jori G. Effect of extracellularly generated singlet oxygen on Gram-positive and Gram-negative bacteria. J Photochem Photobiol B Biol. 1993; **21**(1):81–86. DOI: 10.1016/1011-1344(93)80168-9.

[22] Costerton JW, Stewart PS, Greenberg EP. Bacterial biofilms: a common cause of persistent infections. Science. 1999; **284**(5418):1318–1322. DOI: 10.1126/science.284.5418.1318.

[23] Chokr A, Watier D, Eleaume H, Pangon B, Ghnassia JC, Mack D, Jabbouri S. Correlation between biofilm formation and production of polysaccharide intercellular adhesin in clinical isolates of coagulase-negative staphylococci. Int J Med Microbiol. 2006; **296**(6):381–388. DOI:10.1016/j.ijmm.2006.02.018.

[24] Stewart PS, William Costerton J. Antibiotic resistance of bacteria in biofilms. Lancet. 2001; **358**(9276):135–138. DOI:10.1016/S0140-6736(01)05321-1.

[25] Walters MC, Roe F, Bugnicourt A, Franklin MJ, Stewart PS. Contributions of antibiotic penetration, oxygen limitation, and low metabolic activity to tolerance of *Pseudomonas aeruginosa* biofilms to ciprofloxacin and tobramycin. Antimicrob Agents Chemother. 2003; **47**(1):317–323. DOI: 10.1128/AAC.47.1.317-323.2003.

[26] Saino E, Sbarra MS, Arciola CR, Scavone M, Bloise N, Nikolov P, Ricchelli F, Visai L. Photodynamic action of Tri-meso (N-methyl-pyridyl), meso (N-tetradecyl-pyridyl) porphine on Staphylococcus epidermidis biofilms grown on Ti_6Al_4V alloy. Int J Artif Organs. 2010; **33**(9):636–645.

[27] Sbarra MS, Di Poto A, Arciola CR, Saino E, Sharma M, Bragheri F, Cristiani I, Speziale P, Visai L. Photodynamic action of merocyanine 540 on Staphylococcus epidermidis biofilms. Int J Artif Organs. 2008; 31(9):848–857.

[28] Hegge AB, Bruzell E, Kristensen S, Tønnesen HH. Photoinactivation of Staphylococcus epidermidis biofilms and suspensions by the hydrophobic photosensitizer curcumin—effect of selected nanocarrier: studies on curcumin and curcuminoides XLVII. Eur J Pharm Sci. 2012; **47**(1):65–74. DOI:10.1016/j.ejps.2012.05.002.

[29] Soares BM, da Silva DL, Sousa GR, Amorim JC, de Resende MA, Pinotti M, Cisalpino PS. In vitro photodynamic inactivation of Candida spp. growth and adhesion to buccal epithelial cells. J Photochem Photobiol B Biol. 2009; **94**(1):65–70. DOI:10.1016/j.jphotobiol.2008.07.013.

[30] Biel MA. Photodynamic therapy of bacterial and fungal biofilm infections. Methods Mol Biol. 2010;**635**:175–194. DOI:10.1007/978-1-60761-697-9_13.

[31] Armentano I, Arciola CR, Fortunati E, Ferrari D, Mattioli S, Amoroso CF, Rizzo J, Kenny JM, Imbriani M, Visai L. The interaction of bacteria with engineered nanostructured polymeric materials: a review. Sci World J. 2014; 2014:410423. DOI:10.1155/2014/410423.

[32] Arciola CR, Alvi FI, An YH, Campoccia D, Montanaro L. Implant infection and infection resistant materials: a mini review. Int J Artif Organs. 2005; 28(11):1119–1125.

[33] Wood S, Metcalf D, Devine D, Robinson C. Erythrosine is a potential photosensitizer for the photodynamic therapy of oral plaque biofilms. J Antimicrob Chemother. 2006; **57**(4):680–684. DOI:10.1093/jac/dkl021.

[34] Metcalf D, Robinson C, Devine D, Wood S. Enhancement of erythrosine-mediated photodynamic therapy of *Streptococcus mutans* biofilms by light fractionation. J Antimicrob Chemother. 2006; **58**(1):190–192. DOI:10.1093/jac/dkl205.

[35] Goulart R de C, Thedei G, Souza SLS, Tedesco AC, Ciancaglini P. Comparative study of methylene blue and erythrosine dyes employed in photodynamic therapy for inactivation of planktonic and biofilm-cultivated *Aggregatibacter actinomycetemcomitans*. Photomed Laser Surg. 2010; **28**(1):85–90. DOI:10.1089/pho.2009.2698.

[36] Brown S. Photodynamic therapy: two photons are better than one. Nat Photon. 2008; **2**(7):394–395. DOI:10.1038/nphoton.2008.112.

[37] Henry CH. Theory of the linewidth of semiconductor lasers. J Quant Electron. 1982; 259.

[38] Gould G. The LASER, light amplification by stimulated emission of radiation. In: The Ann Arbor Conference on Optical Pumping, 15-18 June, 1959.

[39] Einstein A. The Quantum Theory of Radiation. Phys Zeitschrift; 1917; 121.

[40] Marshall N, Dumke W, Burns G, Dill GL F. Stimulated emission of radiation from GaAs p-n junctions. Appl Phys Lett. 1962; **1**:62–64.

[41] Hall R, Fenner G, Kingsley J, TSRC. Coherent light emission from GaAs junctions. Phys Rev Lett. 1962; **9**:366–368. DOI: 10.1103/PhysRevLett.9.366

[42] Huang YY. Low-level laser therapy: an emerging clinical paradigm. SPIE Newsroom [Internet]. 2009 [cited 2016 Jul 29]; Available from: http://www.spie.org/x35504.xml

[43] Mauck M. Knife-edge profiling of Q-switched Nd:YAG laser beam and waist. Appl Opt. 1979; **18**(5):599–600. DOI: 10.1364/AO.18.000599.

[44] Perni S, Prokopovich P, Pratten J, Parkin IP, Wilson M. Nanoparticles: their potential use in antibacterial photodynamic therapy. Photochem Photobiol Sci. 2011; **10**(5):712–720. DOI:10.1039/c0pp00360c.

[45] Schwiertz J, Wiehe A, Gräfe S, Gitter B, Epple M. Calcium phosphate nanoparticles as efficient carriers for photodynamic therapy against cells and bacteria. Biomaterials. 2009; **30**(19):3324–3331. DOI:10.1016/j.biomaterials.2009.02.029.

[46] Tsai T, Yang YT, Wang TH, Chien HF, Chen CT. Improved photodynamic inactivation of gram-positive bacteria using hematoporphyrin encapsulated in liposomes and micelles. Lasers Surg Med. 2009; **41**(4):316–322. DOI:10.1002/lsm.20754.

[47] Ferro S, Ricchelli F, Mancini G, Tognon G, Jori G. Inactivation of methicillin-resistant *Staphylococcus aureus* (MRSA) by liposome-delivered photosensitising agents. J Photochem Photobiol B Biol. 2006; **83**(2):98–104. DOI:10.1016/j.jphotobiol.2005.12.008.

[48] Pagonis TC, Chen J, Fontana CR, Devalapally H, Ruggiero K, Song X, Foschi F, Dunham J, Skobe Z, Yamazaki H, Kent R, Tanner AC, Amiji MM, Soukos NS. Nanoparticle-based endodontic antimicrobial photodynamic therapy. J Endod. 2010; **36**(2):322–328. DOI:10.1016/j.joen.2009.10.011.

[49] Nafee N, Youssef A, El-Gowelli H, Asem H, Kandil S. Antibiotic-free nanotherapeutics: hypericin nanoparticles thereof for improved in vitro and in vivo antimicrobial photodynamic therapy and wound healing. Int J Pharm. 2013; **454**(1):249–258. DOI:10.1016/j.ijpharm.2013.06.067.

[50] Liu S, Qiao S, Li L, Qi G, Lin Y, Qiao Z, Wang H, Shao C. Surface charge-conversion polymeric nanoparticles for photodynamic treatment of urinary tract bacterial infections. Nanotechnology. 2015; **26**(49):495602. DOI:10.1088/0957-4484/26/49/495602.

[51] Yin R, Agrawal T, Khan U, Gupta GK, Rai V, Huang YY, Hamblin MR. Antimicrobial photodynamic inactivation in nanomedicine: small light strides against bad bugs. Nanomedicine (Lond). 2015; **10**(15):2379–2404. DOI:10.2217/nnm.15.67.

[52] Sadasivam M, Avci P, Gupta GK, Lakshmanan S, Chandran R, Huang YY, Kumar R, Hamblin MR. Self-assembled liposomal nanoparticles in photodynamic therapy. Eur J Nanomed. 2013; 5(3). DOI:10.1515/ejnm-2013-0010.

[53] Ferro S, Jori G, Sortino S, Stancanelli R, Nikolov P, Tognon G, Ricchelli F, Mazzaglia A. Inclusion of 5-[4-(1-dodecanoylpyridinium)]-10,15,20-triphenylporphine in supramolecular aggregates of cationic amphiphilic cyclodextrins: physicochemical characterization of the complexes and strengthening of the antimicrobial photosensitizing activity. Biomacromolecules. 2009; **10**(9):2592–2600. DOI:10.1021/bm900533r.

[54] Bombelli C, Bordi F, Ferro S, Giansanti L, Jori G, Mancini G, Mazzuca C, Monti D, Ricchelli F, Sennato S, Venanzi M. New cationic liposomes as vehicles of m-tetrahydroxyphenylchlorin in photodynamic therapy of infectious diseases. Mol Pharm. 2008; **5**(4):672–679. DOI:10.1021/mp800037d.

[55] Banfi S, Caruso E, Buccafurni L, Battini V, Zazzaron S, Barbieri P, Orlandi V. Antibacterial activity of tetraaryl-porphyrin photosensitizers: An in vitro study on Gram negative and

Gram positive bacteria. J Photochem Photobiol B Biol. 2006; **85**(1):28–38. DOI:10.1016/j.jphotobiol.2006.04.003.

[56] Ferro S, Ricchelli F, Monti D, Mancini G, Jori G. Efficient photoinactivation of methicillin-resistant *Staphylococcus aureus* by a novel porphyrin incorporated into a poly-cationic liposome. Int J Biochem Cell Biol. 2007; **39**(5):1026–1034. DOI:10.1016/j.biocel.2007.02.001.

[57] Pitsillides CM, Joe EK, Wei X, Anderson RR, Lin CP. Selective cell targeting with light-absorbing microparticles and nanoparticles. Biophys J. 2003; **84**(6):4023–4032. DOI:10.1016/S0006-3495(03)75128-5.

[58] Tang W, Xu H, Kopelman R, Philbert MA. Photodynamic characterization and in vitro application of methylene blue-containing nanoparticle platforms. Photochem Photobiol. 2005; 81(2):242–249. DOI:10.1562/2004-05-24-RA-176.1.

[59] Guo Y, Rogelj S, Zhang P. Rose Bengal-decorated silica nanoparticles as photosensitizers for inactivation of Gram-positive bacteria. Nanotechnology. 2010; **21**(6):065102. DOI: 10.1088/0957-4484/21/6/065102.

[60] Banerjee I, Mondal D, Martin J, Kane RS. Photoactivated antimicrobial activity of carbon nanotube-porphyrin conjugates. Langmuir. 2010; **26**(22):17369–17374. DOI: 10.1021/la103298e.

[61] Gil-Tomás J, Tubby S, Parkin IP, Narband N, Dekker L, Nair SP, Wilson M, Street C. Lethal photosensitisation of *Staphylococcus aureus* using a toluidine blue O-tiopronin–gold nanoparticle conjugate. J Mater Chem. 2007; **17**(35):3739. DOI:10.1039/b706615e.

[62] Yamakoshi Y, Umezawa N, Ryu A, Arakane K, Miyata N, Goda Y, Masumizu T, Nagano T. Active oxygen species generated from photoexcited fullerene (C60) as potential medicines: O2-* versus $^1O_2$. J Am Chem Soc. 2003; **125**(42):12803–12809. DOI:10.1021/ja0355574.

[63] Huang Y-Y, Sharma SK, Yin R, Agrawal T, Chiang LY, Hamblin MR. Functionalized fullerenes in photodynamic therapy. J Biomed Nanotechnol. 2014; **10**(9):1918–1936. DOI:10.1166/jbn.2014.1963.

[64] Foster HA, Ditta IB, Varghese S, Steele A. Photocatalytic disinfection using titanium dioxide: spectrum and mechanism of antimicrobial activity. Appl Microbiol Biotechnol. 2011; **90**(6):1847–1868. DOI:10.1007/s00253-011-3213-7.

[65] Fujishima A, Honda K. Electrochemical photolysis of water at a semiconductor electrode. Nature. 1972; 238(5358):37–38. DOI:10.1038/238037a0.

[66] Chong MN, Jin B, Chow CWK, Saint C. Recent developments in photocatalytic water treatment technology: a review. Water Res. 2010; 44(10):2997–3027. DOI:10.1016/j.watres.2010.02.039.

[67] Dalrymple OK, Stefanakos E, Trotz MA, Goswami DY. A review of the mechanisms and modeling of photocatalytic disinfection. Appl Catal B Environ. 2010; **98**(1–2):27–38. DOI:10.1016/j.apcatb.2010.05.001.

[68] Paspaltsis I, Kotta K, Lagoudaki R, Grigoriadis N, Poulios I, Sklaviadis T. Titanium dioxide photocatalytic inactivation of prions. J Gen Virol. 2006; **87**(10):3125–3130. DOI:10.1099/vir.0.81746-0.

[69] Wang W, Shang Q, Zheng W, Yu H, Feng X, Wang Z, Feng X, Wang Z, Zhang Y, Li G. A novel near-infrared antibacterial material depending on the upconverting property of Er^{3+}-Yb^{3+}-Fe^{3+} tridoped TiO_2 nanopowder. J Phys Chem C. 2010; 114:13663–13669. DOI: 10.1021/jp102320x.

[70] Wu TS, Wang KX, Li GD, Sun SY, Sun J, Chen JS. Montmorillonite-supported Ag/TiO_2 nanoparticles: an efficient visible-light bacteria photodegradation material. ACS Appl Mater Interfaces. 2010; **2**(2):544–550. DOI:10.1021/am900743d.

[71] Wu B, Huang R, Sahu M, Feng X, Biswas P, Tang YJ. Bacterial responses to Cu-doped TiO_2 nanoparticles. Sci Total Environ. 2010; **408**(7):1755–1758. DOI:10.1016/j.scitotenv.2009.11.004.

[72] Musil J, Louda M, Cerstvy R, et al. Two-functional direct current sputtered silver-containing titanium dioxide thin films. Nanoscale Res Lett. 2009; **4**(4):313–320. DOI:10.1007/s11671-008-9244-z.

[73] Hu B, Zhang LP, Chen XW, Wang JH. Gold nanorod-covered kanamycin-loaded hollow SiO_2 (HSKAu(rod)) nanocapsules for drug delivery and photothermal therapy on bacteria. Nanoscale. 2013; **5**(1):246–252. DOI:10.1039/c2nr32457a.

[74] Zharov VP, Mercer KE, Galitovskaya EN, Smeltzer MS. Photothermal nanotherapeutics and nanodiagnostics for selective killing of bacteria targeted with gold nanoparticles. Biophys J. 2006; **90**(2):619–627. DOI:10.1529/biophysj.105.061895.

[75] Khan S, Alam F, Azam A, Khan AU. Gold nanoparticles enhance methylene blue-induced photodynamic therapy: a novel therapeutic approach to inhibit *Candida albicans* biofilm. Int J Nanomed. 2012; **7**:3245–3257. DOI:10.2147/IJN.S31219.

[76] Burygin GL, Khlebtsov BN, Shantrokha AN, Dykman LA, Bogatyrev VA, Khlebtsov NG. On the enhanced antibacterial activity of antibiotics mixed with gold nanoparticles. Nanoscale Res Lett. 2009; **4**(8):794–801. DOI:10.1007/s11671-009-9316-8.

[77] Perni S, Piccirillo C, Pratten J, Prokopovich P, Chrzanowski W, Parkin IP, Wilson M. The antimicrobial properties of light-activated polymers containing methylene blue and gold nanoparticles. Biomaterials. 2009; **30**(1):89–93. DOI:10.1016/j.biomaterials.2008.09.020.

[78] Gu H, Ho PL, Tong E, Wang L, Xu B. Presenting vancomycin on nanoparticles to enhance antimicrobial activities. Nano Lett. 2003; 3(9): 1261–1263. DOI: 10.1021/nl034396z.

[79] Pallavicini P, Donà A, Taglietti A, Minzioni P, Patrini M, Dacarro G, Chirico G, Sironi L, Bloise N, Visai L, Scarabelli L. Self-assembled monolayers of gold nanostars: a convenient tool for near-IR photothermal biofilm eradication. Chem Commun (Camb). 2014; **50**(16):1969–1971. DOI:10.1039/c3cc48667b.

[80] Lim ME, Lee Y, Zhang Y, Chu JJH. Photodynamic inactivation of viruses using upconversion nanoparticles. Biomaterials. 2012; **33**(6):1912–1920. DOI:10.1016/j.biomaterials.2011.11.033.

Chapter 5

Low Level Energy Photodynamic Therapy for Skin Processes and Regeneration

Antonio Tedesco and Priscila Jesus

Additional information is available at the end of the chapter

http://dx.doi.org/10.5772/65344

Abstract

Skin is the largest human organ and displays multiple functions involving structure and protection against external agents that may affect the body. Solar radiation accelerates the normal aging process and may even cause great damage leading to many different cutaneous diseases and skin cancer. Moreover, a wound in the skin may be an open channel for the access of pathogens usually exposing blood vessels for infections and causing serious complications. For many reasons, regulatory skin processes are of great deal in different approaches: basic antiaging, wound healing, and skin cancer. In a good way, photoprocesses with specific wavelength at low energy levels associated with photoactive compounds are known to cause the opposite effect, promoting the healing of cutaneous diseases and leading to well-defined outcomes in rejuvenation and antiaging. This chapter will discuss the most relevant topics in photo skin regeneration using low energy levels associated with photodynamic therapy (PDT), which emerged as a combination to potentialize molecules with the already known effects of PDT and low level laser therapy (LLLT) in the treatment of skin pathologies, known as a photobiomodulation process.

Keywords: skin, wound healing, antiaging, photodynamic therapy, photobiomodulation

1. Introduction

The basic protocol of photodynamic therapy (PDT), the most classic of the photoprocesses applied to health treatment, involves the use of photosensitizer molecules (natural or synthetic) and visible light in a well-suited design for each application. In the presence of molecular oxygen in the medium and under irradiation, reactive oxygen species (ROS) are generated in high amounts or low amounts, depending on the doses of light, promoting either the destruction of malignant cells, in the first case, or the induction of skin cells proliferation, leading to a stimulated wound healing process with promising results in antiaging effects [1, 2]. The effect known as "photobiostimulation," "photobiomodulation," or "biostimulation" is nondestructive at cell levels, in opposition to PDT main effect. Biostimulation has been applied in medical therapies in the treatment of severe wounds and the control of the pain, as well as in basic scientific research [3].

Studies have suggested that sufficiently decreasing the dose of laser light normally used in the basic PDT protocol could lead to a biostimulatory effect in cells, tissue, or organs, similar to what already happens with low level laser therapy (LLLT) [4]. In addition, cells enriched with low amounts of photosensitizer compounds can proliferate better after application of the LED or laser irradiation at the right wavelength and precise window of time, as the low concentration of generated ROS start a cascade of events leading to a proliferative cellular pathway [5]. Another recent approach in this research field is the laser stimulation at extremely low power densities (around 0.15 mW/cm^2) to enhance biological effects, known as ultralow level laser therapy (ULLLT) [6]. However, a laser power under 0.03 mW has not been proven any detectable response, and the effectiveness of ULLLT is only guaranteed when applied together with acupuncture and administered to acupoints. The tinny channels allow photons to be absorbed in the dermal layer, improving the technique [6].

The treatment with PDT requires, by definition, that parameters such as visible light and photosensitizer drug are simultaneously adjusted in a well-defined sequence of time and concentration to induce the desired effect. Important parameters to control *in vivo* studies include the time of drug uptake, time of treatment, number of applications, exposition time of the target tissue, administration route, and doses, which are critical to the success of this procedure. All parameters have been well evaluated during these long years of PDT studies around the world and have been setup under certain restrict intervals. Physical parameters of light include wavelength, irradiated area, power, energy, and frequency of irradiation [7]. The devices used to irradiate (LED, continuous wave laser or pulsed laser) have also been established, for many of the available setup in the market. The combination of all parameters is the major concern and uncertainty in studies of PDT for photoregeneration and may vary considerably when we move from *in vitro* to *in vivo* and clinical trial studies.

2. Mechanisms of PDT at low levels of energy

The mechanisms of light interaction in the organism and its response have been recently quite well understood, despite a long field to be elucidated [8]. An analogy to plants can be made, as via photosynthesis they absorb light energy by the chromophore groups in the chlorophyll and convert CO_2 and water in a sequence of reactions in the Calvin cycle. In eukaryotes, two mechanisms were suggested to be involved during light-cell interaction. One is acceleration of electrons transfer between redox pairs in some sections of the respiratory chain in the mitochondria [9]. The other is the production of small amounts of reactive oxygen species (ROS)

http://dx.doi.org/10.5772/65344

induced by light absorption mainly by cytochrome c oxidase, a photoacceptor molecule in the mitochondria, accelerating ATP production and cellular proliferation [8].

When a photosensitizer molecule is present, as in PDT, it is first photoactivated to the right excited state of the molecule, by classic photochemical and photophysical pathways well defined by Jablonski diagram [10] and then the produced reactive species may accelerate the increments of ATP production. The most common ROS include superoxide anion (O_2^-) and peroxide hydrogen (H_2O_2) [6]. Briefly, the photosensitizer in the ground state (S_0) absorbs photons and is first excited to singlet state (S_1). The S_1 molecule can either return to its ground state as fluorescence emission or move to triplet excited state (T_1) through intersystem crossing, then forming free radical species by Type I reactions or transferring energy (Type II reactions) to molecular oxygen in the triplet state to the singlet state. The T_1 photosensitizer molecule can also return to S_0 through a process that lasts longer than fluorescence known as phosphorescence [7]. All processes are illustrated in **Figure 1**.

Recently, it has been proposed that PDT stimulates proliferation of dermal fibroblasts caused by low amounts of ROS, which activates extracellular signal-regulated kinases (ERK) [11]. ERK contributes in the regulation of critical cell processes, not only in proliferation, but also differentiation, survival, and apoptosis. It is suggested that fibroblast growth factor (FGF) stimulation leads to the reactivation of ERK signaling [12]. This has been most observed for the treatment of acne, as the photobiomodulation (PBM) effect is associated with increased proliferation of extracellular matrix (ECM) components and gene expression of anti-inflammatory cytokines [13]. The ECM cells, such as fibroblasts and macrophages, produce growth factors, cytokines, and chemokines crucial for regeneration and repair [14].

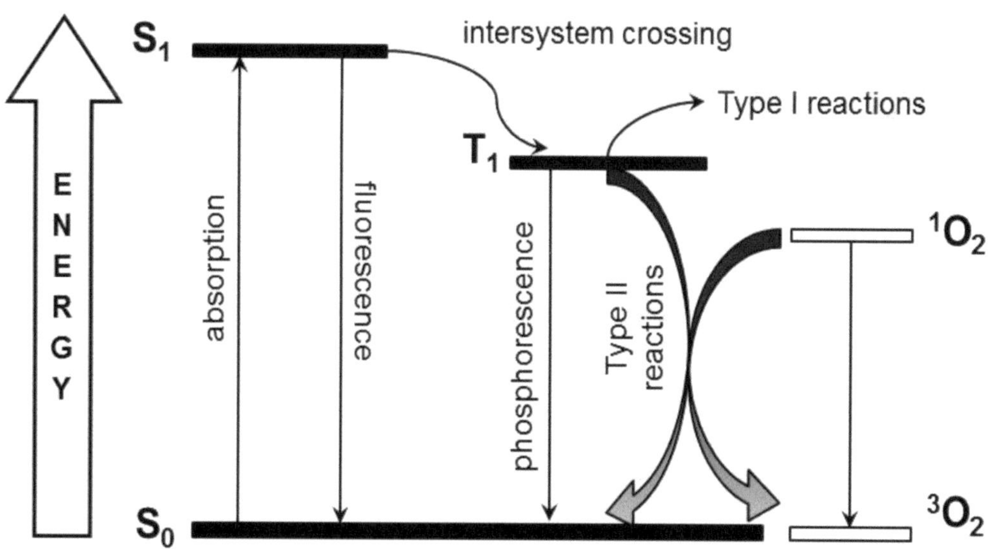

Figure 1. Simplified Jablonski diagram for energy transition between states and from photosensitizers in excited states to molecular oxygen, producing singlet oxygen and other reactive species.

It is important to note that most reactions in the organism are regulated by signaling, altering gene expression. In this concept, the nuclear factor kappa B (NF-kB), a transcription factor, plays an important role, as it regulates the expression of multiple genes and may govern inflammatory and stress-induced responses in the cell [15], activating the mitochondrial cytochrome c oxidase, which will generate ROS. The correlation between NF-kB and the production of ROS happens as NF-kB is activated when the redox state of the mitochondrial membrane is altered. NF-kB is a complex which contains its inhibitory protein, IkB, and for this reason it is inactive in the cytoplasmic medium. ROS are known to stimulate IkB-kinase, which inhibits the production of IkB by ubiquitination and proteasomal degradation with release of NF-kB. NF-kB is then transported to the nucleus and cause the expression of approximately 150 genes possibly involved in defense mechanisms against cell stress. Therefore, the concentration of ROS may contribute to benefit cells proliferation or be cytotoxic [13, 15]. The NF-kB activation can also be stimulated by ROS in other situations involving tumor necrosis factor alpha (TNFa), phorbol ester, and interleukin (IL)-1 [15].

Various signaling routes involved in metalloproteinases (MMPs) transcription control are regulated by redox reactions. This way, researchers propose a relation between MMP activity and production of ROS. It is suggested that ROS acts in the activation or deactivation of some MMPs in transcriptional level, acting in redox signaling routes [16]. Metalloproteinases from the extracellular matrix are calcium-dependent endopeptidases, which contain zinc, and are structural and functionally related to one another [17]. The main function of MMPs is on degradation and/or formation of extracellular matrix. More aspects of MMPs will be discussed in the wound healing section.

3. Topics in photoregeneration

The regeneration process is usually referred to the proliferation of cells and tissues to replace lost structures, as it happens in the growth of an amputated limb in amphibians, as an example. In mammals, whole organs and complex tissues are not fully regenerated; only parts of the liver can grow after partial resection or necrosis, which is known as compensatory growth. Tissues with high proliferative capacity can be continuously renewed after injury, as it happens in the hematopoietic system, the epithelia of the skin, and gastrointestinal tract. However, this is only possible if the stem cells of these tissues are not damaged [14]. These studies belong to the so-called regenerative medicine, an open multidisciplinary field of research involving many different aspects.

Photoregeneration consists in acting direct in the regeneration process using light itself or the combination of a light-based treatment with photoactive compounds in order to restore the lost structures, withhold water loss and decrease the exposition time of a wound or injury, reducing the risk of infection [18]. This is mostly applied in tissue repair in the wound healing process, but the principle can be expanded to regeneration of photodamaged skin, treatment of acne, and other skin pathologies, as well as in antiaging treatment [18]. In the wound healing process, over exposure of a wound can also cause the proliferation of bacteria, as it is an open piece of the organism to the environment. In this context, phototreatment is most considered

http://dx.doi.org/10.5772/65344

due to its antimicrobial properties. This section will discuss important aspects of photoregeneration in anti-aging and wound healing applications. All processes are regarded to skin and, therefore, it is significant to understand the constitution of the skin and its main components.

3.1. Skin

Skin is the largest organ in the human body, comprising about 16% of body weight. An average person can have about 1.8 m^2 of the body covered with skin, which may be submitted to harsh conditions [19]. The same way as other organs, it has the ability to grow, develop, and be repaired. The skin covers the surface of the body and is constituted of an epithelial portion from ectodermal origin, the epidermis, and a connective portion from mesodermal origin, the dermis. The skin plays multiple functions. Due to the corneum layers of epidermis, it protects the organism against water loss and friction, keeping the homeostasis of the system. Besides, the support function is crucial to keep structures such as blood vessels, innervation and muscle, as well as the sensitive function to psycho-emotion reactions, ultraviolet radiation, and endocrine functions [20].

The epidermis can be renewed every 2–3 weeks through the keratinocyte differentiation process [14]. Depending on the thickness of epidermis, varying from 50 to 150 μm, it can be distinguished the thin and thick skin. The thick skin is mostly found in the palms and soles, while the rest of the body is protected by thin skin. The junction between the dermis and epidermis is irregular, as dermis has projections, the dermal papillae, which fit in the indentations in the epidermis, increasing the cohesion between both layers. Hair, nails and sweat and sebaceous glands are attached skin structures [21].

The thickness of the dermis varies from 300 μm in the eyelids to 3 mm in the back. The dermis can be divided in papillary, situated right under the epidermis, and reticular dermis, located between the papillary and hypodermis. The hypodermis, also known as subcutaneous layer, is a loose connective tissue composed primarily by fat cells [22]. The main component of the dermis is the extracellular matrix in the connective tissue. The connective tissue is produced by fibroblasts and is composed of three major classes of biomolecules: glucosaminoglycans (GAGs), proteoglycans, structural proteins (collagen and elastin), and special macromolecules (fibrillin, fibronectin, laminin, and hyaluronan) [23].

3.1.1. Interaction of light in the skin

In PDT, it is important to be able to predict the spatial distribution of light in the target tissue. Light can be scattered or absorbed when it penetrates the tissue, and the extension of both processes depends on the type of tissue and the excitation wavelength. Absorption is mainly due to endogenous chromophores, such as hemoglobin, myoglobin, and cytochromes. Scattering is generally the most relevant factor for the determination of light penetration into the tissue. The combination of light absorption at short wavelengths by important chromophores in the tissue, such as oxy and desoxyhemoglobin and melanin, together with reduced light scattering in longer wavelengths and the occurrence of absorption by water in wavelengths longer than 1300 nm led to the concept of "optical window." In terms of PDT, the effective average of light penetration into the skin is approximately 1–3 mm in 630 nm [1].

The stratum corneum is a protective layer that consists of cells impregnated with keratin and considerably varies in thickness. Except by the scattered light, it is considered optically neutral. In the epidermal layer there is a slight scattering, with low amounts of light that pass through. The result is that all light not absorbed by melanin, main pigment, in the epidermis will pass to the dermis [24]. The dermis is composed by collagen fibers and, different from epidermal layer, it contains sensors, receptors, blood vessels, and nerve endings. Hemoglobin acts as a selective absorber of light. The dermis consists of two structurally different layers, papillary and reticular, which differ mainly in size of collagen fibers. The small size of collagen in the papillary dermis (with diameter smaller in magnitude than the incident light) promotes the back-scattering, in which light is totally directed back to the surface of the skin [24]. **Figure 2** shows an optical microscopy image (10× objective) of human skin biopsy stained by hematoxylin-eosin procedure showing the epidermal and dermal layers and the light pathways.

The blue light penetrates less efficiently into the tissue, while red and infrared radiations penetrate deeper. No source of light is ideal for all indications of PDT, even with the same photosensitizer molecule. The choice of the source of light must be based on the absorption by the photosensitizer drug, the purpose of the action (treatment of a small cancerous lesion or wound healing stimulation), characteristics of the lesion or wound (local, size, accessibility, and characteristics of the tissue) costs and size [7]. A wide number of photosensitizers in different drug delivery systems (DDSs) have been tested for PDT [25–29]. Among them, phthalocyanines

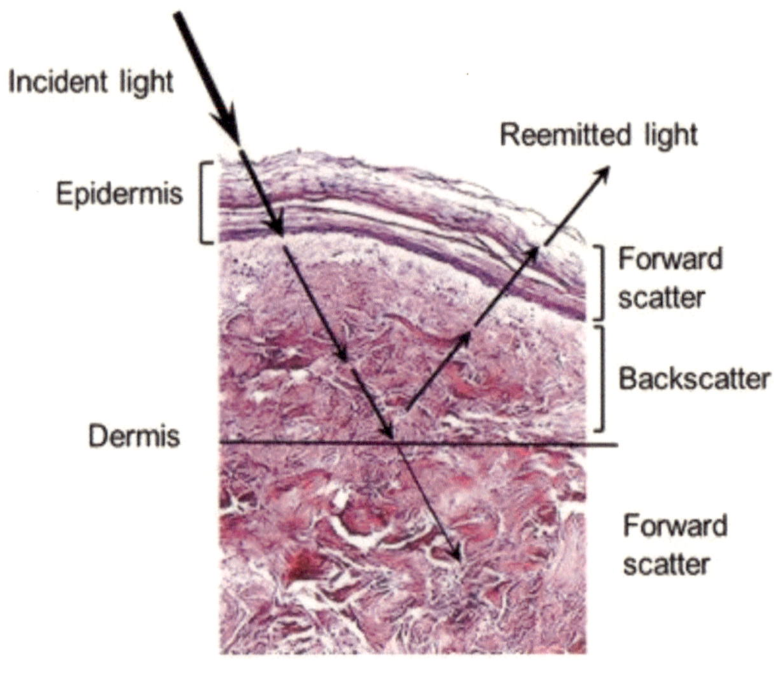

Figure 2. Histological image of human biopsy stained by a hematoxylin-eosin procedure, evidencing the light pathway through epidermal and dermal layers (adapted from Ref. [24]).

(Pc) have been under investigation as promising second-generation photosensitizers, not only for PDT, but also for other applications. Because of their strong red-shifted absorption band, associated with their photophysical response, they are well suited to take advantage of maximal tissue penetration and low-light scattering properties of organelles and tissue at the ideal phototherapeutic window (600–800 nm).For instance, aluminum chloride phthalocyanine presents an intense absorption peak at 670 nm, and, therefore, diode laser operating at this wavelength is required [30, 31].

Mostly, the photobiomodulation effect has been observed when near-infrared light (NIR) is used at low levels; however, there have been reports of red, far-infrared (FIR) [13], green light [32], and specific types of lasers or LED. Normally, PDT requires a source of light in the visible range of light a source of light in the visible range of light spectrum between 600 and 800 nm called "therapeutic window." Today, there are some sources producing visible light in the range of 400–580 nm, due to some natural compounds that absorb light in this range and claim to induce some biological responses, such as curcuminoids and xanthene [33, 34]. Both compounds are phenolic structured in highly conjugated systems and can be used as dyes for drugs, cosmetics, and food. The dyes are primarily photoactivated, affecting enzymes, membrane lipids, and nucleic acids. The ability of these compounds to suppress the superoxide production by macrophages seems to modulate the secretion of protein kinases in tumor cell proliferation and induce the expression of anticarcinogenic enzymes [34, 35]. Recent studies have demonstrated that PDT is not restricted to visible light; deep tissue penetration in PDT could also be achieved with near-infrared (NIR) laser radiation, followed by upconversion to higher-energy visible or ultraviolet light in the biological medium [36, 37].

3.1.2. Collagen and elastin

Collagen constitutes a family of selected proteins during evolution to play different functions, mainly structural. During the organism evolution process, a family from a group of structural proteins influenced by the environment and by organism functional necessities have been modified and acquired variable degrees of stiffness, elasticity, and tensile strength. These proteins are collectively known as collagen, and the main examples of the many types of collagen are the ones found in the skin, bones, cartilage, smooth muscle, and basal lamina [21].

Collagen synthesis was initially associated with a restricted group of cells of the connective tissue, such as fibroblasts, chondroblasts, and osteoblasts. Currently, however, there is sufficient evidence that many types of cells produce this protein. Collagen fibrils are formed by the polymerization of molecular elongated units known as tropocollagen, and various types of collagen result in differences in the chemical structure of these polypeptide chains. In types I, II, and III collagen, the tropocollagen molecules aggregate in subunits to form fibrils. In types I and III collagen, these fibrils associate to form fibers. Type II collagen, present in cartilage, form fibrils but do not form fibers. Type IV collagen, present in basal lamina, form neither fibrils nor fibers [21, 38].

Collagen is the most abundant protein in the organism, representing 30% of its whole dry weight. The types of collagen in vertebrates constitute a family of proteins produced by different cells and are distinguished by their chemical composition, morphological characteristics, distribution, functions, and pathologies. As collagen is the main structural protein and composes 70–80% of the skin dry weight, the modulation of the collagen metabolism in the skin by therapeutic irradiation has clinical importance. The skin collagen synthesized by fibroblasts comprises 80–85% of type I collagen and 10–15% of type III collagen [39]. Type I collagen is easily visualized by optical microscopy after *Picrosirius Red* stain method as long red fibers. However, type III collagen can only be detected by cross-polarized microscopy as short green fibers. **Figure 3** represents both histological procedures [18].

Elastin is the main ECM protein that provides strength and elasticity to many flexible and mechanically active tissues, including skin, lungs, and vocal chords [40]. The most elastin producer cells are fibroblasts and the cells of smooth muscle of blood vessels. Previous to mature elastin, proelastin is formed, a globular molecule of 70 kDa of molecular weight that polymerizes in the extracellular space to form elastin, a rubber-like glycoprotein predominated by elastic fibers. Elastin is resistant to boil, alkaline, and acid extraction and digestion with usual proteinase, but is easily hydrolyzed by pancreatic elastase. The same way as collagen, elastin is rich in glycine and proline. In addition, elastin contains two more uncommon aminoacids, desmosine, and isodesmosine, formed by covalent bonds between four lysine residues. The cross linking seems to be responsible for the elastic consistency of elastin, which is five times more extensible than rubber [21]. Elastin is easily visualized by optical microscopy after *Orcein* stain method as red fibers forming a network, as shown in **Figure 4** [18].

3.2. Antiaging

The aging process of the skin can occur intrinsically and extrinsically. The first refers to chronological changes because of genetic and hormonal modifications with age, and the last is related to external factors, such as UV radiation, smoking, diet, and chemicals [20]. However, among these factors, the most concerning is the prolonged exposure to sunlight during the course of life, promoting serious damage to the skin, and accelerating the regular aging process. This is normally referred to as photoaging, due to the importance of such health care [20]. UV radiation, particularly UVB, is most responsible for direct damage, reaching not only the stratum corneum, but also viable epidermal cells [23]. This way, measures that retard the

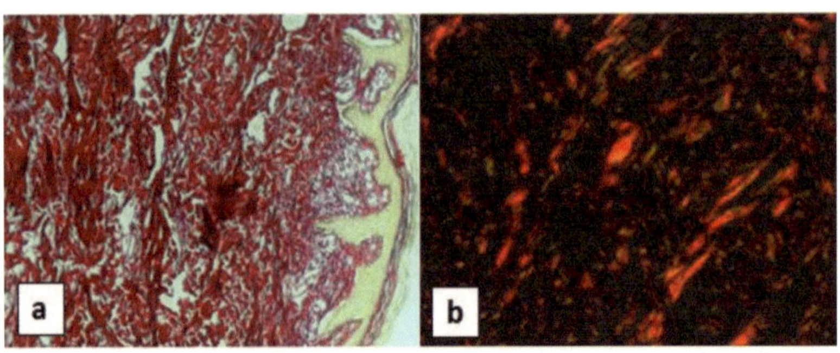

Figure 3. Histological images of human skin biopsies stained by *Picrosirius Red* and visualized by bright field microscopy (a) and cross-polarized microscopy (b).

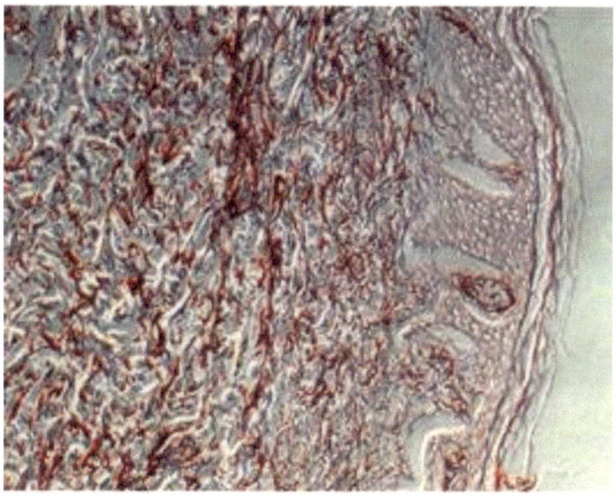

Figure 4. Histological images of human skin biopsies stained by *Orcein* and visualized by bright field microscopy, evidencing elastin fibers.

normal aging process are considered antiaging, and in this context it is relevant to understand the intrinsic changes that happen in the skin during this process.

The first visible and easily recognized aspects that appear in aged skin are the presence of wrinkles, decrease in thickness, transparency, dryness, and irregular hair growth. In deeper level, aged skin has difficulties to sweat and loses subcutaneous fat tissue, which leads to hollowed cheeks and eye sockets [23]. Dermis and epidermis appear to decrease in thickness with age, and their junction may flatten [19]. Despite visible changes, no significant change seems to occur at molecular level, as histology of photoaged skin only presents signs of chronic inflammation [20]. However, at this level it is important to understand the role of stem cells in mitochondria, since stem cell factors regulate mitochondria during aging [41].

The changes in the composition of extracellular matrix constitute an important factor in the aging process. Collagen fibers associated with proteoglycans are important components of dermis, and the healthy skin is dependent on the balance of synthesis and degradation of collagen [42]. In young skin, collagen fibers are more organized, as they are arranged to be extended or stay in the normal configuration. With age, collagen fibers in the skin become denser, decreasing their extensible capacity and being fragmented, disorganized, and less soluble [20].

Not only the fragmentation of ECM occurs, but also in the epidermis the turnover rate of keratinocytes decreases due to decrease of mitotic activity, a process called cellular senescence [23]. This can be explained as the constantly shedding of dead corneocytes in the outer surface and formation of new keratinocytes in the basal layer. Besides, protein composition of cornified envelope, responsible for barrier function, changes. The metabolism of calcium is strictly related to the aging process, especially in the epidermis. Reduction of calcium production with age inhibits full differentiation of keratinocytes in the stratum granulosum [19].

The same way, elastin fibers suffer considerable changes in variation of density, as they are intertwined with collagen forming the ECM. The UV radiation in contact with skin and in the presence of oxygen produces high concentrations of ROS or free radicals, which induce gene expression resulting in collagen degradation and elastin accumulation. The remodeling process of such network is primarily controlled by the activity of matrix metalloproteinase (MMPs). In photodamaged skin, ROS induces the production of MMPs that degrade collagen while the expression of the MMP inhibitors (TIMP) is reduced [20, 23]. These events triggered by ROS can be reduced by the use of antioxidants. In the opposite way, low concentrations of ROS are thought to inactivate MMPs and reduce the formation of wrinkles [43, 44].

Studies examined PDT for the treatment of photoaging in different levels, from *in vitro* assays using fibroblast cells [11] to animal studies using hairless mouse model [45] and clinical assays [43]. There are a few published reviews about photodynamic rejuvenation, most exposing the use of MAL (methyl aminolevulinic acid) or 5-ALA (5-aminolevulinic acid) as photosensitizers [46]. They reported excellent cosmetic effects, sustaining the hypothesis of induction of collagen formation in the dermal layer [44], even in the treatment of patients with severe photodamaged skin [43]. The changes in collagen and skin texture are good parameters for histological examination. The photodynamic rejuvenation technique seems to show excellent short-term efficacy and tolerability.

3.3. Wound healing

In the ancient Egypt, from a paraphysiological perspective, a wound was considered an opening in the body where fiends could enter or leave [47]. With development of medicine, the treatment of wounds consisted in the application of bandages containing medicine, herbs with healing properties, over the lesion. Until not long ago, about 50 years, this was the most used method, considering the advances in medicines and medical techniques.

Wound healing is a natural process to keep the integrity of the skin of those who have been submitted to surgery or that simply have been injured [48, 49]. The concept comprises not only the skin; it can be expanded to treatment of periodontal diseases [50] and cartilage regeneration [51]. Various methods have been adopted to improve the healing of wounds of many types, including the potential use of irradiation at low doses [52]. Some of the biostimulatory effects were confirmed *in vitro* for the proliferation of fibroblasts, collagen synthesis, stimulation of macrophages, and higher rates of extracellular matrix production [53].

Epidermal regeneration in mammals was conventionally described by histologists consisting of three phases: mitosis, migration, and differentiation [54]. Only epidermis is able to regenerate, while complex healing process of dermis and its development can be summarized in three steps: an initial inflammatory stage, followed by proliferation and finally repair, tissue remodeling stage (maturation), although they are not strictly separated from each other [55, 56]. However, regeneration and scar formation depend on the extent of the injury and the ability of the organism to initiate such processes. For instance, a superficial wound only requires reepithelialization, while a deep and extensive wound initiates a series of events essential for the organism survival, which occur right after any indication of tissue destruction [14].

3.3.1. Wound healing phases

The inflammatory phase depends on the inflammatory cells, such as polymorphonuclear leukocytes (PMN), macrophages, and lymphocytes, besides numerous chemical mediators.

PMN acts from the moment of tissue injury for a period that varies from 3 to 5 days, and is responsible for bacteria phagocytosis. Macrophage is the most important cell in this phase and remains in the wound from the 3rd to the 10th day [57, 58]. Besides bacteria phagocytosis, it debrides foreign bodies and directs the development of granulation tissue. Also, they secrete cytokines, compounds that coordinate immune responses, besides recruiting further immune cells to the infection local [50]. Lymphocytes appear in the wound in approximately 7 days and their roles are not fully defined, although lymphokines produced by these cells influence macrophages. In addition to these cells and chemical mediators, the inflammatory phase also counts on the important role of fibronectin, which is synthesized by a variety of cells, such as fibroblasts and endothelial cells, working as an adhesive to strengthen the fibrin clot, the cells, and extracellular matrix components [59].

The cells proliferation phase happens over the 5th to 14th days and initiates the repair process of both dermis and epidermis [59]. It is crucial for the formation of granulation tissue, which is a combination of cell elements, including fibroblasts, inflammatory cells, and endothelial components of ECM, such as fibronectin, glycosaminoglycans, and collagen. The formation of granulation tissue depends on the action of fibroblasts to produce collagen, elastin, fibronectin, glycosaminoglycans, and proteinases, responsible for debridement and physiological remodeling. During proliferation, it also occurs the angiogenesis, essential to oxygen, and nutrients supply for scar formation [60].

The last two phases, contraction and remodeling, are later processes, responsible for maturation of wounds. The first occurs with intense participation of myofibroblasts with consequences on lesion contraction. The latter, provided by bridge formation between collagen fibers, results on the development of mature scar [61]. Synthesis of structural proteins, such as collagen, remains at high levels for 6–12 months, although the scar reaches up to 70% of the tensile strength of intact skin [62].

Fibroblasts play an important role in a series of physiological events, such as the wound healing process. In this case, fibroblasts of the side connective tissue become activated, proliferate, migrate to the clot in reabsorption, and start to synthesize the ECM components, such as collagen and elastin [60]. During wound healing process, the portion of collagen increases with time, and by two weeks their fibers dominate the ECM. Phagocytic cells slightly disappear and the granulation tissue is progressively constituted by a denser and less vascularized tissue, located right under the regenerated epidermis [59]. Collagen degradation initiates early and is more active during inflammatory process. Therefore, the development of ECM is a result of balance between collagen deposition and degradation.

3.3.2. The role of matrix metalloproteinases (MMPs)

Matrix metalloproteinases are a family of secreted or transmembrane endopeptidases with similar structural domains which degrade ECM components. They can be classified in groups based on substrate specificity. One group comprises the interstitial collagenases MMP-1, 8 and 13, that recognize collagen types I, II, and III. Another one is composed of the stromelysins MMP-3, 10, and 11, with specificity for laminin, fibronectin, and proteoglycans. The gelatinases MMP-2 and 9 comprise another group, and cleave collagen types IV and V. Regulation of gene expression of most MMPs occurs by transcription factors [62, 63].

As previously discussed, MMPs can influence various cellular properties, such as growth, death, and migration [64]. In the tissue repair process, MMPs directly interfere in molecular and cell events. In the inflammatory phase, MMP-2 and MMP-9 act as chemical mediators on the stimulation steps in phagocytic phase. In granulation phase (proliferation), MMPs act along with other biomolecules with regulating activity in the formation of collagen and elastin matrix, reepithelialization, and vascularization [65].

Gelatinase B (MMP-9) is a typical MMP, important on the migration of different cell types, such as leucocytes and tumor cells, due to its ability in degrading basal membranes and ECM components, such as collagen and elastin. Gelatinase B promotes migration of new bone marrow leucocytes to blood vessels, and then to the tissue infection sites [66]. MMP-9 expression is normally constant during whole tissue remodeling phase. In addition, it is directly related to the cell migration during morphogenesis and organogenesis processes [67]. Equally, MMP-9 has been considered during creation and development of fibrillar network, associated with the production of elastin network particularly due to the presence of type I fibrillin [68].

Analogous to MMP-9, the expression of MMP-2 (gelatinase A) in the ECM is observed after collagen remodeling phase. Previous studies have demonstrated that dermal fibroblasts promote increase of MMP-2 expression from the first to the 21st day of development [61]. Once such enzymes degrade ECM and are synthesized by cells, there is an important control of their production, which is the latency. These enzymes are synthesized as proenzymes, which are inactive until being activated by (auto)proteolysis. This mechanism initiates a cascade of events in which each enzyme is activated by its precedent and, at the same time, activates the one that succeeds it. This way, the conversion of progelatinase B to its active form is catalyzed by MMP-3 or MMP-2 [66].

Nelson and Melendez [16] demonstrated that the expression and activation of MMPs are regulated via oxidative processes from redox reactions involving ROS in aerobic organisms, by mitochondrial mechanisms and cell modulation. Monochromatic irradiation and photodynamic mechanisms alter ROS intra/intercellular concentration, affecting the electric-physiological metabolism of mitochondria, which leads to acceleration of transcription expression of MMPs and other ECM biomolecules [67].

Studies [44] have demonstrated that ROS generated after UV irradiation initiate the increase of MMPs by a complex signaling mechanism, decreasing the expression of procollagen I and procollagen-III, culminating on reduction of dermal matrix generation. Some physiological processes, such as aging and wound healing, can be evaluated relating collagen synthesis to levels of MMPs expression. The deficiency of collagen due to natural aging derives from its reduced synthesis with increasing of degradation and concomitant elevation of MMP expression. UV radiation induces MMP synthesis in human skin, and the destruction of collagen mediated by MMP counts mostly by the damage in connective tissue with photoaging [69]. It suggests that not only the synthesis of proteins in the ECM, but also their degradation is increased in irradiated skin [39].

The activities of MMP-2 and MMP-9 can be experimentally detected and measured by gelatin zymography followed by data analysis for quantification. As gelatinases are secreted enzymes, the culture media in experiments involving cells proliferation can be collected for the assays, being possible to evaluate the presence of such enzymes during different periods of treatment. The basic procedure consists in electrophoresis in polyacrylamide gels containing gelatin, inoculated with the media samples and revealed by an enzyme substrate buffer (50 mM Tris-HCl pH 8.0, 5 mM $CaCl_2$, 0.02% NaN_3), followed by staining protocols. The non-colored areas are quantitative related to the degradation activity of MMP-2 and MMP-9, in both pro and active forms [18, 70].

3.3.3. PDT on wound healing

Studies have evidenced that the treatment with He-Ne laser in cutaneous lesions would accelerate wound healing process [71]. As no increase of temperature was observed during light irradiation, the effects at cell level were considered more biochemical than thermal. Besides, no stress was expected during irradiation [22]. Combinations of light and drug, such as ALA/He-Ne laser and HpD/He-Ne and Nd:YAG lasers were tested in rats and demonstrated good performance in biostimulation [52].

Tissue stimulation was tested in human skin biopsies using the photosensitizer silicon-naphthalocyanine in lipossomal formulation and irradiation with laser at 670 nm and doses of 0.5, 1, 3, and 5 J/cm^2 [67]. This study has initiated a new approach in the application of photodynamic processes in cutaneous remodeling. It was found that the stimulatory effects were enhanced when PDT at low doses was applied instead of light itself. One study that evaluated the influence of continuous irradiation of diode laser (670 nm), with daily doses of 30 J/cm^2 in rat skin reported that the most significant morphological changes occurred during the first 7 days of wound healing [56]. A recently published study tested the effects of PDT using aluminum chloride phthalcyanine in nanoemulsion as photosensitizer and laser light at doses of 70, 140, and 700 mJ/cm^2 in human skin biopsies [18]. PDT at the intermediary dose promoted the increase of approximately 20% in collagen and elastin, as well as in MMPs expression, which was not reached using only light. The photobiomodulation effect was observed even in the first 7 days after irradiation, but the most prominent was reached after 14 days [72].

Here, we present the results of many photobiological studies evaluating the effects of low visible light at 685 nm, alone or combined with a phthalocyanine-derived photosensitizer dye (NzPC), on the healing process of cutaneous wounds using 3D dermal fibroblast collagen lattice as dermal equivalent (DE). Irradiations were carried out at 685 nm and, first, doses of 5, 10, and 20 J/cm^2 were applied 1 hour after the dye uptake, developed 24 hours after DE preparation. Contraction was reduced in all days of analysis (1, 3, and 7) and the number of cells decreased very fast. Then, lower doses (1, 3, and 5 J/cm^2) were tested and a new parameter was introduced, the effect of a delay time between dye andligth application (1–72 hours). The results showed that for doses higher than 1 J/cm^2 some toxicity were still present (>50%), but the delay in the ligth application seems to be crucial to a positive effect.

In the same studies, gelatin zymography was performed as previously described. Concerning metalloproteinase expressions, interestingly, MMP-9 expression was constant within fibroblasts during the collagen lattice remodeling and its progressive diffusion to the extracellular matrix occured later. The constant value for MMP-9 expression early observed as major lattice remodeling could thus be responsible for the later appearance of type I fibrillin.

Similarly, MMP-2 expression both within the extracellular matrix and the secretion in the culture medium was also observed after the early remodeling phase of the collagen lattice. The observations on the decreasing levels of active MMP-2 are in accordance with the findings of indirect immunodetection analysis comparing the expression of α-actin, fibrillin, and type I and III collagen (data not shown). In addition, it was found that for both types of treatment, the activated form of MMP-2 becomes higher than the proform of the enzyme after 12 days of culture.

Recent publications also reported the use of PDT with different photosensitizers and applications. Regarding oral diseases, PDT with methylene blue (MB) was tested on wound healing of rat buccal mucosa as a promising antimicrobial modality. The study qualitatively showed that MB-mediated PDT would have an inhibitory effect on healing process after 14 days of the wound creation [73]. In the same field, a review study evaluated current evidence and focused on gaps in knowledge to identify potential paths forward for clinical translation with photobiomodulation (PBM) therapy with an emphasis on craniofacial wound healing. They concluded that PBM offers a novel opportunity to examine fundamental nonvisual photobiological processes as well as develop innovative clinical therapies in clinical dentistry [74].

Regarding severe wounds, PDT with MB delayed reepithelialization in rats' wounds on the 7th day and interfered in standard healing. However, when used separately, MB and LLLT had a significant effect in the analyzed periods (1, 3, 14, and 21 days), when compared to control group [75]. Other studies evaluated third degree burns with lesions in mice treated with LED. The results showed that the LED-irradiaton was able to accelerate the wound healing process. In addition, a statistically significant microbial reduction was obtained with photodynamic inactivation compared to chemical decontamination [76]. Other types of model of study have been tested, such as the adult human skin wound healing organ culture (WHOC) treated with PDT. It demonstrated increased reepithelialization and extracellular matrix reconstruction and remodeling [77].

Author details

Antonio Tedesco* and Priscila Jesus

*Address all correspondence to: atedesco@usp.br

Department of Chemistry, Center of Nanotechnology and Tissue Engineering, University of Sao Paulo, USP, Ribeirao Preto, Sao Paulo, Brazil

References

[1] Castano, A.P., Demidova, T.N., Hamblin, M.R. Mechanisms in photodynamic therapy: part one—photosensitizers, photochemistry and cellular localization. Photodiagnosis and Photodynamic Therapy. 2004;**1**:279—293. DOI: 10.1016/S1572-1000(05)00007-4

[2] Primo, F.L., Siqueira-Moura, M.P., Simioni, A.R., Pet, A.P.F., Tedesco A.C. Preparation, characterization and cytotoxicity assays of chloroaluminum phthalocyanine photosensitizer drug loaded in PLGA-nanocapsules. Drugs of the Future. 2007;**32**:74–74.

[3] França, C.M., Anders, J.J., Lanzafame, R.J. Photobiomodulation in wound healing: what are we not considering? Photomedicine and Laser Surgery. 2016;**34**:51–52.

[4] Lubart, R., Eichler, M., Lavi, R., Friedman, H., Shainberg, A. Low-energy laser irradiation promotes cellular activity. Photomedicine and Laser Surgery. 2005;**23**:3–9.

[5] Peplow, P.V., Chung, T.Y., Baxter, G.D. Photodynamic modulation of wound healing: a review of human and animal studies. Photomedicine and Laser Surgery. 2012;**30**:118–148.

[6] Baratto, L., Calza, L., Capra, R., Gallamini, M., Giardino, L. Giulliani, A., et al. Ultra-low-level laser therapy. Lasers in Medical Science. 2011;**26**:103–112.

[7] Agostinis, P., Berg, K., Cengel, K.A., Foster, T.H., Girotti, A.W., Gollnick, S.O., et al. Photodynamic therapy of cancer: an update. Ca—A Cancer Journal for Clinicians. 2011;**61**:250–281.

[8] Passarella, S., Karu, T. Absorption of monochromatic and narrow band radiation in the visible and near IR by both mitochondrial and non-mitochondrial photoacceptors results in photobiomodulation. Journal of Photochemistry and Photobiology B: Biology. 2014;**140**:344–358.

[9] Karu, T., Kolyakov, S.F. Exact action spectra for cellular responses relevant to phototherapy. Photomedicine and Laser Surgery. 2005;**23**:355–361.

[10] Foote, C.S. Definition of Type I and Type II photosensitized oxidation. Journal of Photochemistry and Photobiology. 1991;**54**:659.

[11] Jang, Y.H., Koo, G.B., Kim, J.Y., Kim, Y.S., Kim, Y.C. Prolonged activation of ERK contributes to the photorejuvenation effect in photodynamic therapy in human dermal fibroblasts. Journal of Investigative Dermatology. 2013;**133**:2265–2275.

[12] Joo, D., Woo, J.S., Cho, K.H., Han, S.H., Min, T.S., Yang, D.C. et al. Biphasic activation of extracellular signal-regulated kinase (ERK) 1/2 in epidermal growth factor (EGF)-stimulated SW480 colorectal cancer cells. BMB Reports. 2016;**49**:220–225.

[13] Barolet, D., Christiaens, F., Hamblin, M.R. Infrared and skin: friend or foe. Journal of Photochemistry & Photobiology B: Biology. 2016;**155**:78–85.

[14] Caramella, C., Conti, B., Modena, T., Ferrari, F., Bonferoni, M.C., Genta, I., et al. Controlled delivery systems for tissue repair and regeneration. Journal of Drug Delivery Science and Technology. 2016;**32**:206–228.

[15] Chen, A.C.H., Arany, P.R., Huanh, Y.Y., Tomkinson, E.M., Sharma, S.K., et al. Low-level laser therapy activates NF-kB via generation of reactive oxygen species in mouse embryonic fibroblasts. PLoS One. 2011;**6**(7) e22453

[16] Nelson, K.K., Melendez, J.A. Mitochondrial redox control of matrix metalloproteinases. Free Radical Biology and Medicine. 2004;**37**:768–784.

[17] Bode, W., Maskos, K. Structural basis of the matrix metalloproteinases and their physiological inhibitors, the tissue inhibitors of metalloproteinases. Biological Chemistry. 2003;**384**:863–872.

[18] Jesus, P.C.C., Saeki, S.I.N., Tedesco, A.C. An ex vivo study of photobiostimulation in the treatment of skin pathologies. Journal of Biophotonics. 2016;**9**:1–10. DOI: 10.1002/jbio.201500288

[19] Rinnerthaler, M., Streubel, M.K., Bischof, J., Richter, K. Skin aging, gene expression and calcium. Experimental Gerontology. 2015;**68**:59–65.

[20] Tobin, D.J. Introduction to skin aging. Journal of Tissue Viability. 2017; **26**:37-46 DOI: 10.1016/j.jtv.2016.03.002

[21] Montagna, W., Parakkal, P.F. The structure and function of the skin. 3rd ed. New York: Academic Press; 1974.

[22] Dams, S.D., Liefde-Van Beest, M., Nuijs, A.M., Ooomens, C.W.J., Baaijens, F.P.T. Heat shocks enhance procollagen type I and III expression in fibroblasts in ex vivo human skin. Skin Research and Technology. 2011;**17**:167–180.

[23] Kammeyer, A., Luiten, R.M. Oxidation events and skin aging. Ageing Research Reviews. 2015;**21**:16–29.

[24] Claridge, E., Cotton, S., Hall, P., Moncrieff, M. From colour to tissue histology: physics-based interpretation of images of pigmented skin lesions. Medical Image Analysis. 2003;**7**:489–502.

[25] Vena, F.C.B., Turchiello, R.F., Laville, I., Pigaglio, S., Blais, J., Tedesco, A.C. 5-Aminolevulinic acid ester-induced protoporphyrin IX in a murine melanoma cell line. Lasers in Medical Science. 2004;**19**:119–126.

[26] Turchiello, R.F., Vena, F.C.B., Maillard, Ph., Souza, C.S., Bentley, M.V.B., Tedesco, A.C. Cubic phase gel as a drug delivery system for topical application of 5-ALA, its ester derivatives and m-THPC in photodynamic therapy (PDT). Journal of Photochemistry and Photobiology B: Biology. 2003;**70**:1–6.

[27] Simioni, A.R., Primo, F.L., Tedesco, A.C. Silicon(IV) phthalocyanine-loaded nanoparticles for application in photodynamic process. Journal of Laser Applications. 2012;**24**:012004-1.

[28] Primo, F.L., Bentley, M.V.B., Tedesco, A.C. Photophysical studies and in vitro skin permeation/retention of Foscan®/nanoemulsion (NE) applicable to photodynamic therapy skin cancer treatment. Journal of Nanoscience and Nanotechnology. 2008;**8**:340–347.

[29] Maranho, D.S., De Lima, R.G., Primo, F.L., Da Silva, R.S., Tedesco, A.C. Photoinduced nitric oxide and singlet oxygen release from ZnPC liposome vehicle associated with the nitrosyl ruthenium complex: synergistic effects in photodynamic therapy application. Photochemistry and Photobiology. 2009;**85**:705–713.

[30] Siqueira-Moura, M.P., Primo, F.L., Peti, A.P.F., Tedesco, A.C. Validated spectrophotometric and spectrofluorimetric methods for determination of chloroaluminum phthalocyanine in nanocarriers. Pharmazie. 2010;**65**:9–14.

[31] Barbugli, P.A., Siqueira-Moura, M.P., Espreafico, E.M., Tedesco, A.C. In vitro phototoxicity of liposomes and nanocapsules containing chloroaluminum phthalocyanine on human melanoma cell line. Journal of Nanoscience and Nanotechnology. 2010;**10**:569–573.

[32] Catão, M.H.C.V., Costa, R.O., Nonaka, C.F.W., Albuquerque Junior, R.L.C., Costa, R.R.S. Green LED light has anti-inflammatory effects on burns in rats. Burns. 2016;**42**:392–396.

[33] Cai, Y., Luo, Q., Sun, M., Corke, H. Antioxidant activity and phenolic compounds of 112 traditional Chinese medicinal plants associated with anticancer. Life Sciences. 2004;**74**:2157–2184.

[34] Ritchie, E.E., Princz, J.I., Robidoux, P.Y., Scroggins, R.P. Ecotoxicity of xanthene dyes and a non-chlorinated bisphenol in soil. Chemosphere. 2013;**90**:2129–2135.

[35] Rubya, A.J., Kuttan, G., Babub, D., Rajasekharanb, K.N., Kutta, R. Anti-tumour and antioxidant activity of natural curcuminoids. Cancer Letters. 1995;**94**:79–83.

[36] Kachynski, A.V., Pliss, A., Kuzmin, A.N., Ohulchanskyy, T.Y., Baev, A., Qu, J., et al. Photodynamic therapy by in situ nonlinear photon conversion. Nature Photonics. 2014;**8**:455–461.

[37] Nigoghossian, K., Peres, M.F.S., Primo, F.L., Tedesco, A.C., Pecorarol, E., Messaddeq, Y., et al. Infrared to visible up-conversion in biocellulose-ytrium vanadate nanoparticles composite membranes. Demonstration of Chloroaluminum phthalocyanine light emission under up-converted light excitation. Colloids and Interface Science Communications. 2014;**2**:6–10.

[38] Shoulders, M.D., Raines, R.T. Collagen structure and stability. Annual Review of Biochemistry. 2009;**78**:929–958. DOI: 10.1146/annurev.biochem.77.032207.120833

[39] Riekki, R., Jukkola, A., Sassi, M.L., Hoyhtya, M., Kallioinen, M., Risteli, J., et al. Modulation of skin collagen metabolism by irradiation: collagen synthesis is increased in irradiated human skin. British Journal of Dermatology. 2000;**142**:874–880.

[40] Grieshaber, S.E., Farran, A.J.E., Bai, S., Kiick, K.L., Jia, X.Q. Turning the properties of elastin mimetic hybrid copolymers via a modular polymerization method. Biomacromolecules. 2012;**13**:1774–1786.

[41] Min-Wen, J.C., Jun-Hao, E.T., Shyh-Chang, N. Stem cell mitochondria during aging. Seminars in Cell & Developmental Biology. 2016;**52**:110–118.

[42] Valentini, D.M.Z., Silva, J., Teodoro, W.R., Velosa, A.P., Mello, S.B.V. Effect of topical clay application on the synthesis of collagen in skin: an experimental study. Clinical and Experimental Dermatology. 2012;**37**:164–168.

[43] Bissonnette, R. Treatment of acne with photodynamic therapy. Giornale Italiano di Dermatologia e Venereologia. 2011;**146**:445–456.

[44] Szeimes, R.M., Torezan, L., Niwa, A., Valente, N., Unger, P., Kohl, E., et al. Clinical , histopathological and immunohistochemical assessment of human skin field cancerization before and after photodynamic therapy. British Journal of Dermatology. 2012;**167**(150–159)

[45] Lv, T., Huang, Z.-F., Wang, H.-W., Lin, J.-Q., Chen, G.-N., Chen, X.-W., et al. Evaluation of collagen alteration after topical photodynamic therapy (PDT) using second harmonic generation (SHG) microscopy—in vivo study in a mouse model. Photodiagnosis and Photodynamic Therapy. 2012;**9**:164–169.

[46] Le Pillouer-Prost, A., Hugues, C. Photodynamic photorejuvenation: a review. Dermatologic Surgery. 2016;**42**:21–30.

[47] Sipos, P., Gyory, H., Hagymasi, K., Ondrejka, P., Blazovics, A. Special wound healing methods used in ancient Egypt and the mythological background. World Journal of Surgery. 2004;**28**:211–216.

[48] Coulomb, B., Dubertret, L. Skin cell culture and wound healing. Wound Repair and Regeneration. 2002;**10**:109–112.

[49] Dreifke, M.B., Jayasuriya, A.A., Jayasury, A.C. Current wound healing procedures and potential care. Materials Science and Engineering C. 2015;**48**:651–662.

[50] Morand, D.N., Davideau, J.-L., Clauss, F., Jessel, N., Tenenbaum, H., Huck, O. Cytokines during periodontal wound healing: potential application for new therapeutic approach. Oral Diseases. 2016;12469

[51] Temeno, J.S., Mikos, A.G. Review: tissue engineering for regeneration of articular cartilage. Biomaterials. 2000;**21**:431–440.

[52] Jayasree, R.S., Gupta, A.K., Rathinam, K., Mohanan, P.V., Mohanty, M. The influence of photodynamic therapy on the wound healing process in rats. Journal of Biomaterials Applications. 2001;**15**:176–186.

[53] Gungormus, M., Akyol, U.K. Effect of biostimulation on wound healing in diabetic rats. Photomedicine and Laser Surgery. 2009;**27**:607–610.

[54] Odland, G., Ross, R. Human wound repair. 1. Epidermal regeneration. Journal of Cell Biology. 1968;**39**:135.

[55] Aukhil, I. Biology of wound healing. Periodontology. 2000;**22**:44–50.

[56] Gal, P., Vidinski, B., Toporcer, T., Mokry, M., Mozes, S., Longauer, F., et al. Histological assessment of the effect of laser irradiation on skin wound healing in rats. Photomedicine and Laser Surgery. 2006;**24**(4):480–488.

[57] Leonida, M.D., Kumar, I. Wound healing and skin regeneration. Bionanomaterials for Skin Regeneration. 2016;**3**:17–25.

[58] Synder, R.J., Lantis, J., Kirsner, R.S., Shah, V., Molyneaux, M., Carter, M.J. Macrophages: a review of their role in wound healing and their therapeutic use. Wound Repair and Regeneration. 2016; **24**(4):613-629 DOI: 10.1111/wrr.12444

[59] Shaw, T.J., Martin, P. Wound repair: a showcase for cell plasticity and migration. Current Opinion in Cell Biology. 2016;**42**:29–37.

[60] Kuffler, D.P.. Photobiomodulation in promoting wound healing: a review. Regenerative Medicine. 2015 11(1):107-122.

[61] Chaussain-Miller, C., Septier, D., Bonnefoix, M., Lecolle, S., Lebreton-Decoster, C., Coulomb, B., et al. Human dermal and gingival fibroblasts in a three-dimensional culture: a comparative study on matrix remodeling. Clinical Oral Investigation. 2002;**6**:39–50.

[62] Muzzarelli, R.A.A. Chitins and chitosans for the repair of wounded skin, nerve, cartilage and bone. Carbohydrate Polymers. 2009;**76**:167–182.

[63] Ayuk, S.M., Abrahamse, H., Houreld, N.N. The role of matrix metalloproteinases in diabetic wound healing in relation to photobiomodulation. Journal of Diabetes Research. 2016;2897656.

[64] Couture, C., Zaniolo, K., Carrier, P., Lake, J. The tissue-engineered human cornea as a model to study expression. Biomaterials. 2016;**78**:86–101.

[65] Lazaro, J.L., Izzo, V., Meaume, S., Davies, A.H., Lobmann, R., Uccioli, L. Elevated levels of matrix metalloproteinases and chronic wound healing: an updated review of clinical evidence. Journal of Wound Care. 2016;**25**(5):277–287. DOI: 10.12968/jowc.2016.25.5.277

[66] Van den Steen, P.E., Opdenakker, G., Wormald, M.R., Dwek, R.A., Rudd, P.M. Matrix remodelling enzymes, the protease cascade and glycosylation. Biochimica et Biophysica Acta—General Subjects. 2001;**1528**:61–73.

[67] Simioni, A.R., Coulomb, B., Couty, L., Tedesco, A.C. Photodynamic therapy preserves elastic network from degradation in an ex vivo human skin model. Wound Repair and Regeneration. 2009;**17**:A80.

[68] Coulomb, B., Dubertret, L., Bell, E., Merrill, C., Fosse, M., Bretongorius, J., et al. Endogenous peroxidases in normal human dermis—a marker of fibroblast differentiation. Journal of Investigative Dermatology. 1983;**81**:75–78.

[69] Shin, M.H., Rhie, G.E., Park, C.H., Kim, K.H., Cho, K.H., Eun, H.C., et al. Modulation of collagen metabolism by the topical application of dehydroepiandrosterone to human skin. Journal of Investigative Dermatology. 2005;**124**:315–323.

[70] Damodharan, U., Ganesan, R., Radhakrishnan, U.C. Expression of MMP2 and MMP9 (Gelatinases A and B) in human colon cancer cells. Applied Biochemistry and Biotechnology. 2011;**165**:1245–1252.

[71] Hu, W.P., Wang, J.J., Yu, C.L., Lan, C.C.E., Chen, G.S., Yu, H.S. Helium-neon laser irradiation stimulates cell proliferation through photostimulatory effects in mitochondria. Journal of Investigative Dermatology. 2007;**127**:2048–2057.

[72] Rosique, R.G., Rosique, M.J., Farina Junior, J.A. Curbing inflammation in skin wound healing: a review. International Journal of Inflammation. 2015;316235.

[73] Deyhmi, P., Khademi, H., Birang, R., Akhoondzadeh, M. Histological evaluation of wound healing process after photodynamic therapy of rat oral mucosal ulcer. Journal of Dentistry Shiraz University of Medical Science. 2016;**17**:43–48.

[74] Arany, P.R. Craniofacial wound healing with photobiomodulation therapy: new insights and current challenges. Journal of Dental Research. 2016;**95**(9):977-984.

[75] Carneiro, V.S.M., Catão, M.H.V., Menezes, R.F., Araujo, N.C., Gerbi, M.E.M. Methylene blue photodynamic therapy in rats' wound healing: 21 days follow-up. Biophotonics South America. 2015;**9531.** DOI: 10.1117/12.2181124

[76] Ribeiro, M.S., Nunez, S.C., Sabino, C.P., Yoshimura, T.M., Silva, C.R., Nogueira, G.E.C., et al. Exploring light-based technology for wound healing and appliance disinfection. Journal of Brazilian Chemical Society. 2015;**26**:2583–2589.

[77] Mendonza-Garcia, J., Sebastian, A., Alonso-Rasgado, T., Bayat, A. Optimization of an ex vivo wound healing model in the adult human skin: functional evaluation using photodynamic therapy. Wound Repair and Regeneration. 2015;**23**:685–702.

Chapter 6

Light-Emitting Woven Fabric for Treatment with Photodynamic Therapy and Monitoring of Actinic Keratosis

Yesim Oguz, Vladan Koncar, Cedric Cochrane and Serge Mordon

Additional information is available at the end of the chapter

http://dx.doi.org/10.5772/64997

Abstract

A successful photodynamic therapy (PDT) requires a specific photosensitizer, oxygen and light of a specific wavelength and power. Today photodynamic therapy (PDT) is administered to patients with light-emitting diode (LED) panels. These panels deliver a non-uniform light distribution on the human body parts, as the complex human anatomy is not a flat surface (head vertex, hand, shoulder, etc.). For an efficient photodynamic therapy (PDT), a light-emitting fabric (LEF) was woven from plastic optical fibers (POF) aiming at the treatment of dermatologic diseases such as actinic keratosis (AK). Plastic optical fibers (POF) (Toray, PGR-FB250) have been woven in textile in order to create macro-bendings, and thus emit out the injected light directly to the skin. The light intensity and light-emitting homogeneity of the LEF were improved thanks to Doehlert Experimental Design. During the treatment with PDT, the photosensitizers were activated in the cancerous cells. These cells may be visualized, as they show a characteristic fluorescence under UV light, which is called fluorescence diagnosis (FD). Therefore, it is proposed to modify the developed LEF for PDT to measure the fluorescence amount. For this aim, a part of POFs was cut out to observe the quantity of light that could be collected while the LEF was connected to a light source. The first prototypes showed the possibility of the illumination with the same LEF without losing the efficiency but also imaging the collected light.

Keywords: light emitting fabric (LEF), plastic optical fiber (POF), photodynamic therapy (PDT), weaving, fluorescence diagnosis (FD)

1. Introduction

The actinic keratosis (AK) is a pre-cancerous condition due to chronic UV light exposure that may develop into non-melanoma skin cancer [1, 2]. Thus, the treatment of AK is highly recommended. The AK lesions are characterized by red, scaly and crusty plaques or papules [3, 4]. This skin disease mainly affects fair-skinned individuals (face, bald head, forehead, etc.) [5].

There are many treatment options for AK. Cryosurgery, curettage and photodynamic therapy (PDT) are the common treatments. Cryosurgery is an operation to destroy the tissue by using freezing temperature performed with liquid nitrogen or carbon dioxide. This method is efficient on the thinner lesions but less successful on the thick lesions and may result in scarring [6]. Curettage is used to scrape of larger, hypertrophic lesions with a curette. The drawbacks of this technique are the necessity for a local anesthesia and the scars [7].

Photodynamic therapy (PDT) is a noninvasive method, particularly used to treat pre-cancerous or cancerous lesions with the combination of a photosensitizer and an appropriate light.

PDT has been increasingly used to treat AK, as it is efficient as other techniques given before but also has excellent cosmetic results, repeatable and does not kill the healthy cells (selective cell killing) [8, 9]. This treatment is also suitable for noncancerous lesions such as psoriatic, acne vulgaris, pre-cancerous lesions as AK and Bowen, and cancerous lesions as basal cell carcinoma (BCC) and squamous cell carcinoma (SCC) [9, 10].

The PDT leads to selective destruction of the cancerous cells by activated photosensibilisant agent, methyl aminolevulinate (MAL) in Europe and 5-aminolevulinic acid (ALA) in USA. The photosensitizers (PS) are activated with an appropriate light, which is red light (630 nm) in Europe and blue light (450 nm) in USA in the presence of oxygen [11]. The activation of the PS generates singlet oxygens ($_1O^2$) which causes chemical reactions inside the cancerous cells as they are rich with molecular oxygen [12] (**Figure 1**). This is so-called "selective cells killing."

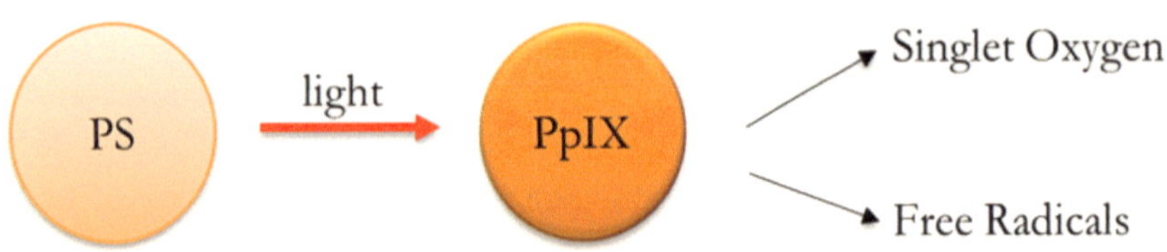

Figure 1. Activation of PS.

In Europe, PDT is performed by using a drug photosensitizer methyl aminolevulinate (MAL by Metvix, Galderma) on cancerous lesions and a 3-hour interval to start enlightenment [13]. The entire treated area is illuminated by a red light source (narrow spectrum around 630 nm) [14]. The activation of Metvix required a dose of 37 J/cm^2 [15, 16]. The light dose is determined by such factors as the size of the light field, the distance between the lamp and the surface of the skin, and the illumination duration. Therefore, it is not possible to treat numerous patients per day since the treatment of a single patient takes about 5 hours. It is possible to reduce the light exposition time by increasing the light dose, but the pain rate will also rise.

http://dx.doi.org/10.5772/64997

Today PDT is administered by light-emitting diode (LED) panels (**Figure 2**) [17]. This is an effective method without side effects with good cosmetic results. However, LEDs do not emit the same light dose over the entire treatment area and do not adapt to the irregularities of the body [13, 18]. Another disadvantage of this method is pain due to the dose of pure light that effective treatment with LED panels [19, 20]. Indeed, if the light output was less, we could limit the pain caused by the PDT.

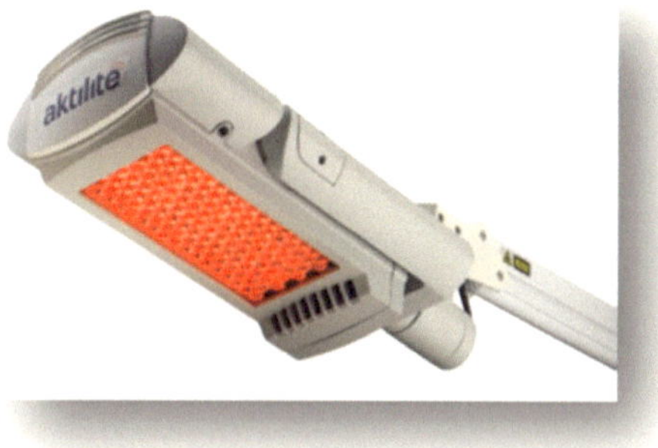

Figure 2. LED panel light source (Aktilite CL 128, Galderma).

PDT needs to evolve despite its benefits, to make this treatment more effective and less painful. The market innovates and proposes inventions that allow surmounting the inconveniences of topical PDT with LED panels.

In order to maximize the comfort of the PDT and remove the disadvantages, Inserm (Institut National de la Santé et de la Recherche Médicale, France) and ENSAIT (École Nationale Supérieure des Arts et Industries Textiles, France) proposed replacing the LED panels by a LEF composed of PMMA optical fibers (POF) [21–23].

2. Development and optimization of a LEF

Optical fibers carry the light between the distal ends but do not emit light laterally in their natural state. There are three methods to bring out the light laterally. Mechanical process consists of creating scratches on the surface of the POF (sandblasting or toothed roll) [24]. Chemical process is by applying a solvent which degrades the outside of the fiber and passes light [25]. And finally the method of creating macro-bends (bindings in macroscopic size), to not satisfy the total internal reflection to create a leakage [26–29].

The optical fiber used in the experiments consists of a Poly MethylMethAcrylate (PMMA) core enveloped by a cladding made of fluorinated polymers. The core of the fiber has a refractive index greater than the cladding's, and therefore the light is confined thus completely reflected

(Snell's Law, Eq. 1). When a macro-bend is formed with an OF, light enters into the OF with an angle larger than the critical angle (Eq. 2). and it undergoes multiple reflections.

$$\sin\alpha\, n_{air} = \sin\theta_1\, n_{core} \tag{1}$$

$$\theta_{critical} = \sin^{-1}(n_{cladding} / n_{core}) \tag{2}$$

As a consequence, when the fiber is bent, the light rays outside of the bend section will be emitted; the others will continue to meet internal reflection as seen in **Figure 3** [30–32].

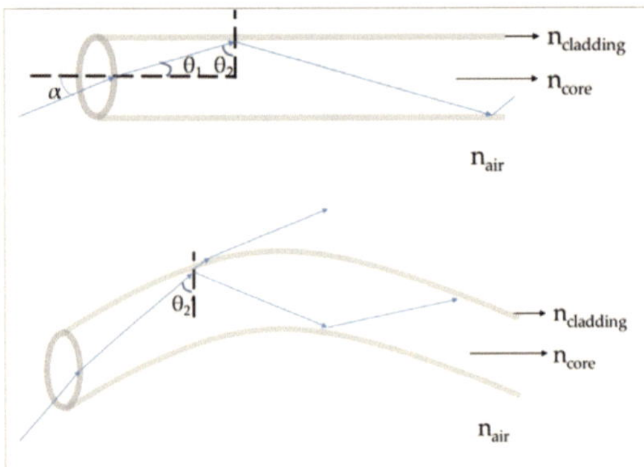

Figure 3. Multiple reflections in a bent optical fiber.

Weaving is a method of textile production which interlaces warp and weft yarns to form a fabric (**Figure 4**).

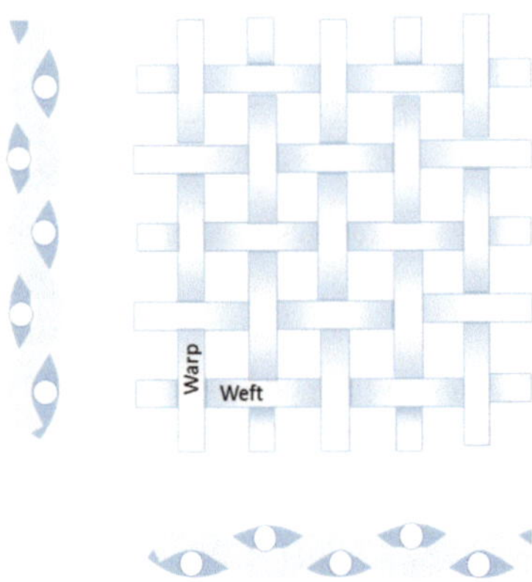

Figure 4. Scheme of a plain weave.

Thanks to the weaving technology, it is possible to create the macro-bends on the POFs as observed on the cross sections of the fabric in **Figure 5**.

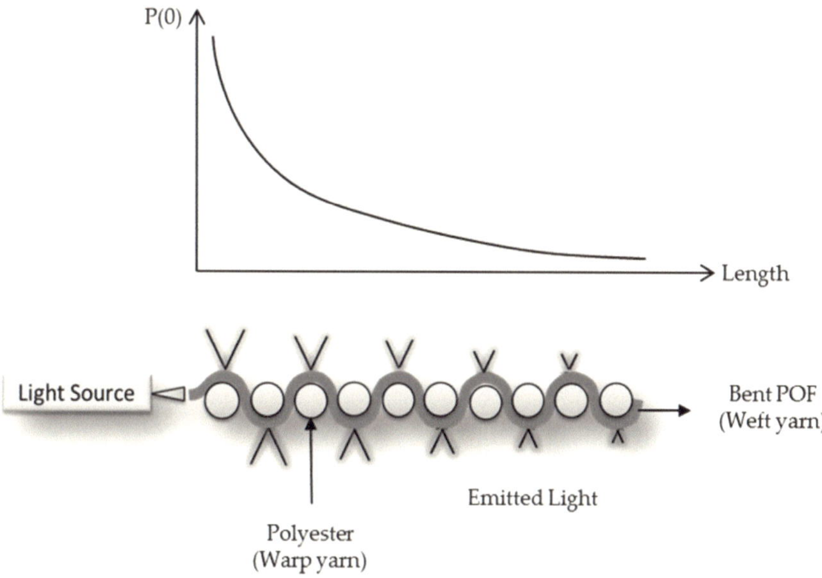

Figure 5. Bending loss in a POF inserted in a woven fabric.

It is possible to use different patterns to change the bending angles of the curvatures. There are three types of fundamental weaving patterns: plain weave, twill weave and satin weave (**Figure 6**) [33].

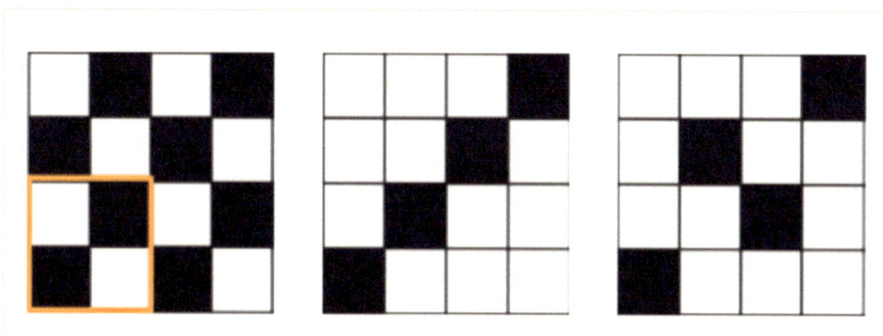

Figure 6. Fundamental Weaves: plain weave, twill 3-1, and satin 4, respectively.

Figure 6 shows the repeating pattern presentations of fundamental weaves. When the warp yarn is on the top of the weft yarn, it is presented in black; in the other case it is white. A weft float is designated as a number of warp yarns under the floating weft yarn between two intersections.

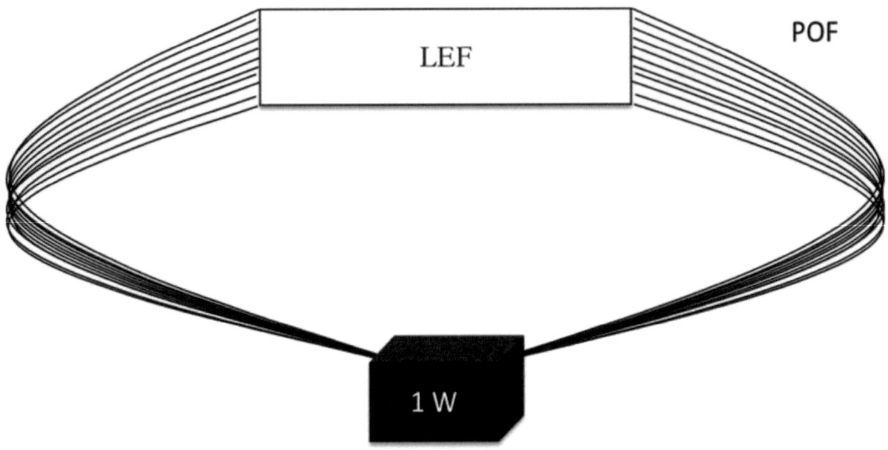

Figure 7. LEF connected to the light source.

The plain weave is the most basic of the three fundamental weaves. The weft thread passes successively above and below the warp yarn, and this order is reversed for each weft line (**Figures 4** and **6**).

The twill weave has a harness number equal to 1, and the crossing points form a diagonal (**Figure 6**). It consists of floats longer than plain weave.

The crossing points of the satin weave are defined with the harness number, and it is higher than 1 (**Figure 6**). Satin weave has longer floats compared to other fundamental weaves. This is the reason that we have used this weave to produce our fabrics. Longer floats prevent covering all the light-emitting POFs with warp yarns.

The quantity of the emitted light decreases with the distance to the light source as seen in **Figure 5**. The light transmission loss in an optical fiber is defined as the following equation according to the scientific literature [34, 35]:

$$\alpha = \frac{10}{L} \log \left[\frac{P(0)}{P(1)} \right] \tag{3}$$

where α represents the light transmission loss (dB/km), the length of the optical fiber (km), P(0) represents optical input power, and P(1) represents optical output power. Based on this formula (Eq. 3), different weaving patterns were woven to measure their attenuation in the same length.

The loss of the light in an OF depends on the radius of the bending curvature, the number of bending points and the wavelength of the signal.

For a successful treatment, a special pattern (patent WO 2012098488 A2) composed of three satin weaves was designed to obtain the same amount of bending, thus a homogenous light distribution on the whole length of the fabric when it is connected to sources from both ends [36–38]. With this new pattern a homogenous light distribution was aimed for a successful PDT. Moreover, the LEF is connected to the light source from the both distal ends.

Polyester Sinterama (330 dTex)was used as warp yarn with a density of 20 per cm. Optical fiber PMMA Toray (250 μm) was used as a weft yarn with a yarn density of 37 per cm. The size of the luminous fabric is 21.5 × 5 cm. The total length of POF is about 60 cm but only 21.5 cm of POFs are woven in the middle. The both ends of the LEF were connected to the laser (1 W from both sides) as demonstrated in **Figure 7** and the light intensity (mW.cm^{-2}) was measured for each cm^2 of LEF length. For the medical application, it was important to obtain the light intensity values change within the limits of -/+ 20%, for a homogenous light distribution.

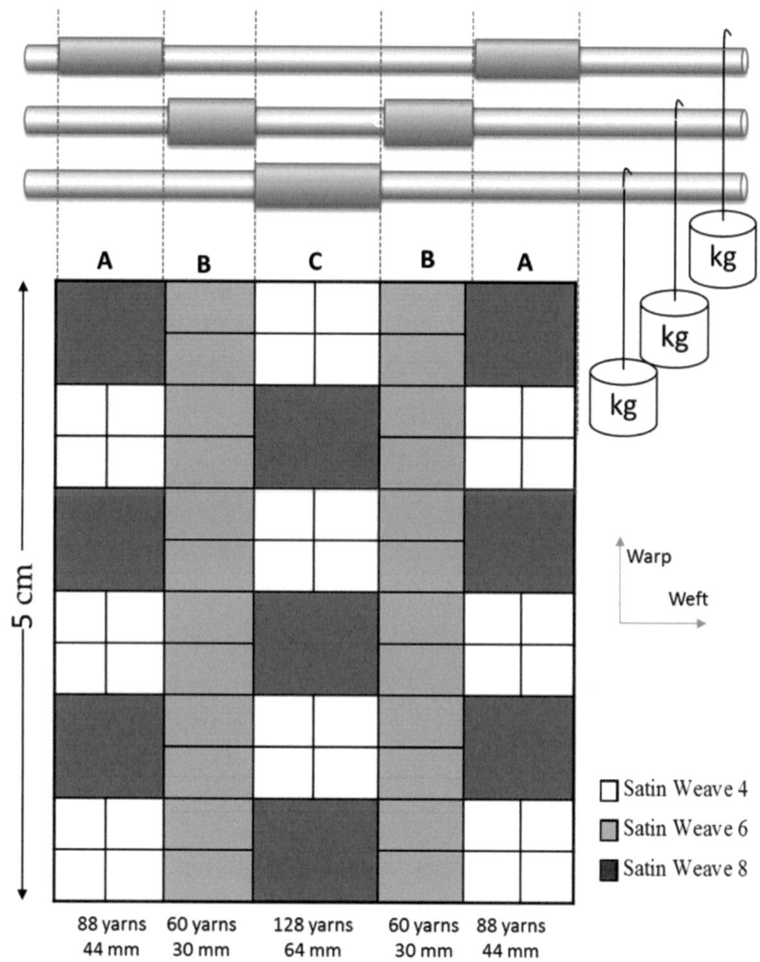

Figure 8. Scheme of the optimized weaving system.

An LEF which diffuses homogeneously light was obtained by using the designed pattern. However, it was also important to optimize the light intensity ($mW.cm^{-2}$) for a successful PDT. To improve the lateral light intensity and obtain an LEF that emits a consistent and powerful light at the same time, tension is added on the warp yarns during weaving [39]. Thanks to the added tension during weaving, it was possible to modify the curvatures of the optical fibers inserted into the LEF.

It is also very important to maintain the low light from the connectors on both sides to avoid feedback light toward the laser. This injection can increase the temperature of the laser sources, which can cause damage to the devices.

Three warp beams were prepared for three different weaving zones A, B, C and the loads were added on the beams, which were calculated with Doehlert experimental design. The samples are woven with the weaving machine (Dornier, HTVS8-SD). The optimized weaving system is shown diagrammatically below **Figure 8**.

In order to reduce the number of experiments, a three-factor Doehlert design was used in this work. This experimental design allows to find out the best parameters to optimize the results. The three weaving zones with different pattern combinations (A, B, C) were chosen as variables, and the three levels are chosen 40, 70 and 100 g/warp yarn, respectively. Fifteen samples were studied with the calculated tension parameters.

Furthermore, response surface methodology (RSM) graphics were generated with a Doehlert matrix design results. The graphics showed the emplacement of best results for the light intensity and light distribution homogeneity. Five more experiments were woven based on these parameters which should give the compromise result with a good light intensity and less heterogeneity (12.8 +/- 3 $mW.cm^{-2}.W^{-1}$). The sample number 15 gave the best result as predicted and proved the reality of this approach (**Figure 9**). This was the optimal sample with given pattern, warp/weft material and density.

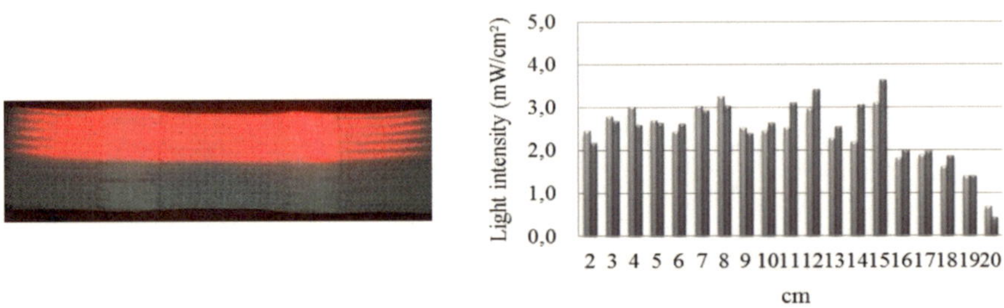

Figure 9. Light distribution of the optimized with Doehlert Experimental Design.

This diffuser light textile meets the basic requirements for PDT: uniform distribution of light and flexibility. The great light diffusers (500 cm^2) textiles can be easily manufactured and can be used not only on the skin but also in the peritoneal or pleural cavities.

PDT administrated with LEF will improve the effectiveness of treatment and make the procedure almost painless. Clinical trials were started (at CHR and Klinikum Vest) on 55

http://dx.doi.org/10.5772/64997

patients. For each patient, half of lesions were treated with conventional therapy, and the other half with the smart textiles, to compare the pain and the effectiveness on the same patient. The results are expected before 2017. Whenever the convincing results are provided, this method will replace the current treatments with the LED panels.

In addition, the new procedure will allow to treating multiple patients simultaneously, with less pain, under the supervision of doctors. Thanks to miniature laser sources and their decreasing prices, this procedure may also be transformed into a portable medical device that will allow patients to be active (**Figure 10**).

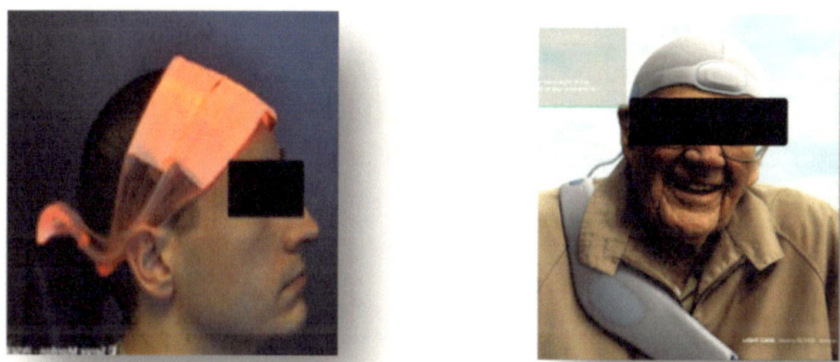

(a) (b)

Figure 10. The PDT with woven LEF by ENSAIT (a), LEF inserted helmet design (b).

As the phototherapy has a good future, there are many concurrences developed to improve the procedure existent. Philips has developed a new technology called "BlueControl" which is a portable light therapy device for the treatment of Psoriasis Vulgaris. This device provides a treatment of 30 minutes per lesion, through the benefits of blue LED light without UV (453 nm) [40, 41].

Philips also developed the "Bilirubin blanket," made of woven fabric consisting of stitched tiny blue LED lights. This device is used for the treatment of jaundice which is a condition caused by high levels of bilirubin in the blood.

And Metvix Galderma has proposed PDT daylight as an alternative to the PDT conventional. The daylight PDT allows patients to be active and under the sun during treatment, contrary to illumination with a fixed wavelength in clinical place [42, 43]. Daylight PDT has a good efficiency and is less painful thanks to low light output compared to the conventional method. However, this new method has several disadvantages. Allowing the patient to prepare the area to be treated may cause a lack of control of the light dose and time of exposure. In addition, the patient is dependent on the season and weather conditions.

In conclusion, PDT with flexible woven LEF by ENSAIT overcomes the obstacles of the other alternatives. One of the most important advantages of this technology is the possibility of using different wavelengths and dose of light by just changing the light source, thus allowing the treatment of different diseases (red for AK, blue for Jaundice, etc.). Also the possibility of using miniature lasers prevents the lack of control of the light dose or time exposure. That makes the treatment applicable any time or anywhere without depending on the weather conditions.

3. Future prospects of monitoring the cancerous cells with an LEF

During the PDT, the accumulated MAL is converted into active Protoporphyrine IX (PpIX) with the light exposure in cancerous cells. These PpIX are characterized by a red fluorescent color when viewed with a Wood lamp which uses ultraviolet (UV) light to examine the skin ([13, 44–47]; **Figure 11**). It is therefore possible to monitor the amount of PpIX in tissues by measuring the fluorescence before or during treatment. This procedure is called fluorescence diagnosis (FD) [13, 45, 48].

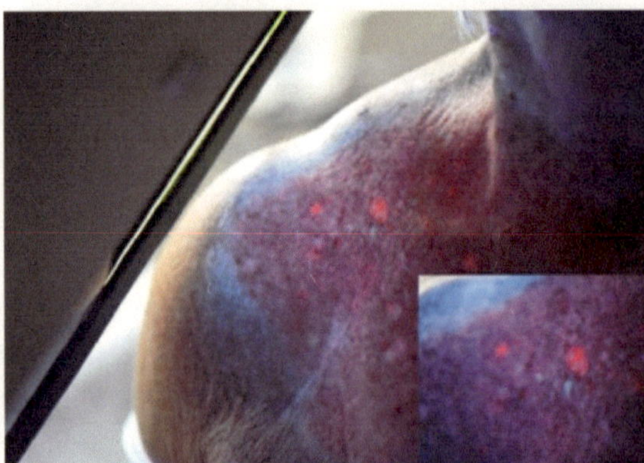

Figure 11. Imaging of PpIX after illumination with Wood Lamp to monitor the cancerous cells.

The use of LEF already developed in our research as a tool for FD is also investigated in this work. The aim was to use the same LEF for not only treating but also monitoring the cancerous cells. For this purpose, first of all, 1 fiber out of every 20 fiber is cut out from the connector on both edges as in **Figure 12**, and 1 W light is injected inside the both connectors. Secondly, the collected light from the fibers cut out (shown with second power meter sensor in **Figure 12**, and the light puissance of LEF were measured (shown with first power meter sensor in **Figure 12**).

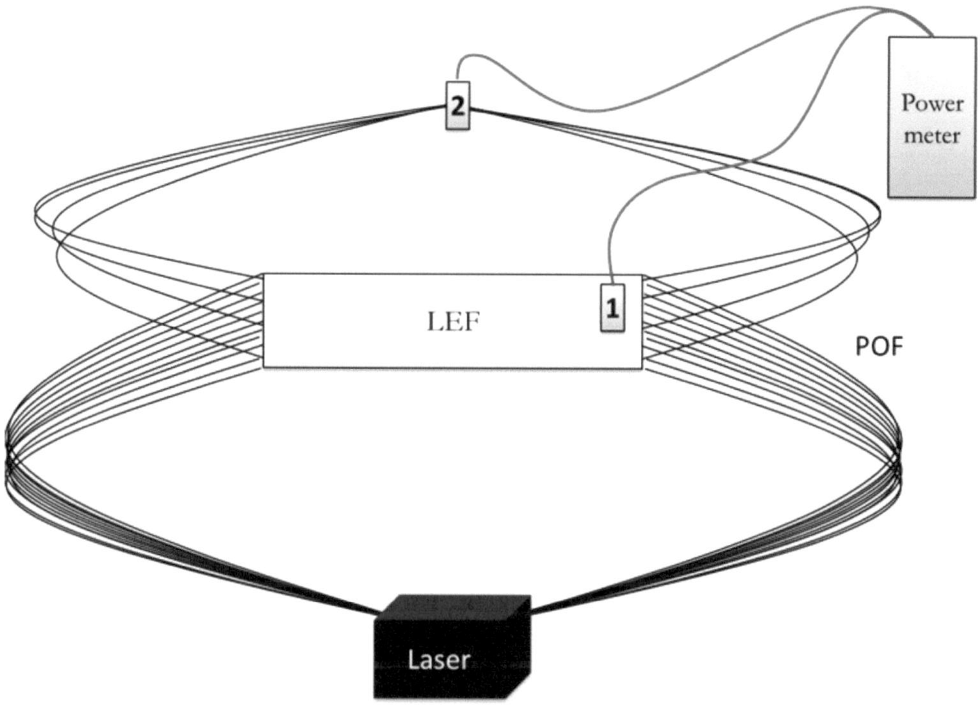

Figure 12. Measure method for monitoring application.

Furthermore, with the aim of finding the best ratio between the number of POF for the treatment and for the monitoring, the measures were repeated on the same LEF by cutting out 1 of 10 POF, 1 of 5 POF and 1 of 2 POF for using as a monitor. The results are given below for each experience.

As given in **Figure 13**, the collected information from the POFs cut out for the monitoring was increased with the number of the monitoring POFs. In the same time, there was no significant decrease of light power on the LEF, except for the last trial with one of two POFs. This could be explained by the light transmission of the neighbor POFs. On this wise, the emitted light from the neighbor POFs may penetrate inside the concerning fiber and keep stable the light intensity of the LEF in a 1 cm^2 area.

However, the monitoring sample with one of two POFs showed low light output from the LEF surface and the monitoring fibers. It shows that the monitoring POFs which are not covered with several bended fibers may not accumulate enough quantity of scattered light from the neighbor POFs.

The results were obtained from an LEF woven with 37 POFs/cm. The best compromise was using one of fivePOFs as monitoring fibers which showed a good light output from the monitoring fibers without losing the lateral light emission power.

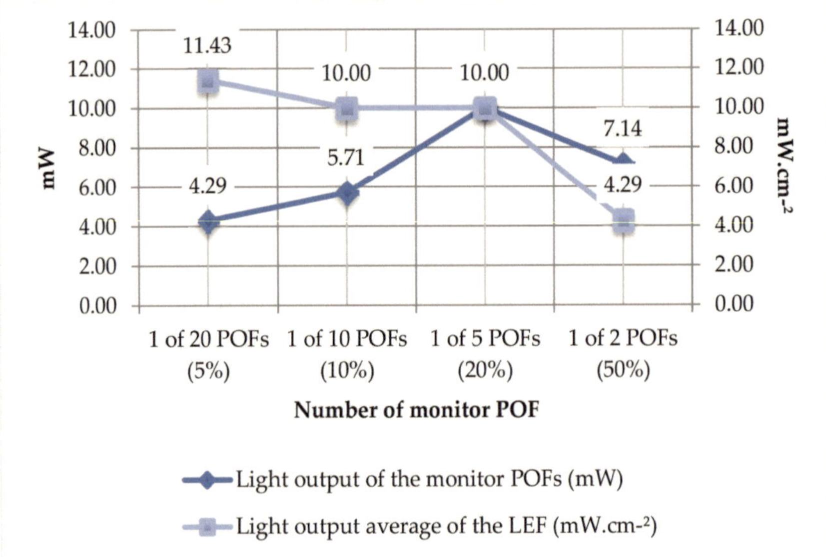

Figure 13. Monitoring measure results.

4. Conclusion

An LEF has been developed and optimized to use in PDT, thanks to the weaving technology and Doehlert experimental design. Furthermore, it is proposed to use the LEF to observe the cancerous cells that are visualized as red fluorescent after illuminated with UV light. The procedure requires a treatment with red light for a specific time period, and then diffuses a UV light to measure the fluorescence quantity to observe if there are more cancerous cells. The trials to prove the possibility of using a part of POFs as a monitoring tool were experienced successfully and worked well.

This work has demonstrated the possibility of treating and then controlling the amount of remaining tumor cells with the same LEF. There are similar examples in dentistry, such as fluorescence signal detection with polymeric optical fiber. The next step will be a simulation of the fluorescence diagnosis by injecting fluorescence light to the surface of LEF and measuring the output from the monitor optical fibers.

Acknowledgements

This work was supported by the GEMTEX Laboratory, European Commission grant PHOSISTOS in the Framework Programme 7, and INSERM for the development and test of a light-emitting textile for the treatment of skin disease actinic keratosis.

Author details

Yesim Oguz[1,2*], Vladan Koncar[1,2], Cedric Cochrane[1,2] and Serge Mordon[1,3]

*Address all correspondence to: yesim.oguz@ensait.fr

1 University Lille Nord de France, Lille, France

2 ENSAIT, GEMTEX, Roubaix, France

3 INSERM 1189 ONCO-THAI, Lille University Hospital—CHRU, France

References

[1] Zalaudek I, Giacomel J, Schmid K, Bondino S, Rosendahl C, Cavicchini S, et al. Dermatoscopy of facial actinic keratosis, intraepidermal carcinoma, and invasive squamous cell carcinoma: A progression model. J Am Acad Dermatol. 2012;66(4):589–97.

[2] Krouse RS, Alberts DS, Prasad AR, Yozwiak M, Bartels HG, Liu Y, et al. Progression of skin lesions from normal skin to squamous cell carcinoma. Anal Quant Cytol Histol [Internet]. 2009;31(1):17–25. Available from: http://www.ncbi.nlm.nih.gov/pubmed/19320189

[3] Anwar J, Wrone DA, Kimyai-Asadi A, Alam M. The development of actinic keratosis into invasive squamous cell carcinoma: Evidence and evolving classification schemes. Clin Dermatol. 2004;22(3):189–96.

[4] Moy RL. Clinical presentation of actinic keratoses and squamous cell carcinoma. J Am Acad Dermatol [Internet]. 2000;42(1):S8–10. Available from: http://www.sciencedirect.com/science/article/pii/S019096220027494X

[5] Smits T, Moor ACE. New aspects in photodynamic therapy of actinic keratoses. J Photochem Photobiol B Biol [Internet]. 2009;96(3):159–69. Available from: http://dx.doi.org/10.1016/j.jphotobiol.2009.06.003

[6] Ceilley RI, Jorizzo JL. Current issues in the management of actinic keratosis. J Am Dermatology [Internet]. 2013;68(1):S28–38. Available from: http://dx.doi.org/10.1016/j.jaad.2012.09.051

[7] Sheridan AT, Dawber RP. Curettage, electrosurgery and skin cancer. Australas J Dermatol [Internet]. 2000;41(1):19–30. Available from: http://doi.wiley.com/10.1046/j.1440-0960.2000.00383.x

[8] Kawczyk-Krupka A, Bugaj AM, Latos W, Zaremba K, Wawrzyniec K, Sieroń A. Photodynamic therapy in colorectal cancer treatment: The state of the art in clinical trials. Photodiagnosis Photodyn Ther. 2015;12(3):545–53.

[9] Lee Y, Baron E. Photodynamic therapy: Current evidence and applications in dermatology. Semin Cutan Med Surg [Internet]. 2011;30(4):199–209. Available from: http://www.ncbi.nlm.nih.gov/pubmed/22123417 [cited 2014 Oct 1].

[10] Svanberg K, Bendsoe N. Photodynamic therapy for human malignancies with superficial and interstitial illumination [Internet]. Lasers for Medical Applications. 2013:760–778. Available from: http://linkinghub.elsevier.com/retrieve/pii/B9780857092373500254

[11] Buggiani G, Troiano M, Rossi R, Lotti T. Photodynamic therapy: Off-label and alternative use in dermatological practice. Photodiagnosis Photodyn Ther. 2008;5(2):134–8.

[12] Dinehart SM. The treatment of actinic keratoses. J Am Acad Dermatol [Internet]. 2000;42(1):S25–8. Available from: http://dx.doi.org/10.1067/mjd.2000.103338

[13] Kalka K, Merk H, Mukhtar H. Photodynamic therapy in dermatology. J Am Acad Dermatol [Internet]. 2000;42(3):389–413. Available from: http://linkinghub.elsevier.com/retrieve/pii/S0190962200902093

[14] Allison RR, Sibata CH, Downie GH, Cuenca RE. A clinical review of PDT for cutaneous malignancies. Photodiagnosis Photodyn Ther. 2006;3(4):214–26.

[15] Salvio AG, Ramirez DP, de Oliveira ER, Inada NM, Kurachi C, Bagnato VS. Evaluation of pain during large area photodynamic therapy in patients with widespread actinic keratosis of upper limbs. Photodiagnosis Photodyn Ther [Internet]. 2015;12(3):326–7. Available from: http://dx.doi.org/10.1016/j.pdpdt.2015.07.013

[16] Gholam P, Denk K, Sehr T, Enk A, Hartmann M. Factors influencing pain intensity during topical photodynamic therapy of complete cosmetic units for actinic keratoses. J Am Acad Dermatol [Internet]. 2010;63(2):213–8. Available from: http://dx.doi.org/10.1016/j.jaad.2009.08.062

[17] Kuonen F, Gaide O. Nouvelle lumière sur la thérapie photodynamique cutanée. Rev Med Suisse. 2014;10:754–9.

[18] Khan T, Unternährer M, Buchholz J, Kaser-Hotz B, Selm B, Rothmaier M, et al. Performance of a contact textile-based light diffuser for photodynamic therapy. Photodiagnosis Photodyn Ther [Internet]. 2006;3(1):51–60. Available from: http://linkinghub.elsevier.com/retrieve/pii/S1572100005001821

[19] Warren CB, Karai LJ, Vidimos A, Maytin EV. Pain associated with aminolevulinic acid-photodynamic therapy of skin disease. J Am Acad Dermatol [Internet]. 2009;61(6):1033–43. Available from: http://dx.doi.org/10.1016/j.jaad.2009.03.048

[20] Attili S, Lesar A, McNeill A, Camacho-Lopez M, Moseley H, Ibbotson S, et al. An open pilot study of ambulatory photodynamic therapy using a wearable low-irradiance

organic light-emitting diode light source in the treatment of nonmelanoma skin cancer. Br J Dermatol [Internet]. 2009;161(1):170–3. Available from: http://doi.wiley.com/10.1111/j.1365-2133.2009.09096.x

[21] Daniel M. Light emitting fabric [Internet]. US Patent 4,234,907, 1980. Available from: http://www.google.com/patents/US4234907 [cited 2014 Sep 24].

[22] Koncar V. Optical fiber fabric displays. Opt Photonics News. 2005;16(4):40–4.

[23] Meunier L, Kell FM, Cochrane C, Koncar V. Flexible displays for smart clothing: Part I—Overview. Indian J Fibre Text Res. 2011;36(December):422–8.

[24] Bernasson A, Peuvergne H. Optical fiber with multiple point lateral illumination. US 5737472, 1998.

[25] Brochier C, Malhomme D, Deflin E. Fabric web having photocatalysis-based pollution control properties. US 2010/0029157 A1, 2010.

[26] Nishii Y. Glass material for carrying a photocatalyst, filter device using the same and light irradiating method. EP0823280 A1, 1998.

[27] Potter BG. Module 3—Attenuation in Optical Fibers. Mater Sci Eng Dept, Univ Arizona; 2010: 1–16.

[28] Zubia J, Arrue J. Plastic optical fibers: An introduction to their technological processes and applications. Opt Fiber Technol [Internet]. 2001;7(2):101–40. Available from: http://www.sciencedirect.com/science/article/pii/S1068520000903559

[29] Kovacevic MS, Nikezic D. Influence of bending on power distribution in step-index plastic optical fibers and the calculation of bending loss. Appl Opt [Internet]. 2007;46(22):4867–8; discussion 4869–70. Available from: http://www.ncbi.nlm.nih.gov/pubmed/17676088

[30] Jay J. An overview of macrobending and microbending of optical fibers. White Pap WP1212, Corning [Internet]. 2010. Available from: http://www.corning.com/assets/0/433/573/637/639/1bea48ac-d675-44c7-aa18-11a3a1a0adbd.pdf [cited 2014 Oct 2].

[31] Selm B, Gurel EA, Rothmaier M, Rossi RM, Scherer LJ. Polymeric optical fiber fabrics for illumination and sensorial applications in textiles. J Intell Mater Syst Struct [Internet]. 2010;21(11):1061–71. Available from: http://jim.sagepub.com/cgi/doi/10.1177/1045389X10377676 [cited 2014 Sep 22].

[32] Kuang KSC, Quek ST, Koh CG, Cantwell WJ, Scully PJ. Plastic optical fibre sensors for structural health monitoring: A review of recent progress. J Sensors. 2009;2009.

[33] Goerner D. Woven Structure and Design. Wira Technology Group Ltd; 1986.

[34] Spigulis J, Pfafrods D, Stafeckis M, Jelinska-Platace W. The glowing optical fibre designs and parameters. In: Krumins A, Millers DK, Sternberg AR, Spigulis J, editors. 1997;231–

6. Available from: http://proceedings.spiedigitallibrary.org/proceeding.aspx?articleid=1027053 [cited 2014 Sep 30].

[35] Sasaki I, Nishida K, Morimoto M, Yamamoto T. Light-transmitting fiber. EP 0 155 567 B1, 1991.

[36] Cochrane C, Mordon SR, Lesage JC, Koncar V. New design of textile light diffusers for photodynamic therapy. Mater Sci Eng C [Internet]. 2013;33(3):1170–5. Available from: http://dx.doi.org/10.1016/j.msec.2012.12.007

[37] Oguz Y, Cochrane C, Mordon SR, Lesage JC, Koncar V. Light-emitting fabrics for photodynamic therapy. Adv Smart Med Text [Internet]. 2016:177–94. Available from: http://linkinghub.elsevier.com/retrieve/pii/B9781782423799000086

[38] Mordon S, Cochrane C, Lesage J, Koncar V. Innovative engineering design of a textile light diffuser for photodynamic therapy. Photodyn Ther [Internet]. 2011. Available from: http://scholar.google.com/scholar?hl=en&btnG=Search&q=intitle:Innovative+engineering+design+of+a+textile+light+diffuser+for+photodynamic+therapy#0 [cited 2014 Sep 30].

[39] Oguz Y, Cochrane C, Koncar V, Mordon SR. Doehlert experimental design applied to optimization of light emitting textile structures. Opt Fiber Technol [Internet]. 2016;30:38–47. Available from: http://www.sciencedirect.com/science/article/pii/S1068520016000237

[40] philips. Philips BlueControl—Traitement du psoriasis—Philips BlueControl [Internet]. 2015. Available from: http://www.psoriasis-bluecontrol.com/accueil/8-philips-bluecontrol-traitement-du-psoriasis.html [cited 2016 Feb 11].

[41] Kleinpenning MM, Otero ME, van Erp PEJ, Gerritsen MJP, van de Kerkhof PCM. Efficacy of blue light vs. red light in the treatment of psoriasis: A double-blind, randomized comparative study. J Eur Acad Dermatology Venereol [Internet]. 2012;26(2):219–25. Available from: http://doi.wiley.com/10.1111/j.1468-3083.2011.04039.x

[42] Wiegell SR, Wulf HC, Szeimies RM, Basset-Seguin N, Bissonnette R, Gerritsen MJP, et al. Daylight photodynamic therapy for actinic keratosis: An international consensus: International Society for Photodynamic Therapy in Dermatology. J Eur Acad Dermatology Venereol. 2012;26(6):673–9.

[43] Braathen LR. Daylight photodynamic therapy in private practice in Switzerland: Gain without pain. Acta Derm Venereol. 2012;92(6):652–3.

[44] Huang Y-Y, Mroz P, Hamblin MR. Basic photomedicine [Internet]. Photobiology. 2009. Available from: http://www.photobiology.info/Photomed.html [cited 2016 May 24].

[45] Rollakanti KR, Kanick SC, Davis SC, Pogue BW, Maytin EV. Techniques for fluorescence detection of protoporphyrin IX in skin cancers associated with photodynamic therapy.

Photonics Lasers Med [Internet]. 2013;2(4):287–303. Available from: http://www.degruyter.com/view/j/plm.2013.2.issue-4/plm-2013-0030/plm-2013-0030.xml

[46] Babilas P, Kohl E, Maisch T, Bäcker H, Groß B, Branzan AL, et al. In vitro and in vivo comparison of two different light sources for topical photodynamic therapy. Br J Dermatol. 2006;154(4):712–8.

[47] Mitton D, Ackroyd R. A brief overview of photodynamic therapy in Europe. Photodiagnosis Photodyn Ther. 2008;5(2):103–11.

[48] Bäumler W, Abels C, Szeimies R-M. Fluorescence diagnosis and photodynamic therapy in dermatology. Med Laser Appl [Internet]. 2003;18(1):47–56. Available from: http://www.thieme-connect.de/DOI/DOI?10.1055/s-2007-980149

Chapter 7

Nurses and Pharmacists in Interdisciplinary Team of Health Care Providers in Photodynamic Therapy

Tomasz Kocki, Beata Czarczynska-Goslinska,
Katarzyna Kocka, Magdalena Stolarska,
Daria Wachowska, Sebastian Lijewski,
Tomasz Koczorowski and Tomasz Goslinski

Additional information is available at the end of the chapter

http://dx.doi.org/10.5772/65975

Abstract

Background: The modern treatment is based on wide cooperation between diverse representatives of medical professions. The photodynamic therapy is a noninvasive method of treatment both neoplastic diseases and miscellaneous noncancerous illnesses. It is complementary and competitive in some way to various traditional treatment techniques, including chemotherapy, radiotherapy, and surgery. This review emphasizes the significance of collaboration between specialists engaged in research, development, and practical use of photodynamic therapy.

Methods: A literature search of electronic bibliographic databases and scientific publishers was performed. The relevant literature was analyzed to identify articles on the involvement of nurses, pharmacists, physicians, and other representatives in photodynamic therapy treatment.

Results: In the photodynamic therapy, the overall success is not only dependent of a single unit. Coordinated actions of representatives possessing expertise in various fields of medical, and natural sciences are necessary both during joint research, development, and during the course of the photodynamic therapy treatment in clinics.

Conclusions: The effective interaction between professionals and the division of responsibilities at different stages of therapy can guarantee the successful treatment. During therapy, the most important role belongs to the patient who is responsible for acting in accordance with schedules elaborated by physicians, nurses, and pharmacists.

Keywords: hospital pharmacy, nursing, photodynamic therapy, photosensitizer, treatment

1. Introduction

Photodynamic therapy (PDT) is a low-invasive therapeutic method, which allows the selective destruction of diseased tissue. This is complementary to various traditional treatment techniques, including chemotherapy, radiotherapy, and surgery. It is used for the treatment of both neoplastic diseases and miscellaneous noncancerous illnesses. Although many ancient civilizations utilized phototherapy, it appeared again as the treatment procedure in the last century [1–3]. It seems that the success of this particular treatment procedure depends on both the further development of novel photosensitizers and light sources as well as schemes of cooperation between specialists and an interdisciplinary team. **Figure 1** presents the professions of which expertise is essential for photodynamic therapy and which are able to undertake various actions to increase the effectiveness of treatment.

PDT is based on a multi-stage procedure, and its success depends upon a number of procedure components. In addition, successful treatment requires the cooperation of an interdisciplinary team of specialists belonging to different fields of medical sciences: physicians, nurses, and

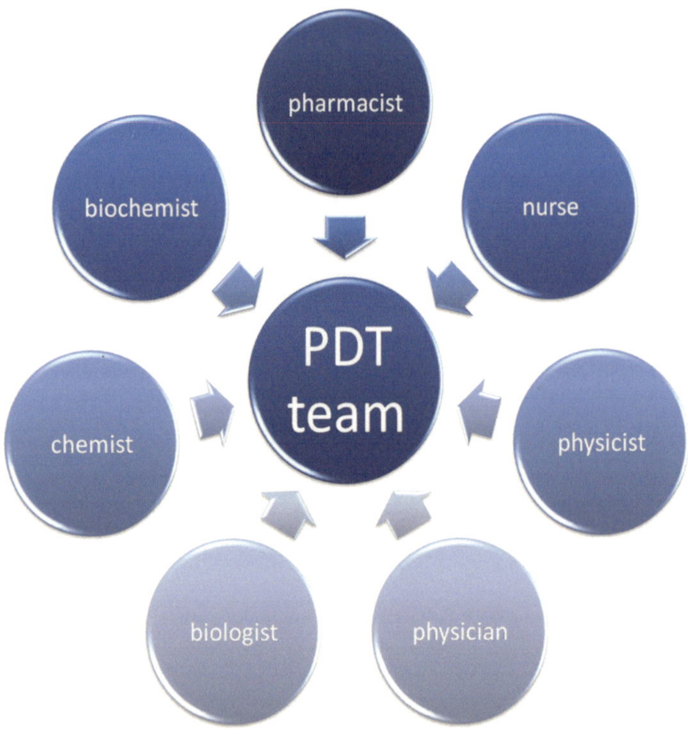

Figure 1. Professionals indispensable for carrying out PDT, based on Ref. [4].

pharmacists, but also at certain stages: chemists, physicists, biophysicists, and biologists [4]. Many advantages resulting from cooperation between laboratory and clinical researchers have been raised by Sieroń and Kwiatek [5], who summarized laboratory and clinical research on PDT and photodynamic diagnosis (PDD) in Poland. Benefits resulting from cooperation between various specialists have been noted for several years of PDT treatment in Brazil, stressing that the cooperation between specialists helps to improve the results and the quality of treatment. The patient potential for PDT treatment in Brazil needed to be initially assessed by the physician, nurse, and a physicist. The role of nurses is of great importance in this system, as they participate in the PDT procedures and have the closest contact with patients. Each case is discussed by specialists in order to assess potential benefits and consequences of therapy [4]. Researchers implementing the photodynamic therapy in patients with lung cancer have described an effective collaborative team consisting of a surgeon, oncologist, nurse, and pharmacist. For each patient, they elaborated the so-called schedule of photodynamic therapy. As light delivery requires special skills, during PDT treatment the presence of a "laser specialist" was found necessary [6].

The nurse's role in PDT treatment of patients is apparent and for example might be given a procedure utilized in the treatment of patients with neovascular (wet) age-related macular degeneration which was summarized in excellent review by Rich et al. [7]. Moreover, Collins and Garner stressed at least two points when nurse-pharmacist cooperation would be beneficial for patient in PDT therapy: (i) in the planning of PDT therapy before the patient arrives in the acute care environment, (ii) and in the prevention of medication being exposed to light and its dilution before administration [6].

On the one hand, access to PDT is often insufficient. On the other hand, operating costs would be astronomical for each hospital. Therefore, a mobile PDT unit designed to be put into operation by the Yorkshire Laser Centre is the solution to this problem. This unit allows more patients to benefit from PDT treatment. The personnel in such units consist of a driver/technician, a PDT physician, a nurse or a carer, and coordinator [8].

2. Photodynamic reaction

The legitimacy of the established interdisciplinary team justifies the photodynamic reaction mechanism, which is the basis of PDT. It is well known that PDT is a suitable combination of three components: the drug—photosensitizer, light, and oxygen. Photosensitizer is a drug, which, when introduced to the body, accumulates in the tissue. Drugs used in PDT treatments belong to different chemical classes and are of different structures and properties. After the tissue has been irradiated with light in an appropriate wavelength and intensity, the photosensitizer is activated. Reactive oxygen species are generated, which effectively causes apoptotic or necrotic death of the diseased tissues [9–11].

Photosensitizer and light are both necessary for PDT. After parenteral or topical application, photosensitizers are mainly present in cancer cells and also to some extent in surrounding healthy tissue (**Figure 2**). The subcellular localization of the photosensitizers in cells embraces various organelles including plasma membranes, endoplasmic reticulum, mitochondria,

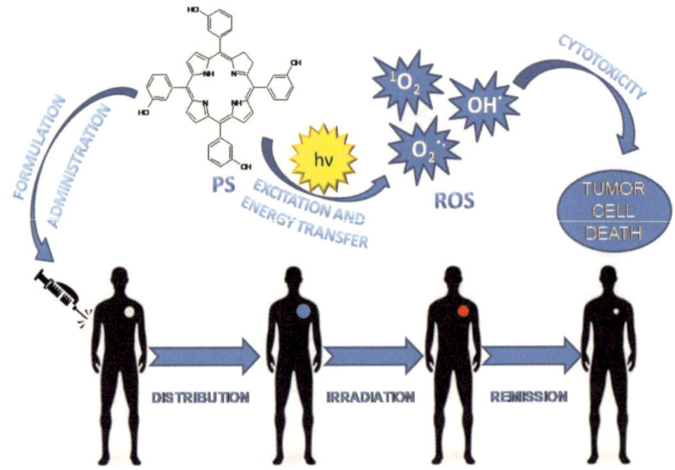

Figure 2. Mechanism of photodynamic reaction and photodynamic therapy.

lysosomes, and Golgi apparatus [12, 13]. Up to that point, photosensitizer occurs in an unexcited singlet state which has two electrons with different spins in the low energy orbital. Light is necessary for the activation of the photosensitizer and the induction of the photodynamic reaction [14]. For this reason, the photosensitizer is irradiated with light in an appropriate wavelength generated by precise sources, e.g., diode lasers or, considering the relatively high cost of lasers, the much cheaper, and portable light emitting diodes (LED). Fiber optics, or LED portable arrays illuminating light, are used for various types of cancer, including pulmonary tumors and fit through a bronchoscope or CT-guided needle or catheters [15]. A very important problem to be addressed is the suitable drug-light interval: as the photosensitizer is introduced into the body, and the vascular supply circulates as long as it accumulates in the tumor. Early illumination, after photosensitizer introduction, causes predominantly vascular effects, whereas later illumination favors tumor-cell effect. As a result, the photosensitizer when illuminated is "boosted" from its ground state to a higher energy state singlet-excited state. This state is an extremely short-lived, so an excess of accumulated energy has to be released in two different ways: the first one, which is the basis of PDD, involves the emission of light called fluorescence and corresponding to the relaxation of a molecule from the excited to ground state. The second alternative is an intersystem crossing which undergoes without energy emission and results in the formation of the triplet-excited state of the photosensitizer. Note that the half-life of the triplet-excited state is much longer than that of the singlet-excited state. In this case, photosensitizers can very rarely return to their ground state through the emission of energy called phosphorescence. In the comparison of the singlet and triplet excited states, it can be ascertained that both of them are utilized in photodynamic therapy. However, the contribution of the triplet state is much greater. As the energy is released by the excited photosensitizer, the initiation of the photodynamic reaction processes may result in the formation of reactive oxygen species (ROS) which are known to be toxic to neoplastic cells [12, 16].

The three main types of photodynamic reactions can be identified, among which two are extremely important in PDT. In the first type of reaction, energy from the excited photosensitizer is transferred to an electron or hydrogen atom of a substrate or another molecule and anion or cation radicals may be obtained. Afterwards, they interact with the surrounding oxygen which is transformed into toxic oxygenated species. Water molecules are the main target of this attack with a hydroxyl radical and superoxide anion radical formed as the products of the reaction. The mechanism of the second type of photodynamic reaction consists of a reaction of the photosensitizer with molecular oxygen ($^3O_2$) and singlet oxygen ($^1O_2$) formation. As singlet oxygen is thought to play a main role in destroying cancer cells, the type II PDT mechanism is known as an appropriate photodynamic reaction (PDR). Although in both types, I and II, reactions may occur simultaneously, in most cases, one of them is more common, depending on the structure and physicochemical properties of photosensitizers. The newest photosensitizers are designed to generate as much singlet oxygen as possible (preferring type II). There is also another type of photodynamic therapy mechanism called the type III PDT mechanism. However, it is based on the direct interaction of excited photosensitizers, which is toxic to the target cancer cells without oxygen species being involved [12, 15, 17].

The singlet oxygen obtained during PDT is thought to be a very reactive derivative of the oxygen species. It is able to initiate a cascade of molecular effects resulting in the selective destruction of lesions, indirect vascular damaging effects (vascular shutdown), and the influence on immune systems (inflammation induction and other tumor-specific immune reactions) [10]. Its half-life is 40 ns and the range of action is 20 nm [9, 18]. The amount of singlet oxygen species produced by photosensitizers has to be sufficient to destroy even large lesions. The toxic character of radicals and singlet oxygen species results in apoptotic (via signal transduction pathways) and/or necrotic cell death. The destructive influence on the vascular system is a result of vasoconstriction, thrombosis, ischemia or necrosis connected with the singlet oxygen lethal effect to the nearest cells [19].

3. Modern photosensitizers—drugs—applied in therapy nowadays

There are few important requirements that chemical compound meets to serve as a photosensitizer for PDT. One of the first requirements is its synthetic purity and stability. A photosensitizer should be water-soluble and easily distribute in the body. It should not exhibit toxicity or mutagenicity in the human organism without light activation; therefore, it should be inert until activation by light. Ideal photosensitizers should also selectively accumulate in tumor tissue and be characterized by the clearance from healthy tissue, so therapy would only involve pathologically altered cells. In addition, they should be non-toxic to non-illuminated bystander regions. Photosensitizers should be activated by light in an appropriate wavelength that penetrates tissue deeper, and efficiently generates reactive oxygen species (especially singlet oxygen). Therefore, the repeated generation of type II reactions with a clinically successful photosensitizer is very important. The ideal photosensitizer does not induce pain during and after therapy and may be used in outpatient care. The drug, photosensitizer, should be transported in a stable state and its reconstitution should be performed by trained pharmacists without specialized laboratories. Generally, clinicians and chemists have different views concerning the ideal photosensitizer. Chemists put more stress on a high extinction coefficient and a high quantum yield of singlet oxygen, whereas clinicians emphasize low toxicity and high selectivity [3, 15, 17, 20, 21].

Most of the currently used photosensitizers in clinical PDT belong to the porphyrinoid family. These aromatic, macrocyclic compounds consist usually of four pyrrole rings linked together by methine or azomethine bridges. The first clinically applied photosensitizer and, parallel to which, a representative of the first generation of photosensitizers approved for photodynamic therapy, is Photofrin®. It is a complex mixture of porphyrin monomers, dimers, and oligomers obtained by chemical processing of hematoporphyrin with a Q1 band at 630 nm in phosphate buffered saline (PBS) and a very low singlet oxygen generation φ_Δ value of 0.01 in PBS. This photosensitizer is administered by intravenous route to achieve concentration in the lesion and/or clear healthy tissue ca. 48 h prior to illumination. It was found that illumination, 2–4 h post infusion to the target tissue, is possible but the preservation of healthy tissue is not achieved. It was found that this photosensitizer was evident to a certain degree in all tissues for 4–8 weeks post infusion due to a long clearance time. It possesses wide applications in PDT, e.g., in the early and late stages of lung cancer, superficial and advanced esophageal cancer, bladder cancer, cervical dysplasia and early stage cervical cancer, cancers of head and neck, brain, and skin [15, 17, 22, 23]. However, this photosensitizer has many crucial defects. Most important is its long-elimination time reaching 8 weeks, which causes long-lasting photosensitivity. Patients can experience skin burns when exposed to strong light, e.g., sunlight. Based on chlorine structure, Temoporfin 1 (**Figure 3**) belongs to the second generation photosensitizers and can be obtained in high purity and chemical identity. Moreover, it exhibits better photosensitizing properties than Photofrin® and is used under Foscan® brand name. PDT

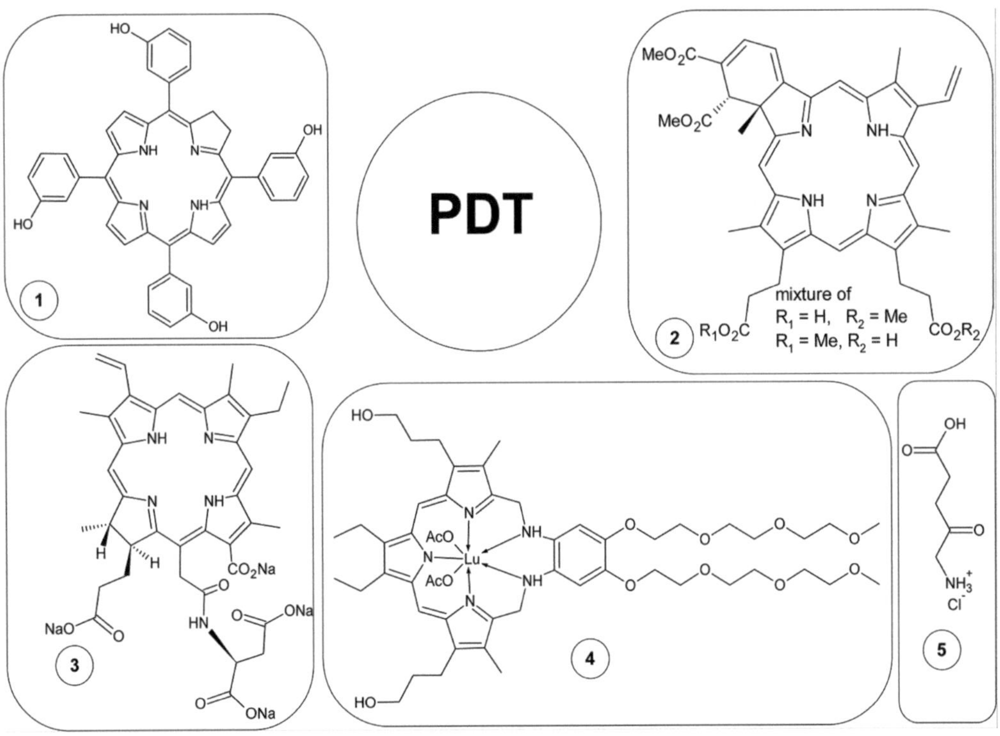

Figure 3. Chemical structures of clinically used photosensitizers: (**1**) Foscan, (**2**) Visudyne, (**3**) Talaporfin sodium, (**4**) Lutetium texaphyrin, (**5**) 5-Aminolevulinic acid.

with Foscan® is 100 times more effective due to its absorption maximum shifted toward longer wavelengths (Q1 band appears at 652 nm), higher molar absorption coefficient, and singlet oxygen generation yield (φ_Δ value is 0.43 in aerated methanol). These features enable the use of a lower dose of administered photosensitizer ca. 0.15 mg/kg intravenously, in comparison to 2–5 mg/kg, as in the case of Photofrin®. Temoporfin has been applied against, e.g., esophageal cancer, lung cancer, gastric cancer, prostate cancer, and skin cancer. However, the elimination time of this photosensitizer is still very long (about 4–6 weeks). Another synthetic chlorine-based photosensitizer is mono aspartyl chlorine e6 (MACE), which possesses improved characteristics as compared to Photofrin®. Its sunlight photosensitivity skin reaction is in fact 2–3 weeks, but it is activated 4 h post infusion, which enables the convenient treatment in a single one day session. It possesses potential in ophthalmic lesions [11, 15, 20]. In the case of Verteporfin (Visudyne®) **2**, the accumulation and elimination times are 20 times shorter than that of Foscan®. Other advantages of **2** as a photosensitizer are the strong absorption band shifted even further into longer wavelengths (Q1 band at 686 nm) than those of Foscan® and Photofrin®. In addition, the ability to generate singlet oxygen by Visudyne® is extremely strong. This photosensitizer is used as the liposomal formulation in the PDT of age-related macular degeneration. It is also used in rheumatoid arthritis due to its immunomodulatory properties. Visudyne® has been also considered against psoriasis and cutaneous tumors [24]. Talaporfin sodium **3**, known as Laserphyrin® is a water-soluble second generation photosensitizer. It exhibits all desired features of an ideal photosensitizer, including good light absorption (Q1 band at 654 nm), efficient singlet oxygen generation (φ_Δ value is 0.43 in PBS), and fast accumulation and elimination. In Japan, Lutrin®, which is a brand name of **4**, has been used in therapy at early-stage lung cancer. Lutetium texaphyrin (Lutrin®) **4** possesses significantly lower singlet oxygen generation yield (φ_Δ value is 0.11 in methanol) than other second generation photosensitizers. However, its absorption maximum wavelength is shifted toward 732 nm. It can be administered in lower doses than Photofrin® and irradiated with lower light doses 3 h after injection. Lutrin®, which is a brand name of **4**, can be successfully used in PDT in cervical and prostate cancer. It undergoes clinical trials against melanomas, breast cancer, and Kaposi's sarcoma. Moreover, some animal *in vivo* study revealed an increase in damage to tumor blood vessels during Lutetium texaphyrin-PDT through the use of low fluence rates [11, 25].

Aside from the photosensitizers described above, which are commercially available and participate directly in the photodynamic reaction, there is also another approach to PDT. 5-Aminolevulinic acid (ALA, Levulan®) **5** mediated PDT has received much attention of researchers and physicians. Unlike other photosensitizers ALA is a prodrug (pro-metabolite). When administered intravenously, it enters metabolically, which physiologically leads to heme formation. However, in tumor tissue, this enzyme conducts the last step in heme synthesis, ferrochelatase, and is less active; therefore, the metabolic pathway stops at protoporphyrin IX (Pp IX). This endogenous porphyrin possesses photosensitizing activity and can be employed as a PDT agent. ALA-PDT has shown promising potential in animal testing and early clinical trials in many tumors, including epithelial nonmelanoma skin cancers [26]. Recently, the efficacy and safety of topical ALA-PDT in the treatment of extramammary Paget's disease (EMPD) and its role in surgical improvements have been discussed [27].

Although second generation photosensitizers are effective PDT agents, there is a constant need for further development and improvements. Many potential PDT active pharmaceutical substances are under clinical trials, as well as many research reports, and embrace the very promising properties of the newly obtained compounds. The main paths of research have involved the elaboration of tumor selective agents by conjugating photosensitizers with biologically active moieties, e.g., carbohydrates [28], folate molecules [29], or antibodies targeting cancer cells [30]. This can increase the uptake of photosensitizers in cancerous cells and make PDT more effective and less harmful to healthy tissue. A huge challenge may bring the development of nanosized carriers for photosensitizers, including polymeric nanoparticles, liposomes, niosomes, micelles, nanocrystals, microcapsules, and dendrimers. It should improve the efficiency of photodynamic activity and, in this way, overcome many side effects associated with classic PDT. Huge success noted in this field is connected with two liposomal formulations of photosensitizers, such as Verteporfin (Visudyne®) and Temoporfin (Foslip®) [31, 32].

4. The expertise of the health care providers and associated specialists working collaboratively with patients during photodynamic therapy

4.1. The role of associated specialists in preclinical trials

Interdisciplinary team, including medicinal chemists, chemists, biologists, biochemists, and physicists conducts preliminary step of photodynamic therapy (**Figure 4**). Medicinal chemists and chemists are engaged in the design and chemical synthesis of compounds that may have the potential for photodynamic therapy. The production process should be efficient and easy to reproduce. As far as PDT is concerned, an important measurement is also the assessment of light absorption and emission by a photosensitizer, solubility, aggregation tendency, its chemical, and photostabilities (photobleaching). This research is usually performed by physicist and chemical physicist. In the area of biochemistry, biology, and molecular pharmacology,

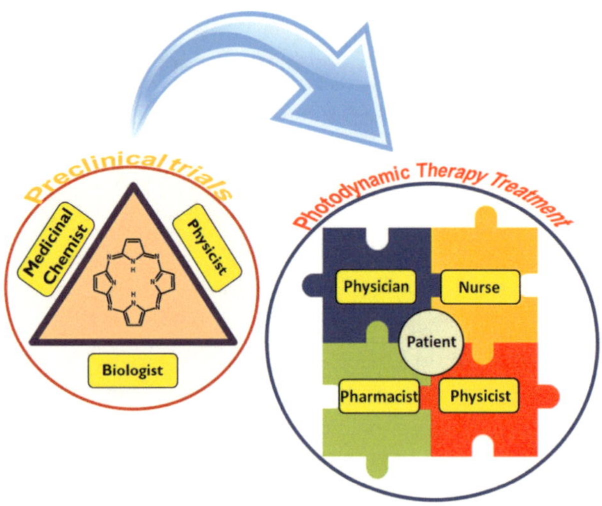

Figure 4. Health care providers and associated specialists in photodynamic therapy team.

researchers look into the activity of the compounds. They conduct tests on cell cultures *in vitro* and using animals *in vivo* experiments [4, 21].

The role of team members listed herein is, therefore, to produce a medicine, that, when used during PDT should possess features such as: chemical purity, chemo- and photostability, a lack of activity in the dark, selective accumulation in target tissue (e.g., neoplasms), a lack of toxicity, and mutagenicity in healthy tissues. The rate of the elimination of the substances from the body and its availability to patients are apparent. One of the most important issues is also the reduction or overcoming of the adverse effects caused by photosensitizers such as photosensitivity lasting up to several weeks after treatment or elimination of pain associated with treatment [20]. Sieroń and Kwiatek [5] discussed the work carried out by an interdisciplinary team consisting of physicists and chemists, whose aim was to develop an optimal structure of a novel photosensitizer. They performed chemical synthesis in a novel potential photosensitizer and its physicochemical characterization with the detailed assessment of spectroscopic properties. Part of the team consisted of physicists focused on the determination of crystalline and electronic structures and the chemical composition of novel photosensitizers. The presence of physicists in the PDT team is recommended also for another reason. The necessary condition for the photodynamic therapy is the activation of the photosensitizer through light in the appropriate wavelength. In practice, laser and nonlaser light sources are used. Physicists are responsible for providing a source of light, establishing the wavelength, and dose of the photosensitizer suitable for irradiation during treatment. Further studies on cell and molecular aspects of PDT action with the newly elaborated photosensitizers are necessary on various cells *in vitro* and *in vivo* tumor models. All these studies can help to explore cytotoxicity, photocytotoxicity, and genotoxicity of novel photosensitizers [5, 33]. Considering the relevant aspects of medicinal chemistry and pharmaceutical chemistry important in various stages of preclinical trials, the pharmacist's expertise can also be very useful. In particular, it concerns problems arising from limited solubility and the aggregation of various photosensitizers prepared for initial preclinical biological study. Many limitation appearing in such a stage may be overcome by both chemical modification in the periphery of the photosensitizer and/or suitable pharmaceutical formulation, e.g., by entrapping the photosensitizer in liposomes or polymeric nanoparticles [32, 34].

4.2. The role of health care providers in clinical trials

Health care providers, such as physicians, nurses, and pharmacists, work closely with patients in photodynamic therapy processes.

4.2.1. Physicians

Among specialists in the interdisciplinary team of health care providers conducting photodynamic therapy, an important task falls on the doctor's shoulders. His knowledge and skills are used in each stage of PDT in the treatment of neoplastic and nonneoplastic diseases. His main task is to carry out the treatment itself and to take responsibility for the whole therapy. The doctor assesses the patient's state of health before treatment and decides on the patient's qualification for PDT, informs about the procedure and possible adverse effects [6, 7]. In Brazil, a physician consults a nurse and physicist and considers the potential benefits and consequences of therapy for each patient. Doctors and nurses spend a lot of time in explaining details with the patient and answering his questions [4].

The cooperation within the interdisciplinary PDT team has been professionally elaborated by researchers from the Laser Center, Thompson Cancer Survival Center of Knoxville. Their conclusions concerned the treatment of Barrett's esophagus using endoscopic ablation of Barrett's esophagectomy with PDT. The method applied is based on the medication followed by the endoscopy procedure during which the laser light is emitted to the so-called Barrett's esophagus through an endoscope. This technique requires the coordinated work of a physician, an endoscopic nurse, a laser expert, and, an endoscopic assistant. The authors of this paper, Overholt and Panjehpour [35] clearly demonstrated that the proposed construction of the "PDT team of excellence" is necessary for professional and successful treatment of the patient.

4.2.2. Nursing personnel

Nurses are professionally active and involved in the care of patients treated through phototherapy following tasks resulting from four functions of nursing: (i) health care provision, (ii) patient education, (iii) active action in health care team, and (iv) the development of nursing practice standards (**Figure 5**). As far as the above-mentioned nursing features are concerned, a nurse performs a number of tasks that contribute to improving the quality of services provided through which the most dominant feature is the provision of nursing care. The term health service means measures to strengthen, maintain, restore, or improve health, resulting from the process of diagnosis, treatment, and rehabilitation. In order to optimize health care services, specific tasks performed by nurses need to be taken on: (i) assessing the needs of patients treated with phototherapy, and the recognition of their condition and existing health problems, (ii) creation of conditions for aware patient participation in the planned form of treatment, (iii) planning and implementing nursing care during treatment and after its completion, and (iv) documenting the activities of nursing (medical history, results of preclinical examinations such as the BP intervals, heart rate, body weight, height, respiratory-rate) [36–39]. Particularly important is the provision of health care to chronically ill patients whose bio-psycho-social welfare has

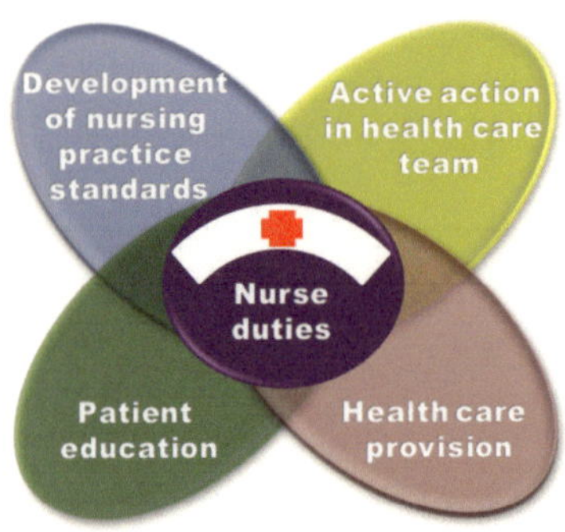

Figure 5. General duties of nurses during PDT [39].

been violated. Therefore, the principal activity carried out by nurses as health care providers is to conduct an interview with a person who is to undergo photodynamic therapy. The interview should include elements concerning the health and social situation of the family. Before the provision of health services prior to therapy, a nurse takes the height and weight measurements of patient, assesses visual acuity, heart-rate, blood pressure, and the respiratory-rate. The tasks of the nurse participating in the therapy are drug administration and observation of the patient to acute allergic reactions or other adverse effects during the course of treatment. As an essential topic in the interview, it should cover the kind of existing treatment and possibilities of occurrence of contraindications to phototherapy i.e., existing allergy, liver diseases, hypersensitivity to sunlight or pregnancy. Noteworthy, as porfimer sodium is classified as a chemotherapy agent, only a registered nurse can administer the medication [6, 40, 41]. Excellent examples concerning PDT as a treatment option for two groups of patients utilizing its curative or palliative effect for lung cancer (nonsmall cell lung cancer) patients were discussed by Collins and Garner [6]. They presented the cooperation model in a PDT team consisting of a nurse, a surgeon, an oncologist, and a pharmacist. As emphasized by Rich et al. [7], included in the nurses' tasks before treatment, a detailed interview with the patient aimed at obtaining a medical history of treatment is necessary. It is important to collect a complete medical and surgical history, including current medications used and an ophthalmologic history. Particular attention should be paid to the presence of contraindications to photodynamic therapy with Verteporfin (Visudyne), such as allergies, hypersensitivity to sunlight, liver disease, or pregnancy. Prior to the surgery, nursing personnel tests the visual acuity, blood pressure, pulse, respirations, and body weight and height of the patient for BSA (body surface area).

During surgery, the nurse, according to the doctor's recommendation, administers medication (eye drops) to the patient and starts the infusion line with use of a No. 22 angio safety catheter. The nurse also has to make sure that the patient has knowledge of the entire procedure. It is also important for the patient throughout the procedure to remain in the correct position, so that the doctor can accurately direct the laser light on the treated area. After treatment, the patient receives detailed instructions about potential side effects, the optimization of pain management, and precautions that must be taken. Mainly the patient should be told to protect skin and eyes from sunlight and other so-called sources of bright light and warned that nonadherence to these instructions may result in skin burns or eye damage. It is very important to assure that patient understands the necessity for light precautions for 5 days, even in terms of avoiding bright lights, like surgical and dental lighting. Thus, nurses are significant members of the professional team and fulfill an important role in the patient assessment including pretreatment and posttreatment teaching [7, 42].

Similarly, the nurse's role is depicted in disease therapy of lung or esophageal cancers. Also, in this case, they are responsible for informing the patient about the effects of photosensitivity and explaining how and for how long patient's skin and eyes should be protected, as the illumination is connected with extreme photosensitivity, including ocular sensitivity. It is also worth mentioning that education about the procedure, side effects, and precautions should be extended to all patient family members. These subjects are of immense interest for nurses and have been included in many oncology nursing treatment schemes [6, 42, 43]. Allison et al. [44]

while discussing PDT for chest wall recurrence from breast cancer analyzed many specific precautions accompanying this kind of treatment, including photosensitivity, illumination, pain control, photosensitivity reaction, posttreatment, patient selection, curing wounds, and retreatment. Some of them are under the direct control of a physician, but many need the supervision of other medical team members. Although photosensitivity is a common problem, patients must be informed that even minimal light levels as those coming from a light bulb or fireplace or light reflected from a car window can cause photosensitivity reaction. Interestingly, giving consent to PDT therapy according to information about sunlight precautions has not prevented any patient from photosensitivity, Therefore, patients found to be unable to accept sunlight precautions should not be offered PDT. Pain may accompany the PDT therapy, therefore patient should be given narcotic or nonnarcotic pain pills prior to illumination. In some cases, patients subjected to PDT for the recurrence of breast cancer in the chest wall, pain control resulting from lesion diminishment can be seen within 2 weeks of the PDT session. Nevertheless, even at that time continued narcotic or nonnarcotic analgesia is recommended. It is very important as to how the problem is recognized when the photosensitivity reaction occurs. Although the treatment of the sign and symptoms of skin burns may be easily treated with, e.g., steroids, ice/cold compresses, the treatment of, e.g., airway and neck is more complicated and a proper intensive care approach may be required, often on an inpatient basis. Posttreatment patient management is a major therapeutic challenge. Patients need to drink plenty of fluids and be protected from light. Some patients may need steroids, while others oral narcotic and nonnarcotic analgesia, and many, in the course of treatment, antibiotics [44, 45].

Nurses take on many tasks in the PDT treatment procedure; therefore, they should know the principles of photodynamic therapy. Later after treatment, the nurse actively participates in the patient recovery process or motivating patients to continue therapy using PDT and other health procedures [40, 41]. Meticulous patient monitoring and the evaluation of the effectiveness of nursing care taken will allow the nurse to implement the next health service function, which is health education. The purpose of health education is for people with disabilities and the chronically ill to be motivated to take responsibility for their own health and to prepare for self-care. Educational activities are closely linked with health promotion, the main objective of which is to strengthen and enhance health, and, without a doubt, improve their quality of life. The concept of health promotion in relation to chronic diseases may often be as a contradiction misunderstood, in other words illogical. However, it must be kept in mind that the purpose of the promotion is to improve and control one's own health. Therefore, especially those who are ill should take care of the development of their bio-psycho-social opportunities, because no illness limits human functioning to the extent that it was impossible to creatively use the remaining potential [46]. It is important that nurses use their knowledge of health promotion to motivate patients in the field of their health protection and restoring them to health by activating compensatory mechanisms. In the nursing care process, it is important to have permanent psychotherapeutic impact, by which a positive effect on the patient and the creation of a therapeutic relationship nurse-patient is meant. An important element is to establish a relationship between the nurse and the patient and sends a "positive support message" containing, uplifting and at the same time mobilizing to action. Mutual understanding, creating an atmosphere of releasing a suffering person from negative feelings allows the nurse to establish efficient communication, as it was discussed during the PDT lung cancer treatment and AMD patients. Moreover, a nurse acts not only as the patient's teacher, but also an advocate [6, 47].

Considering their educational activities, nurses conduct the following tasks: (i) they collect information at the request of patients for educational and advisory activities, (ii) they set targets for educational activities, and preventional promotion actions involving the provision of behavioral information after PDT treatment. The topic of education regards behavior after illumination. Nurses should recommend avoiding sunlight, wearing headgear, clothing with long sleeves, and sunglasses. Patient should be informed that their entire skin must be covered and that daily activities, including driving should be done at night. In the case of some photosensitizers, patients should be house-bound up to 3 months. Nurses should also report any reactions to medication. Significant to patient education is learning how to cope with any stress resulting from the disease and how to control stress. Some emotional problems experienced by patients are not symptoms of their disease, but are related to a manifestation of some "adaptation efforts" arising from attempts to cope with the existing situation. It should be emphasized that all educational activities undertaken by the nurse should be tailored to the level of the recipient, and so communicated in a clear and simple manner without medical jargon. In fulfilling the role, the nurses should work with other members of the therapeutic team, who will help them and give advice. In Brazil, nurses participate not only in the whole procedure at each stage of therapy but are also in very close contact with the patient. They are responsible for education concerning the course of treatment and risk minimization of side effects. They also observe the patient during surgery for adverse events [4, 6, 48].

Another feature of nursing is the active involvement in health care organization. Care for patients undergoing photodynamic therapy is exercised by different professionals (physician, nurse, and pharmacist) and therefore their close cooperation is required, including the exchange of experiences and information on patients. This is important because of the deliberate planning and organizing health care. Due to the frequent contact of nurses to patients, it is advisable for them to function as a link between patients and other members of the therapeutic team. Nurses cooperate with other professionals, the patient's family, and the local community. This allows them to work together with a team to come up with the optimum therapeutic care plan for the patient treated with PDT and to provide comprehensive assistance in line with the expectations of the patient. In order to fulfill this function, nurses begin work with both the team caring for the patient and with his family (through contact with a health visitor, primary care physician). The consequence of cooperation with such people is the exchange of insights and experiences on the patient's health and social situation in order to improve the quality of health services [6, 7].

Based on these experiences and research conducted on persons undergoing phototherapy, nurses should develop innovative ways of working with patients, in order to achieve better care results. It should allow them to fulfill the fourth nursing function which is the development of nursing skills. In carrying out this function, nurses should undertake the following tasks: (i) take an active part in training through participation in conferences and courses on phototherapy, which will enable them to broaden their knowledge, (ii) keeping up to date through the self-study and analysis of the latest medical reports in the field of PDT, (iii) develop standard of nursing care for patients being treated with photodynamic therapy, implement the above-mentioned standards, and evaluate the effectiveness of nursing actions taken. Photodynamic therapy of age-related macular degeneration is a stage process, which includes intravenous administration of the photosensitizer followed by the use of lasers to activate the drug. The role of the care providers consists in administration, evaluation, and monitoring of the patient for acute drug reactions during the procedure or patient education. It is noteworthy that the implementation of formalized, proactive interdisciplinary approaches in treating other diseases, like chronic kidney disease, was found to have a positive impact on patients' well-being [49, 50].

4.2.3. Pharmacists

Many pharmacists have expressed a desire to become more involved in patient care and in providing services traditionally offered by physicians and nurse practitioners [51]. The role of the pharmacists in patient-centered medical home practices revealed knowledge and skills that can complement the care provided by other health care team members [52]. Moreover, many studies emphasize that the cooperation between general practitioners, pharmacists, and nurses is necessary to effectively dispense drugs to the patient [53]. A very interesting report concerning approaches in improving the outcome of the patient and health care system through advanced pharmaceutical experience and have recently been reviewed by Giberson et al. [54]. Moreover, Makowsky et al. [55] recently discussed working relationships in the inpatient medical setting between pharmacists, physicians, and nurse practitioners. The integration of pharmacists into the nurse practitioners and physicians teams was positively felt in terms of patient well-being (drug-therapy decision-making, continuity of care, patient safety).

Pharmacists as specialist—team players in the field of medicinal chemistry, pharmacology, and toxicology—are responsible for the preparation of drugs for both topical and systemic administration. They are also responsible for the proper drug storage, i.e., temperature control and protection against solar radiation and other light sources. Pharmacists cooperate with physicians and nurses during the procedure to ensure the adequate preparation of the drug directly before the administration to the patient [4, 6]. In this regard, it is especially important that the specialized team cooperates on the various aspects of specific medications at various stages of the procedure, such as narcotic and nonnarcotic medications including nonsteroidal anti-inflammatory drugs analgesics, acetaminophen, metamizole or topical pain relievers, antibiotics, steroids, and nausea-suppressing agents. Moreover, some patients require parenteral nutrition or hydration. Hypersensitivity to light requires specific precautions. Failure to comply with these rules may result in skin burns, peeling of the treated skin, local edema, erythema, dysuria, urethral irritation which requires the use of additional therapeutic agents [6, 20, 35, 56].

The researchers emphasize the important role of pharmacists and cooperation with the pharmacy. The application of each drug should be preceded by their compatibility studies with other medications. It is also used to assess the properties of the drug formulations considering patient's light hypersensitivity. Scientists dealing with modifications of oral drug forms turned their attention to the possibility of cooperation of physicians, pharmacists, and nurses. They conducted the survey among representatives of these three professions. It turned out that the personnel working in the public health centers employing specialists in various fields, for example hospitals often cooperate with each other discussing and exchanging views and experiences [6, 53].

Another expertise area of pharmacists includes drug formulation. It seems that the development of novel photosensitizers depends on both the development of novel photosensitizers, as well as novel formulations including the latest achievements of nanomedicine. Very interesting pharmaceutical studies were conducted for 5-aminolevulinic acid (5-ALA) that is a photosensitizer with broad applications in photodynamic therapy and photodynamic diagnosis. This compound is a prodrug/prometabolite which is converted into protoporphyrin IX (PpIX) and possesses photosensitizing properties [44]. Its topical formulations are used in the treatment of neoplastic and nonneoplastic diseases. Unfortunately, ALA-PDT treatment has certain drawbacks. One of them is low skin permeability, limiting this treatment only to surface skin lesions, e.g., malignant skin tumors [5, 20]. Researchers, who rely on their knowledge and clinical experience, are attempting to modify the drug formulations containing this compound [57]. Therefore, a 20% topical solution of 5-aminolevulinic under the brand name of Levulan® Kerastick® is being used. A lack in the stability of the substance in solution requires combining the drug with a solvent just before application. Another product called Metvix® is a 16% cream containing the methyl ester of 5-aminolevulinic acid (methyl aminolevulinate) as hydrochloride, which in comparison to the parent compound should penetrate the skin more effectively. In searching for another stable formulation, a precise dose to the affected area was provided by Donnelly et al. [57] and E.P. Patent No. 1467706 B1 [58]. They described an adhesion patch based on Eudragit® NE that contains ALA dispersed in the adhesive matrix and requires moisture for activation. It is also of interest that mucoadhesive Carbopol® 941- and Poloxamer® PF127-based polymeric mucoadhesive thermoresponsive gel containing ALA was described by Tsui-Min [59]. Promising data was obtained for 20% oil-in-water emulsion formulations of 5-aminolevulinic acid. These drugs were administered topically to patients with various types of skin diseases [60]. Interesting experiments that compared the efficacy of 5-aminolevulinic acid (5-ALA) and its methyl ester (mALA) were performed for Lutrol F-127-based thermolabile gel 10% formulation in treatment of basal cell carcinomas of the skin [61].

A very interesting study on pharmaceutical development, composition, and quantitative analysis of the phthalocyanine photosensitizer for cancer photodynamic therapy has recently been presented by Jiang et al. [62]. The authors discussed phthalocyanine derivatives in terms of pharmaceutical development and molecular modification in order to enhance drug effectiveness and to improve its intracellular localization. Therefore, various approaches concerning the conjugation of photosensitizers to various antibodies, proteins, and peptides have also been described. In addition, various strategies concerning an improvement of pharmaceutical properties utilizing direct formulations of phthalocyanines were discussed.

5. Perspectives

The aim of this short review was to present the topic of photodynamic therapy and activities taken by health care providers and associated specialists working together with patients during the photodynamic therapy. The expert literature indicates that the effective implementation of photodynamic therapy requires intensive cooperation within the interdisciplinary team and possesses a broad knowledge in various fields. Coordinated actions of representatives possessing expertise in various fields of medical and natural sciences, especially doctors, nurses, pharmacists, chemists, physicists, biologists, and biochemists, are necessary both during joint research, development and during the course of the PDT procedure.

During therapy, the patient plays the most important role and is responsible for acting in accordance with the schedule set by the physician, nurse, and pharmacist. Activities aimed to increase the effectiveness of treatment conducted by the physician or surgeon, minimizing side effects, and ensuring of the comprehensive care to patients also require the participation of physicians, nurses, and pharmacists. In conclusion, only the effective interaction between professionals and clear sharing of responsibilities at different stages of therapy should guarantee successful treatment.

Acknowledgements

Tomasz Goslinski and Magdalena Stolarska acknowledge the Polish National Science Centre for the Grant No. 2012/05/E/NZ7/01204.

Author details

Tomasz Kocki[1]*, Beata Czarczynska-Goslinska[2], Katarzyna Kocka[3], Magdalena Stolarska[2,4], Daria Wachowska[4], Sebastian Lijewski[4], Tomasz Koczorowski[4] and Tomasz Goslinski[4]

*Address all correspondence to: tomasz.kocki@umlub.pl

1 Department of Experimental and Clinical Pharmacology, Medical University of Lublin, Lublin, Poland

2 Department of Pharmaceutical Technology, Poznan University of Medical Sciences, Poznan, Poland

3 Chair of Oncology and Environmental Health, Medical University of Lublin, Lublin, Poland

4 Department of Chemical Technology of Drugs, Poznan University of Medical Sciences, Poznan, Poland

References

[1] Ackroyd R, Kelty C, Brown N, et al. The history of photodetection and photodynamic therapy. Photochem Photobiol. 2001;74:656–669. http://dx.doi.org/10.1562/0031-8655(2001)0740656THOPAP2.0.CO2

[2] Brown SB, Brown EA, Walker I. The present and future role of photodynamic therapy in cancer treatment. Lancet Oncol. 2004;5:497–508. http://dx.doi.org/10.1016/S1470-2045(04)01529-3

[3] Huang Z. A review of progress in clinical photodynamic therapy. Technol Cancer Res Treat. 2005;4:283–293. http://dx.doi.org/10.1177/153303460500400308

[4] Bagnato VS, Kurachi C, Ferreira Jet, et al. PDT experience in Brazil: A regional profile. Photodiagn Photodyn Ther. 2005;2:107–118. http://dx.doi.org/10.1016/S1572-1000(05)00058-X

[5] Sieroń A, Kwiatek S. Twenty years of experience with PDD and PDT in Poland – Review. Photodiag Photodyn Ther. 2009;6:73–78. http://dx.doi.org/10.1016/j.pdpdt.2009.07.003

[6] Smith Collins A, Garner M. Caring for lung cancer patients receiving photodynamic therapy. Crit Care Nurse. 2007;27:53–60.

[7] Rich D, Lane AM, Miller JW. Photodynamic therapy: The nurse's role. Insight. 2001;26:44–48. http://dx.doi.org/10.1067/min.2001.113401

[8] Moghissi K, Dixon K. Yorkshire Laser Centre mobile photodynamic therapy unit: For service to district general hospitals. Photodiag Photodyn Ther. 2005;2:169–174. http://dx.doi.org/10.1016/S1572-1000(05)00102-X

[9] Buytaert E, Dewaele M, Agostinis P. Molecular effectors of multiple cell death pathways initiated by photodynamic therapy. BBA. 2007;1776:86–107. http://dx.doi.org/10.1016/j.bbcan.2007.07.001

[10] Kudinova NV, Berezov TT. Photodynamic therapy of cancer: search for ideal photosensitizer. Biochem (Moscow) Suppl B: Biomed Chem. 2010;4:95–103. http://dx.doi.org/10.1134/S1990750810010129

[11] Yano S, Hirohara S, Obata M, et al. Current states and future views in photodynamic therapy. J Photochem Photobiol C. 2011;12:46–67. http://dx.doi.org/10.1016/j.jphotochemrev.2011.06.001

[12] Robertson CA, Hawkins Evans D, Abrahamse H. Photodynamic therapy (PDT): a short review on cellular mechanisms and cancer research applications for PDT. J Photochem Photobiol B. 2009;96:1–8. http://dx.doi.org/10.1016/j.jphotobiol.2009.04.001

[13] Skupin-Mrugalska P, Sobotta L, Kucińska M, et al. Cellular changes, molecular pathways and the immune system following photodynamic treatment. Curr Med Chem. 2014;21:4059–4073. http://dx.doi.org/10.2174/0929867321666140826120300

[14] Kübler AC. Photodynamic therapy. Med Laser Appl. 2005;20:37–45. http://dx.doi.org/10.1016/j.mla.2005.02.001

[15] Allison RR, Moghissi K, Downie G, et al. Photodynamic therapy (PDT) for lung cancer. Photodiagn Photodyn Ther. 2011;8:231–239. http://dx.doi.org/10.1016/j.pdpdt.2011.03.342

[16] Allison RR, Moghissi K. Oncologic photodynamic therapy: Clinical strategies that modulate mechanisms of action. Photodiagn Photodyn Ther. 2013;10:331–341. http://dx.doi.org/10.1016/j.pdpdt.2013.03.011

[17] Sharman WM, Allen CM, van Lier JE. Photodynamic therapeutics: basic principles and clinical applications. Drug Discov Today. 1999;4:507–517. http://dx.doi.org/10.1016/S1359-6446(99)01412-9

[18] Moan J., Berg K. The photodegradation of porphyrins in cells can be used to estimate the lifetime of singlet oxygen. Photochem Photobiol. 1991;53:549–553. http://dx.doi.org/10.1111/j.1751-1097.1991.tb03669.x

[19] Plaetzer K, Kiesslich T, Verwanger T, et al. The modes of cell death induced by PDT: an overview. Med Laser Appl. 2003;18:7–19. http://dx.doi.org/10.1078/1615-1615-00082

[20] Allison RR, Downie GH, Cuenca R, et al. Photosensitizers in clinical PDT. Photodiagn Photodyn Ther. 2004;1:27–42. http://dx.doi.org/10.1016/S1572-1000(04)00007-9

[21] Allison RR, Sibata CH. Oncologic photodynamic therapy photosensitizers: a clinical review. Photodiagn Photodyn Ther. 2010;7:61–75. http://dx.doi.org/10.1016/j.pdpdt.2010.02.001

[22] Dougherty TJ. Hematoporphyrin as a photosensitizer of tumors. Photochem Photobiol. 1983;38:377–379. http://dx.doi.org/10.1111/j.1751-1097.1983.tb02687.x

[23] Dougherty TJ. A brief history of clinical photodynamic therapy development at Roswell Park Cancer Institute. J Clin Laser Surg Med. 1996;14:219–221. http://dx.doi.org/10.1089/clm.1996.14.219

[24] Gryziewicz L. Regulatory aspects of drug approval for macular degeneration. Adv Drug Deliver Rev. 2005;57:2092–2098. http://dx.doi.org/10.1016/j.addr.2005.09.009

[25] Busch TM, Wang HW, Wileyto EP, et al. Increasing damage to tumor blood vessels during Motexafin Lutetium-PDT through use of low fluence rate. Radiat Res. 2010;174:331–340. http://dx.doi.org/10.1667/RR2075.1

[26] Nokes B, Apel M, Jones C, et al. Aminolevulinic acid (ALA): photodynamic detection and potential therapeutic applications. J Surg Res. 2013;181:262–271. http://dx.doi.org/10.1016/j.jss.2013.02.002

[27] Gao Y, Zhang XC, Wang WS, et al. Efficacy and safety of topical ALA-PDT in the treatment of EMPD. Photodiagn Photodyn Ther. 2015;12:92–97. http://dx.doi.org/10.1016/j.pdpdt.2014.11.004

[28] Hirohara S, Obata M, Alitomo H, et al. Synthesis, photophysical properties and sugar-dependent in vitro photocytotoxicity of pyrrolidine-fused chlorins bearing S-glycosides. J Photochem Photobiol B. 2009;97:22–33. http://dx.doi.org/10.1016/j.jphotobiol.2009.07.007

[29] Gravier J, Schneider R, Frochot C, et al. Improvement of meta-tetra(hydroxyphenyl) chlorin-like photosensitizer selectivity with folate-based targeted delivery. Synthesis and in vivo delivery studies. J Med Chem. 2008;51:3867–3877. http://dx.doi.org/10.1021/jm800125a

[30] van Dongen GAMS, Visser GWM, Vrouenraets MB. Photosensitizer-antibody conjugates for detection and therapy of cancer. Adv Drug Deliver Rev. 2004;56:31–52. http://dx.doi.org/10.1016/j.addr.2003.09.003

[31] Klajnert B, Rozanek M, Bryszewska M. Dendrimers in photodynamic therapy. Curr Med Chem. 2012;19:4903–4912. http://dx.doi.org/10.2174/092986731120902490 3

[32] Paszko E, Ehrhardt C, Senge MO, et al. Nanodrug applications in photodynamic therapy. Photodiag Photodyn Ther. 2011;8:14–29. http://dx.doi.org/10.1016/j.pdpdt.2010.12.001

[33] Allison RR, Mota HC, Sibata CH. Clinical PD/PDT in North America: an historical review. Photodiagn Photodyn Ther. 2004;1:263–277. http://dx.doi.org/10.1016/S1572-1000(04)00084-5

[34] Skupin-Mrugalska P, Piskorz J, Goslinski T, et al. Current status of liposomal porphyrinoid photosensitizers. Drug Discov Today. 2013;18:776–784. http://dx.doi.org/10.1016/j.drudis.2013.04.003

[35] Overholt BF, Panjehpour M. Photodynamic therapy techniques for ablation of Barrett's esophagus. Tech Gastrointest Endosc. 2000;2:203–208. http://dx.doi.org/10.1053/tgie.2000.8944

[36] Castner J. Emergency Nursing Decisions: a proposed system of nursing diagnosis, J Emerg Nurs. 2008;34:33–36. http://dx.doi.org/10.1016/j.jen.2006.12.020

[37] Ciechaniewicz W: Dawca i biorca pielęgnowania. In: Ślusarska B, Zarzycka D, Zahradniczek K, editors. Podstawy pielęgniarstwa. Założenia teoretyczne. Lublin: Czelej; 2004. pp. 293–326.

[38] Lee T, Mills ME. The relationship among medical diagnosis, nursing diagnosis, and nursing intervention and the implications for home health care. J Prof Nurs. 2000;16:84–91. http://dx.doi.org/10.1016/S8755-7223(00)80020-4

[39] Salvage J. Nursing in action. Strengthening nursing and midwifery to support health for all. WHO Reg Publ Eur Ser. 1993;48:1–123.

[40] Goodell TT, Muller PJ. Photodynamic therapy: a novel treatment for primary brain malignancy. J Neurosci Nurs. 2001;33:296–300.

[41] Oliver P. Topical photodynamic therapy: an introduction for nurses. Br J Nurs. 2006;15:811–813. http://dx.doi.org/10.12968/bjon.2006.15.15.21686

[42] Minnich DJ, Bryant AS, Dooley A, et al. Photodynamic laser therapy for lesions in the airway. Ann Thorac Surg. 2010;89:1744–1748. http://dx.doi.org/10.1016/j.athoracsur.2010.02.025.

[43] Schulmeister L. Integrating new information and technology in oncology nursing practice. Clin J Oncol Nurs. 2000;4:185–186.

[44] Allison RR, Sibata C, Mang TS, et al. Photodynamic therapy for chest wall recurrence from breast cancer. Photodiagn Photodyn Ther. 2004;1:151–171. http://dx.doi.org/10.1016/S1572-1000(04)00039-0

[45] Allison RR, Cuenca RE, Downie GH, et al. Clinical photodynamic therapy of head and neck cancers – a review of applications and outcomes. Photodiagn Photodyn Ther. 2005;2:205–222. http://dx.doi.org/10.1016/S1572-1000(05)00092-X

[46] Kaplun A. (Ed.). Health promotion and chronic illness. Discovering a new quality of health. WHO Reg Publ Eur Ser. 1992;44:1–461.

[47] Sahota B, Potter MJ. The nursing process in photodynamic therapy. J Ophthalmic Nurs Technol. 2000;19:252–254.

[48] Karski JB. Ed. Promocja zdrowia. Warszawa: Ignis; 1999. pp. 349–366.

[49] Stokkermans TJW. Treatment of age-related macular degeneration. Clin Eye Vis Care. 2000;12:15–35. http://dx.doi.org/10.1111/j.1444-0938.2005.tb06716.x

[50] Wojtaszek E, Matuszkiewicz-Rowińska J. The role of nurse in the multidisciplinary therapeutic team in the treatment of patients with chronic kidney disease. Nefrologia i Dializoterapia Polska 2008;12:44–46.

[51] Apollonio DE. Political advocacy in pharmacy: challenges and opportunities. Integr Pharm Res Pract. 2014;3:89–95. http://dx.doi.org/10.2147/IPRP.S47334

[52] Lewis NJW, Shimp LA, Rockafellow S, et al. The role of the pharmacist in patient-centered medical home practices: current perspectives. Integr Pharm Res Pract. 2014;3:29–38. http://dx.doi.org/10.2147/IPRP.S62670

[53] Nguyen T, Lau ETL, Steadman KJ, et al. Pharmacist, general practitioner, and nurse perceptions, experiences, and knowledge of medication dosage form modification. Integrat Pharm Res Pract. 2014;3:1–9. http://dx.doi.org/10.2147/IPRP.S53797

[54] Giberson S, Yoder S, Lee MP. Improving patient and health system outcomes through advanced pharmacy practice. A report to the U.S. Surgeon General. Office of the Chief Pharmacist. U.S. Public Health Service 2011.

[55] Makowsky MJ, Schindel TJ, Rosenthal M, et al. Collaboration between pharmacists, physicians and nurse practitioners: A qualitative investigation of working relationships in the inpatient medical setting. J Interprof Care. 2009;23:169–184. http://dx.doi.org/10.1080/13561820802602552

[56] Zawislak A, Donnelly RF, McCluggage WG, et al. Clinical and immunohistochemical assessment of vulval intraepithelial neoplasia following photodynamic therapy using a novel bioadhesive patch-type system loaded with 5-aminolevulinic acid. Photodiagn Photodyn Ther. 2009;6:28–40. http://dx.doi.org/10.1016/j.pdpdt.2009.03.004

[57] Donnelly RF, McCarron PA, Woolfson D. Drug Delivery Systems for photodynamic therapy. Recent Pat Drug Deliv Formul. 2009;3:1–7. http://dx.doi.org/10.2174/18722110 9787158319

[58] Lee G, Sziemies RM, Kosciessa U. Dermal application system for aminolevulinic acid-derivatives. European Patent No. EP 1467706 B1. 2007 Mar 14.

[59] Tsui-Min T, inventor; Pharma Power Biotec Co. Ltd., assignee. Mucoadhesive thermoresponsive medicament-carrier composition. US Patent No. US20040009212 A1. 2004 Jan 15.

[60] Sieroń A, Kawczyk-Krupka A, Adamek M, et al. Photodynamic therapy (PDT) using topically applied δ-aminolevulinic acid (ALA) for the treatment of malignant skin tumors. Photodiag Photodyn Ther. 2004;1:311–317. http://dx.doi.org/10.1016/S1572-1000(04)00069-9

[61] Schleier P, Berndt A, Kolossa S, et al. Comparison of aminolevulinic acid (ALA)-thermogel-PDT with methyl-ALA-thermogel-PDT in basal cell carcinoma. Photodiag Photodyn Ther. 2007;4:197–201. http://dx.doi.org/10.1016/j.pdpdt.2007.04.004

[62] Jiang Z, Shao J, Yang T, et al. Pharmaceutical development, composition and quantitative analysis of phthalocyanine as the photosensitizer for cancer photodynamic therapy. J Pharmaceut Biomed. 2014;87:98–104. http://dx.doi.org/10.1016/j.jpba.2013.05.014

Section 2

Photobiology and Phototherapies

Chapter 8

Effectiveness and Safety of Topical Phototherapy in the Treatment of Dermatological Diseases

Giorgio Delrosso and Paola Savoia

Additional information is available at the end of the chapter

http://dx.doi.org/10.5772/65712

Abstract

Phototherapy consists in the use of ultraviolet (UV) radiation from artificial sources for therapeutic purposes. Despite the introduction of new and powerful drugs (including biological and target therapies), phototherapy remains an established, lower cost, and effective option for the treatment of many common skin diseases.

In systemic photochemotherapy or PUVA, photosensitizing agents of the family of Psoralens are used in combination with UVA, i.e. with long wave ultraviolet radiation . Psoralens strongly enhance the effect of UVA alone, as they interact with biological macromolecules, causing the production of oxygen free radicals within the photoactivated cells. However, systemic administration of psoralens can be problematic, causing possible negative interactions with other drugs and the onset of serious side effects.

To counteract these limitations, it has been developed the bath-PUVA therapy, which consists in the topical administration of psoralens by bathing the whole body surface in an alcoholic solution of 8-methoxypsoralen (8-MOP); immediately afterwards this pretreatment, the patient is UVA-irradiated. This technique has several advantages over conventional PUVA, including the use of a reduced UVA dosage, thus resulting in minimal skin damage with complete elimination of skin photosensitivity within three hours after the treatment; furthermore, it virtually eliminates systemic side effects and drug interference due to the very limited percutaneous absorption of psoralens. Bath-PUVA is indicated and effective in the treatment of many chronic inflammatory dermatoses (including psoriasis, atopic and allergic dermatitis, lichen ruber planus, chronic urticaria, and mastocitosis), autoimmune skin diseases (including vitiligo, and alopecia aerata), and premalignant/malignant lymphoproliferative conditions (including actinic reticulosis, parapsoriasis, and early stages of mycosis fungoides). Chronic and refractory pruritus and graft-versus-host diseases can also benefit from bath-PUVA.

Another emerging PUVA technique is gel-PUVA, which is based on the application of a gel-based formulation of 8-MOP on affected skin areas , followed by UVA radiation. The formulation of 8-MOP-containing gels is conceived to increase bioavailability, limit its spread to adjacent skin and improve cosmetic aspects, while making negligible the systemic absorption of the psoralen. Ultraviolet A (UVA) irradiation is administered by cabins or partial devices according to the extension of the body areas to be treated. Gel-PUVA has produced its best responses in morfea, palmo-plantar psoriasis, contact dermatitis and vitiligo.

The purpose of this chapter is to provide a detailed description of the various phototherapy techniques and discuss their possible applications to the treatment of specific acute and chronic skin diseases.

Keywords: phototherapy, dermatological diseases, bath-PUVA, gel-PUVA, psoralen

1. Introduction

Phototherapy consists in the use of ultraviolet (UV) radiation from artificial sources for therapeutic purposes and remains an established, lower cost, and effective option for the treatment of many common skin inflammatory and immune-related diseases [1–5]. **Table 1** displays the major dermatological diseases and skin conditions in which phototherapy has been proven to be an effective therapeutic strategy. In the systemic photochemotherapy (PUVA), UVA radiation occurs after the oral administration of photosensitizing agents of the family of Psoralens.

Indications	
Inflammatory dermatoses	Atopic dermatitis
	Actinic prurigo
	Contact dermatitis
	Hydroa vacciniforme
	Lichen ruber planus
	Physical and chronic urticaria
	Pruritus
	Psoriasis
	Seasonal and polymorphic light eruption
Premalignant and malignant skin diseases	Actinic reticulosis
	Lymphomatoid papulomatosis
	Mastocytosis
	Mycosis fungoides (Stage 1A–IIB)
	Patch or plaque parapsoriasis
Others	Alopecia areata
	Erytropoietic protoporphyria
	Vitiligo

Table 1. Indication to UVA and PUVA therapy.

http://dx.doi.org/10.5772/65712

2. Psoralens

Psoralen (also called psoralene) is the progenitor of a family of natural organic compounds known as linear furanocoumarin, that is, derivatives of coumarin by the addition of a furan ring. Its methoxylated derivatives are commonly used in phototherapy and comprise the 5-methoxypsoralen (5-MOP) and the 8-methoxypsoralen (8-MOP). 5-MOP (or 4-methoxy-furo[3,2-*g*]benzopyrane-7-one, Bergaptene) is generally extracted from bergamot and many other citrus essential oils, including those from lemon, sweet orange, bitter orange, and mandarin, whereas the 8-MOP (or 9-methoxyfuro[3,2-g][1]benzopyran-7-one, ammoidin, methoxsalen, and xanthotoxin) is extracted from *Ammi majus*, a plant of the Ammi Umbelliferae family [6]. The absorption spectrum of psoralens ranges between 320 and 360 nm, *in vitro*; *in vivo*, due to the interaction with biological structures, the spectrum extends toward a longer wavelength, around 400 nm. Using artificial sources with a conventional emission spectrum (such as Philips TL/09 lamps), the peak of sensitivity for 8-MOP is between 335 and 355 nm.

Photosensitization determined by psoralen occurs by means of two mechanisms [7, 8]:

i. *Photoaddition reactions*: In the dark, psoralens intercalate between base pairs of the DNA double helix. Upon UVA excitation, intercalated psoralens get photoactivated; as a result of this reaction, they form [2 + 2]-cycloadducts, primarily with adjacent thymine bases, involving either their furan or pyrone moiety; more precisely, the [2 + 2]-type photoconjugation occurs between the 3,4-pyrone and/or 4',5'-furan double bond of the intercalated psoralen and the pyrimidine 5,6 double bond. The furan adduct is then capable of absorbing another UVA photon, resulting in interstrand cross-links [9]. DNA interstrand cross-links are among the most cytotoxic types of DNA damage; their repair is extraordinarily difficult for the cell since it requires the coordination of proteins from several pathways, including nucleotide excision repair, base excision repair, mismatch repair, homologous recombination, translation synthesis, and proteins involved in Fanconi anemia [10]. Monoadducts and cross-links inhibit DNA-readout processes, thus leading to necrosis or apoptosis of the photodamaged cells [11]. Psoralens are highly soluble in body fluids, and therefore they can form photoadducts with a variety of other molecules besides DNA, including RNAs, proteins, and polyunsaturated fatty acids; actually, most of the administered 8-MOP have been found to be conjugated to proteins rather than to nucleic acids or lipids [12]. Psoralen photoadducts to those molecules result in disruption and silencing of a variety of metabolic and signaling pathways, thus exerting a broad range of phototoxicity.

ii. *Photodynamic reactions*: Photoactivation of psoralens in the presence of oxygen results in the formation of reactive oxygen species (ROS), including singlet oxygen and superoxide radical anions. Thus, psoralens activate both type 1 photodynamic mechanisms (i.e., the production of superoxide, hydrogen peroxide, and hydroxyl radical (HO•) by electron transfer) and type 2 mechanisms (i.e., the production of singlet oxygen (1O2) by energy transfer) [13]. Reactive oxygen species are extremely unstable and react with other molecules, causing a variety of cell damages, including lipid peroxidation, DNA breaks, and DNA-protein cross-links (PMID: 24721421). To counteract oxidative damage/stress, cells rely on a number of antioxidative defense systems, including natural radical scavengers (e.g., tocopherol and vitamin A) and different enzymes (e.g., superoxide dismutase, glutathione peroxidase, and catalase).

Adducted DNA by psoralens is also implicated in melanogenesis: modified nucleotides, in particular oligonucleotides composed by two thymidine residues, stimulate cells to express tyrosinase, a known key enzyme in melanin production, with variable effects in patients with vitiligo vulgaris [14–17]. The demonstrated ability of furocoumarines to bind proteins, including those of the lens, can induce cataract in long-term therapy. Finally, it has to be noticed that PUVA has also the ability to induce apoptosis of Langerhans cells, activated T-lymphocytes, neutrophils, macrophages, NK cells, fibroblasts, endothelial cells, and mast cells, thus exerting a beneficial effect for the most common dermatoses [18].

2.1. Dosage

Pharmacokinetic studies have shown that psoralens absorption is subject to individual variations, in terms of both mean plasma concentration and timing for reaching the maximum peak. In addition, in the same individual, plasma concentration varies during the day, although the maximum peak represents a constant [19–21].

Recommended doses are the following:

i. 8-MOP: 0.6 mg/kg (or 25 mg/m^2, for subjects weighing less than 60 kg) 2 h before exposure if in a micronized form or 1 h before if in liquid or gelatinous form. The dosage should then be adjusted according to the response.

ii. 5-MOP: 1.2 mg/kg, 3.5 h before the treatment.

8-MOP administration results in a photosensitization which reaches its maximum, 2–4 h after the intake and disappears in 6–8 h. Psoralens are transported in the blood by serum proteins (mainly albumin), and are predominantly catabolized in the liver by cytochrome P450 (CYP450)-triggered oxidation. CYP450s make a large superfamily of heme-containing monooxygenases, which take care of the detoxification of many drugs [22]. Recent studies have shown that CYP3A11 is the major target cytochrome for psoralens metabolism in mice [23]. Another key cytochrome for detoxification or activation of many toxicologically important substrates is CYP2B1 [24]. Psoralens are oxidized by CYP3A11 at the furan ring to form a furan epoxide that binds to CYP 2B1 with a high stoichiometry [25]; after biding, CYP 2B1 produces dihydrodiols, which are the final catabolic products of linear fucocoumarins [25]. In addition, 8-MOP up-regulates CYP1A1 expression, and can be a substrate for this CYP450 [26]. CYP450s are encoded by highly polymorphic genes [27] and their expression varies among individuals, in relation with alcohol intake and drug use; both these facts provide an easy explanation for individual variations in response to psoralen-related therapies. About 75% of furanocoumarins catabolic products produced by the liver are excreted in the urine as inactive hydroxylated- or glucurono-conjugates derivatives within

12 h; key proteins for this excretory function are the solute carrier (SLC) 22A family organic cation/carnitine transporters (OCTs/OCTNs) and the organic anion transporters (OATs). More specifically, the administration of furocoumarins up-regulates renal OCT1, OCT2, OCTN2, and OAT3 protein levels, as a result of increased gene expression in mice; in addition, oxidized linear furocoumarins induce high expression of mURAT1, mMRP4, and mGLUT9, which may also play important roles in renal transportation, and accumulation of psoralen metabolites as well as in related kidney injury. Notably, 8-MOP clearance in the lens is rather slow, it being detectable in this organ for 18 h after oral intake [28].

2.2. Cautions

In view of the prolonged photosensitivity induced by 8-MOP [29], it is mandatory to avoid exposition to the sunlight after the treatment; to this purpose, eyes and lips should be protected with glasses and sunscreen.

During treatment with psoralens, regular evaluation of liver function is needed and drug should be reduced or discontinued if there is any sign of liver damage. The most frequent pharmacological interactions are with other topical or systemic photoactive drugs (e.g., phenothiazine, chlorothiazide and derivatives, sulfonylureas, sulfonamides, neomycin, and bergamot essence). Diet with low (or free) coumarins should also be recommended, which are mainly contained in fig, cedar, lime, parsley, mustard, carrots and celery, and parsnips.

The most frequently observed side effects related to 8-MOP administration include severe burns, gastric distress, nausea, nervousness, insomnia, and depression.

Major contraindications to PUVA therapy are summarized in **Table 2**.

Contraindications		
Absolute	**Major**	**Relative**
Autoimmune diseases	Age >10 years	Age >16 years
Basal cell carcinoma syndrome	Actinic keratosis	Bullous skin diseases
Dysplastic nevus syndrome	Personal history of nonmelanoma skin cancer	Cataract
Personal history of melanoma	Previous exposure to UVA >1500 J/cm^2	Photosensitization
Porphyry	Previous exposure to X-ray or arsenic	Photo type I
Pregnancy and lactation	Systemic immunosuppressive therapy	Poor compliance
Severe heart failure		Renal and/or hepatic failure
Systemic lupus erythematosus; Dermatomyositis		
Xeroderma pigmentosum and other congenital defects of DNA repair mechanisms		

*Photo type I is characterized by pale white skin, blue or hazel eyes, and blond or red hair; patients with photo-type I always have burns, does not tan.

Table 2. Contraindications to PUVA therapy.

3. UV irradiation

The most frequently used lamps for phototherapy are fluorescent, low-pressure mercury vapor tubes (e.g., Philips TL/09, Philips CLEO-UVA or Sylvania F 85 tubes) with an emission spectrum ranging from 320 to 450 nm, and an emission peak at 352 nm. PUVA units are either whole-body cabins or small-panel irradiators for the treatments of hands and feet or other restricted areas of the body. To provide consistency and repeatability of treatment doses, it is fundamental to measure the emission by calibrated radiometers-photometers, sensitive to the spectrum emitted by the lamps. Treatment times are automatically calculated on the basis of variables such as (i) total or daily usage time of the lamps, (ii) environmental and patient's conditions (temperature, humidity, dust, and distribution of adipose tissue), and (iii) presence of other UV sources. When devices devoid of dosimeters are used, the dosage should be calculated according to the formula: Dose (mJ/cm^2) = irradiance (mW/cm^2) × time (seconds); special tables are then used to calculate the appropriate dosage, according to patient's phototype. In any case, it is recommended a semiannual or annual assessment of the UVA cabin or panel with external radiometer-photometer calibrated to the National Physics Laboratory, which will provide an adjustment for timing and doses [5, 6].

3.1. Dose assessment

Dose assessment, according to the different published protocols, is based on (i) evaluation of the Fitzpatrick phototype, (ii) calculation of the minimal phototoxic dose (MPD), that is, the lowest UVA dose that produces a perceptible erythema after psoralen administration, and (iii) assessment of an attack dosage equal to 50% of MPD.

The sessions are initially carried out three to four times a week and then reduced to two times a week after a clinical improvement has been obtained. The possibility of performing one session every 7–10 days as maintenance therapy can be considered. Side effects are resumed as shown in **Table 3**.

Side effects	
Early	**Late**
Gastric intolerance	Anti-DNA and antinucleus antibodies (low title)
Hypertrichosis or alopecia	Carcinogenesis (actinic keratosis, NMSCs, melanomas)
Neomelanogenesis and stratum corneum thickening	Cataract
Pain	Disorder of pigmentation
Photo-inducted dermatitis	Idiopathic guttate hypomelanosis
Phototoxic exanthema	Melanocytes dystrophies
Skin dryness and pruritus	
Teratogenicity	

Table 3. Side effects related to PUVA therapy.

4. Topical photochemotherapy: bath-PUVA

Bath-PUVA therapy consists in the immersion of the whole body in a bath containing an 8-MOP alcoholic solution, at concentrations ranging from 1 to 3 mg/L, for a time varying from 15' to 20'. Then, the patient is exposed to increasing doses of UVA, which varies in relation to the phototype, with a minimal initial doses of 0.25–0.50 J/cm^2 and progressive increments of 0.25 J/cm^2 up to a maximum of 5–7 J/cm^2 .

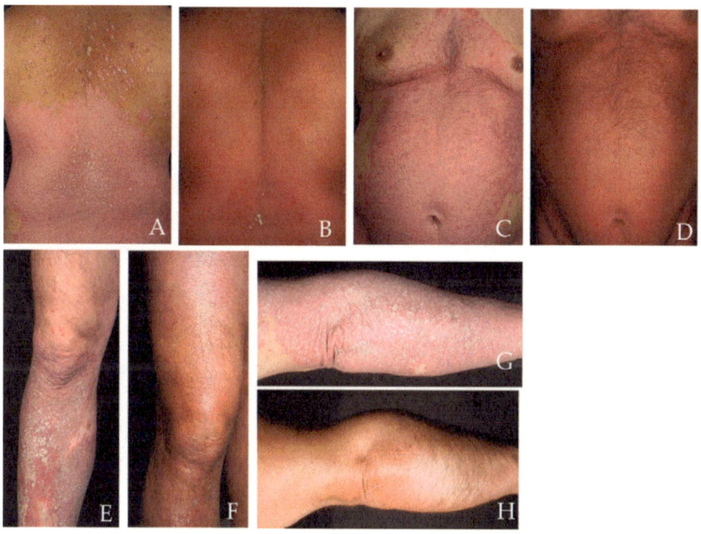

Figure 1. Plaque psoriasis before (A, C, E, G) and after (B, D, F, H) bath-PUVA therapy.

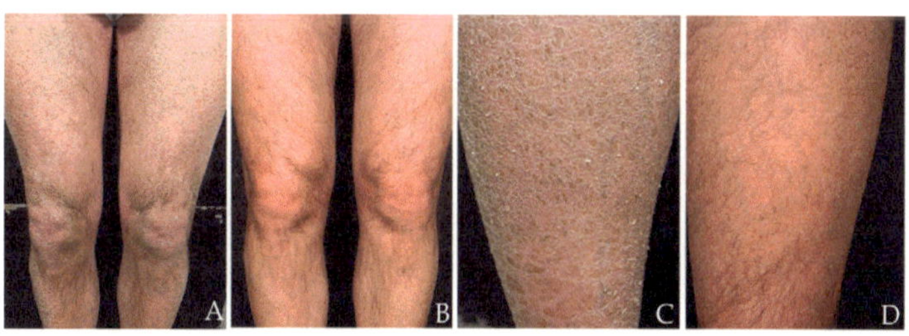

Figure 2. Ichthyosis-like atopic dermatitis before (A and C) and after (B and D) bath-PUVA therapy.

This modality of treatment minimizes short- and long-term side effects due to the systemic administration of the drug [19, 30–33]. Three hours after treatment, photosensitivity is negligible, due to the low systemic absorption of 8-MOP; thus, patients can avoid the use of photoprotections, including sunglasses [34, 35]. Gas chromatography and mass spectrometry analyses have shown that plasmatic trixolaren concentrations range between 0.27 and 12.5 ng/ml after the ingestion of a 0.6 mg/kg dose and between 9 ng/ml and 25 pg/ml after bath-PUVA [20, 36].

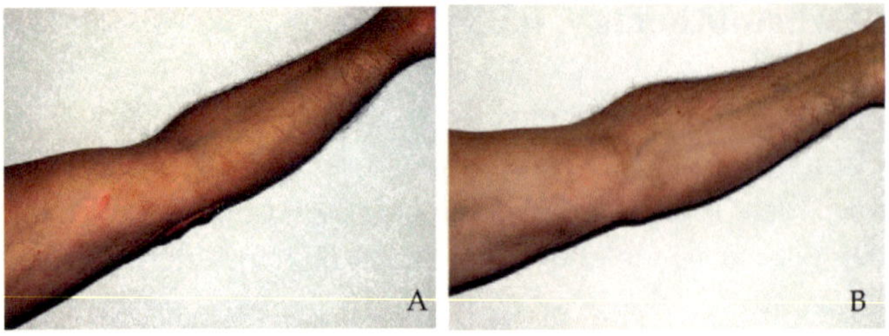

Figure 3. Stage I mycosis fungoides before (A) and after (B) bath-PUVA therapy.

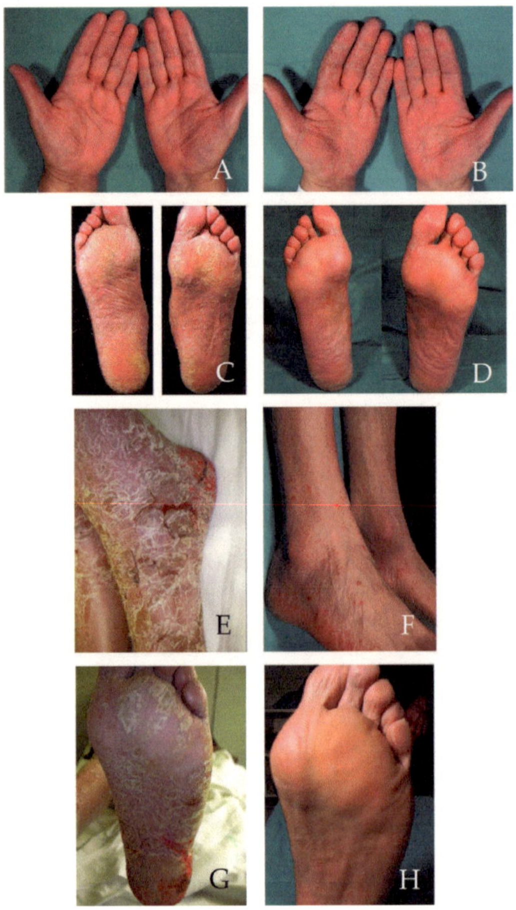

Figure 4. Palmoplantar psoriasis before (A and C) and after (B and D) gel-PUVA therapy; eczematized psoriasis before (E and G) and after (F and H) gel-PUVA therapy.

In the skin, the drug absorption peak occurs within 15–35 min; the maximum concentration is reached in the stratum corneum and the removal of this cell layer (by "stripping") significantly enhances the possibility of drug penetration to the underlying layers. The higher psoralen concentration in superficial layers of the epidermis justifies the increased effectiveness of this type of treatment in those diseases in which the epidermal involvement is massive [30, 36, 37]. The concentration measured by microanalytical techniques is instead of 1.7–6.6 ng/ml after oral intake and of 200–520 ng/ml after the bath.

Literature reports encourage results obtained with bath-PUVA in the treatment of several inflammatory [38–47] and lymphoproliferative skin diseases [48–52]. **Figures 1–4** report same examples of results obtained with bath-PUVA at our center.

4.1. Treatment

Before treatment, an accurate collection of clinical data is mandatory; patient should be informed about the treatment modality, its potential benefits and risks, and the need to avoid other potentially photosensitizing agents. Skin should be carefully examined and nevi should be covered with high-protection sunscreen, as well as the lips and genital areas; patient should also wear sunglasses during treatment and up to 3 h afterwards. At the end of treatment, we recommended also a shower, to remove residual traces of the drug from the skin, and the application of topical emollients [53, 54]. The treatment requires special attention and the protocol described above must necessarily be adapted to each patient, on the basis of the phototype and other clinical characteristics.

5. Topical photochemotherapy: gel-PUVA therapy

The gel-PUVA therapy is a variant of the cream-PUVA therapy and consists in the application of a 0.05% of 8-MOP gel on restricted skin areas, 20–30 min before the irradiation. The preparation of the 8-MOP gel is galenical; the psoralen is dissolved, in order to obtain a higher bioavailability and better cosmetic aspects and to avoid the "border effect." The UVA radiation could be realized through cabin or panels according to the extent of the body areas affected by the disease, with an irradiation spectrum of 320–370 nm. Dose calculation is performed manually, because panels are not equipped with dosimeter; hence, every 6 months, their calibration is mandatory. Usually, an initial dose of 0.25–0.50 J/cm^2 is used, with a progressive increase in 0.25–0.50J/cm^2 for each session, up to a maximal dose of 9 J/cm^2. Treatment sessions are performed three times/week for the first month of treatment and then reduced to two times/week in the second month and to one time/week in the third month. A weekly maintenance session could also be proposed.

Best responses to gel-PUVA treatment are described for morphea, palmoplantar psoriasis, contact dermatitis, and vitiligo [43, 55–57]. Inclusion and exclusion criteria are those described for systemic PUVA.

The amount of 8-MOP that is absorbed with this method is negligible [21, 58] and the only side effects that have been described are transitory erythema and pruritus, which can be easily managed with topical moisturizing creams. In a few cases, peripheral hyperpigmentation of the treated areas has also been reported [59].

In literature, also a topical psoralen-narrow-band UVB therapy has been described, based on the association of topical 8-MOP and narrow-band UVB irradiation [60–62].

6. Conclusions

Phototherapy and especially topic phototherapy are efficient treatment methods for a variety of dermatological diseases, able to induce complete and durable responses in several inflammatory, immune-mediated, and neoplastic skin diseases. Relapses are rare, due to the absence of tachyphylaxis. Although the cost of phototherapy is low, the relative discomfort and the time required to reach the site of the treatment should be considered.

For the risk of carcinogenesis, a number of factors should be taken into account, including dose, age at the treatment, other potentially carcinogenic drugs, photodamaged skin areas, and the type of treatment (a lower carcinogenetic potential has been reported for bath-PUVA in respect to systemic PUVA). The analysis of 11 clinical trials, 10 of which were conducted on psoriatic patients (for a total of about 3400 patients), did not show an increased risk of melanoma [63–66] or of nonmelanoma skin cancer after UVA phototherapy [60, 66, 67]. However, another study [63, 66] conducted on patients previously treated with PUVA therapy and subsequently exposed to a high amount of UVB (for more than 300 treatments) demonstrated a small but significant increased risk of both squamous (relative risk (RR): 1.37) and basal cell carcinomas (RR: 1.45). The risk was further increased for patients who received less than 100 PUVA but more than 300 UVB treatments (RR: 2.75 for SCC and 3.00 per BCC). An increased risk to develop malignant melanoma has also been reported, based on the phototype and on the number of treatments; melanoma could arise more than 20 years after the start of therapy, showing a greater aggressiveness than in the general population. An increased risk to develop other cancers (colon, lung, pancreas, and kidney) has not been documented. The putative carcinogenetic risk of narrow-band UVB is higher than for UVA, but its increased effectiveness requires lower cumulative doses, resulting in a reduced actual risk [60].

In summary, an accurate follow-up of patients is essential, in order to detect precancerous skin lesions, and identify suspicious melanocytic lesions, which must be excised. Accurate calculation of cumulative doses, number of treatments and their cumulative dosage, represents an absolute requirement for a correct planning of phototherapy. In addition, alternating PUVA therapy with other topical or systemic treatments can significantly reduce the carcinogenic potential of phototherapy.

Author details

Giorgio Delrosso[1,2] and Paola Savoia[1,2*]
*Address all correspondence to: paola.savoia@med.uniupo.it

1 Azienda Ospedaliero-Universitaria "Maggiore della Carità" di Novara, Novara, Italy

2 "A. Avogadro" University of Eastern Piedmont, Novara, Italy

References

[1] Bie V: Remarks on Finsen's phototherapy. Br Med J. 1899; 2:825–830. PMID: 20758681

[2] Benedetto AV, Roenigk HH Jr: Photochemotherapy (PUVA) in psoriasis. J Am Osteopath Assoc. 1976; 75:885–892. PMID: 777077

[3] Roenigk HH Jr: Photochemotherapy for mycosis fungoides: Long term follow up study. Cancer Treat Rep. 1979; 63:669–673. PMID: 445519

[4] Molin L, Skogh M, Volden G: Successful PUVA-treatment in the tumour stage of mycosis fungoides associated with the appearance of lesions in organs other than the skin. Acta Derm Venereol. 1978; 58:189–190. PMID: 76405

[5] Rajatanavin N, Scharf MJ, Bernhard JD: Phototherapy and photochemotherapy in dermatologic diseases. Compr Ther. 1988; 14:11–18. PMID: 3053012

[6] Bethea D, Fullmer B, Syed S, Seltzer G, Tiano J, Rischko C, Gillespie L, Brown D, Gasparro FP: Psoralen photobiology and photochemotherapy: 50 years of science and medicine. J Dermatol Sci. 1999; 19:78–88. PMID: 10098699

[7] Cimino GD, Shi YB, Hearst JE: Wavelength dependence for the photoreversal of a psoralen-DNA cross-link. Biochemistry. 1986; 25:3013–3020. PMID: 3718936

[8] Shi YB, Hearst JE: Wavelength dependence for the photoreactions of DNA-psoralen monoadducts. 2. Photo-cross-linking of monoadducts. Biochemistry. 1987; 26:3792–3798. PMID: 3651414

[9] Noll DM1, Mason TM, Miller PS: Formation and repair of interstrand cross-links in DNA. Chem Rev. 2006; 106:277–301. PMID: 16464006

[10] Vasquez KM: Targeting and processing of site-specific DNA interstrand crosslinks. Environ Mol Mutagen. 2010; 51:527–539. doi: 10.1002/em.20557. PMID: 20196133

[11] Bethea D, Fullmer B, Syed S, Seltzer G, Tiano J, Rischko C, Gillespie L, Brown D, Gasparro FP: Psoralen photobiology and photochemotherapy: 50 years of science and medicine. J Dermatol Sci. 1999; 19:78–88. PMID: 10098699

[12] Beijersbergen van Henegouwen GM1, Wijn ET, Schoonderwoerd SA, Dall'Acqua F: A method for the determination of PUVA-induced in vivo irreversible binding of 8-methoxypsoralen (8-MOP) to epidermal lipids, proteins and DNA/RNA. J Photochem Photobiol B. 1989; 3:631–635. PMID: 2477521

[13] Garcia-Diaz M, Huang YY, Hamblin MR: Use of fluorescent probes for ROS to tease apart type I and type II photochemical pathways in photodynamic therapy methods. 2016 Jun 30. pii: S1046-2023(16)30200-6. doi: 10.1016/j.ymeth.2016.06.025. [Epub ahead of print]. PMID: 27374076

[14] Szekeres E, Török L, Szücs M: Appearance of disseminated hyperpigmented lesions during PUVA therapy. Hautarzt. 1981; 32:33–35. PMID: 7228659

[15] Schneider B, Vogel A, Zisiadis S, Panizzon R, Groh V: Hyperpigmented small spots induced by long-term PUVA therapy. A clinical, light and electron microscopic study. Dermatologica. 1982; 165:330–341. PMID: 7152069

[16] Jung EG, Obert W: The incidence of PUVA lentigines. Photodermatol. 1986; 3:46–47. PMID: 3703703

[17] Cruz A, Sánchez JL: Acral PUVA-induced pigmented macules. Bol Asoc Med P R. 1990; 82:460–462. PMID: 2080960

[18] Situm M, Bulat V, Majcen K, Dzapo A, Jezovita J: Benefits of controlled ultraviolet radiation in the treatment of dermatological diseases. Coll Anthropol. 2014; 38:1249–1253. PMID: 25842770

[19] Lowe NJ, Weingarten D, Bourget T, Moy LS: PUVA therapy for psoriasis: Comparison of oral and bath-water delivery of 8-methoxypsoralen. J Am Acad Dermatol. 1986; 14:754–760. PMID: 3711379

[20] Thomas SE, O'Sullivan J, Balac N: Plasma levels of 8-methoxypsoralen following oral or bath-water treatment. Br J Dermatol. 1991; 125:56–58. PMID: 1873204

[21] Tegeder I, Bräutigam L, Podda M, Meier S, Kaufmann R, Geisslinger G, Grundmann-Kollmann M: Time course of 8-methoxypsoralen concentrations in skin and plasma after topical (bath and cream) and oral administration of 8-methoxypsoralen. Clin Pharmacol Ther. 2002; 71:153–161. PMID: 11907489. doi: 10.1067/mcp.2002.121908

[22] Guengerich FP: Cytochrome P450s and other enzymes in drug metabolism and toxicity. AAPS J. 2006; 8:E101–E111. doi: 10.1208/aapsj080112

[23] Wang X1, Lou YJ, Wang MX, Shi YW, Xu HX, Kong LD: Furocoumarins affect hepatic cytochrome P450 and renal organic ion transporters in mice. Toxicol Lett. 2012; 20:67–77. doi: 10.1016/j.toxlet.2011.11.030. Epub 2011 Dec 7.

[24] Cederbaum AI1, Wu D, Mari M, Bai J: CYP2E1-dependent toxicity and oxidative stress in HepG2 cells. Free Radic Biol Med. 2001; 31:1539–1543. PMID: 11744327

[25] Koenigs LL, Trager WF: Mechanism-based inactivation of cytochrome P450 2B1 by 8-methoxypsoralen and several other furanocoumarins. Biochemistry. 1998; 37:13184–38193. doi: 10.1021/bi981198r

[26] Baumgart A1, Schmidt M, Schmitz HJ, Schrenk D: Natural furocoumarins as inducers and inhibitors of cytochrome P450 1A1 in rat hepatocytes. Biochem Pharmacol. 2005; 69:657–667. Epub 2005 Jan 12. PMID: 15670584.

[27] Tverdohleb T, Dinc B, Knezevic I, Candido KD, Knezevic NN: The role of cytochrome P450 pharmacogenomics in chronic non-cancer pain patients. Expert Opin Drug Metab Toxicol. 2016 Jul 7 [Epub ahead of print]. PMID: 27388970

[28] Wamer W, Giles A Jr, Kornhauser A: Kinetics of 8-methoxypsoralen and 5-methoxypsoralen distribution in guinea pig serum, epidermis and ocular lens. Photodermatol. 1987; 4:236–239. PMID: 3697346

[29] Bech-Thomsen N, Wulf HC: A polychromatic action spectrum for photosensitivity to orally administered 8-methoxypsoralen in humans. Clin Exp Dermatol. 1994; 19:12–15. PMID: 8313631

[30] Anigbogu AN, Williams AC, Barry BW: Permeation characteristics of 8-methoxypsoralen through human skin; relevance to clinical treatment. J Pharm Pharmacol. 1996; 48:357–366. PMID: 8794983

[31] Reuther T, Gruss C, Behrens S, von Kobyletzki G, Neumann N, Lehmann P, Altmeyer P, Kerscher M: Time course of 8-methoxypsoralen-induced skin photosensitization in PUVA-bath photochemotherapy. Photodermatol Photoimmunol Photomed. 1997; 13:193–196. PMID: 9542757

[32] von Kobyletzki G, Hoffmann K, Kerscher M, Altmeyer P: Plasma levels of 8-methoxypsoralen following PUVA-bath photochemotherapy. Photodermatol Photoimmunol Photomed. 1998; 14:136–138. PMID: 9779504

[33] Delrosso G. Photodermatology and phototherapy. Interlinea Ed, Novara, Italy, 2016. ISBN 97888-6857-078-1

[34] Dolezal E, Seeber A, Hönigsmann H, Tanew A: Correlation between bathing time and photosensitivity in 8-methoxypsoralen (8-MOP) bath PUVA. Photodermatol Photoimmunol Photomed. 2000; 16:183–185. PMID: 11019944

[35] Tanew A, Kipfelsperger T, Seeber A, Radakovic-Fijan S, Hönigsmann H: Correlation between 8-methoxypsoralen bath-water concentration and photosensitivity in bath-PUVA treatment. J Am Acad Dermatol. 2001; 44:638–642. PMID: 11260539. doi: 10.1067/mjd.2001.112360

[36] David M, Lowe NJ, Halder RM, Borok M: Serum 8-methoxypsoralen (8-MOP) concentrations after bath water delivery of 8-MOP plus UVA. J Am Acad Dermatol. 1990; 23:931–932. PMID: 2254480

[37] Löffler H, Aramaki J, Friebe K, Happle R, Effendy I: Changes in skin physiology during bath PUVA therapy. Br J Dermatol. 2002; 147:105–109. PMID: 12100191

[38] Grundmann-Kollmann M, Ochsendorf FR, Zollner TM, Tegeder I, Kaufmann R, Podda M: Cream psoralen plus ultraviolet A therapy for granuloma annulare. Br J Dermatol. 2001; 144:996–999. PMID: 11359387

[39] Hannuksela M, Karvonen J: Trioxsalen bath plus UVA effective and safe in the treatment of psoriasis. Br J Dermatol. 1978; 99:703–707. PMID: 737133

[40] Väätäinen N, Hollmen A, Fräki JE: Trimethylpsoralen bath plus ultraviolet A combined with oral retinoid (etretinate) in the treatment of severe psoriasis. J Am Acad Dermatol. 1985; 12:52–55. PMID: 3980803

[41] Kerscher M, Volkenandt M, Meurer M, Lehmann P, Plewig G, Röcken M: Treatment of localised scleroderma with PUVA bath photochemotherapy. Lancet. 1994; 343:1233. PMID: 7909904

[42] Hawk JL, Grice PL: The efficacy of localized PUVA therapy for chronic hand and foot dermatoses. Clin Exp Dermatol. 1994; 19:479–482. PMID: 7889668

[43] Schiener R, Gottlöber P, Müller B, Williams S, Pillekamp H, Peter RU, Kerscher M: PUVA-gel vs. PUVA-bath therapy for severe recalcitrant palmoplantar dermatoses. A randomized, single-blinded prospective study. Photodermatol Photoimmunol Photomed. 2005; 21:62–67. PMID: 15752122. doi: 10.1111/j.1600-0781.2005.00134.x

[44] Batchelor R, Clark S: Clearance of generalized papular umbilicated granuloma annulare in a child with bath PUVA therapy. Pediatr Dermatol. 2006; 23:72–74. PMID: 16445418

[45] Vongthongsri R, Konschitzky R, Seeber A, Treitl C, Hönigsmann H, Tanew A: Randomized, double-blind comparison of 1 mg/L versus 5 mg/L methoxsalen bath-PUVA therapy for chronic plaque-type psoriasis. J Am Acad Dermatol. 2006; 55:627–631. PMID: 17010742. doi: 10.1016/j.jaad.2006.05.024

[46] Delrosso G, Bornacina C, Farinelli P, Bellinzona F, Leigheb G, Colombo E: Bath PUVA and psoriasis: Is a milder treatment a worse treatment? Dermatology 2008; 216:191–193. PMID: 18182808. doi: 10.1159/000112924

[47] Ghoreschi K, Thomas P, Penovici M, Ullmann J, Sander CA, Ledderose G, Plewig G, Kolb HJ, Röcken M: PUVA-bath photochemotherapy and isotretinoin in sclerodermatous graft-versus-host disease. Eur J Dermatol. 2008; 18:667–670. PMID: 18955201. doi: 10.1684/ejd.2008.0517

[48] Weber F, Schmuth M, Sepp N, Fritsch P: Bath-water PUVA therapy with 8-methoxypsoralen in mycosis fungoides. Acta Derm Venereol. 2005; 85:329–332. PMID: 16191854. doi: 10.1080/00015550510032814

[49] Hoetzenecker W, Guenova E, Hoetzenecker K, Yazdi A, Röcken M, Berneburg M: Successful treatment of recalcitrant lymphomatoid papulosis in a child with PUVA-bath photochemotherapy. Eur J Dermatol. 2009; 19:646–647. PMID: 19797036. doi: 10.1684/ejd.2009.0790

[50] Friedland R, David M, Feinmesser M, Fenig-Nakar S, Hodak E: Idiopathic guttate hypomelanosis-like lesions in patients with mycosis fungoides: A new adverse effect of phototherapy. J Eur Acad Dermatol Venereol. 2010; 24:1026–1030. Epub 2010 Feb 17. PMID: 20180893. doi: 10.1111/j.1468-3083.2010.03571.x

[51] Errichetti E, Piccirillo A, Ricciuti F, Ricciuti F: Steroid-resistant localized lymphomatoid papulosis treated with local bath-PUVA therapy. Indian J Dermatol. 2013; 58:163. PMID: 23716855 PMCID: PMC3657265. doi: 10.4103/0019-5154.108109

[52] Kato H, Saito C, Ito E, Furuhashi T, Nishida E, Ishida T, Ueda R, Inagaki H, Morita A: Bath-PUVA therapy decreases infiltrating CCR4-expressing tumor cells and regulatory T cells in patients with mycosis Fungoides. Clin Lymphoma Myeloma Leuk. 2013; 13:273–280. PMID: 23332394. doi: 10.1016/j.clml.2012.12.002

[53] Halpern SM, Anstey AV, Dawe RS, Diffey BL, Farr PM, Ferguson J, Hawk JL, Ibbotson S, McGregor JM, Murphy GM, Thomas SE, Rhodes LE: Guidelines for topical PUVA: A report of a workshop of the British photodermatology group. Br J Dermatol. 2000; 142:22–31. PMID: 10651690

[54] Rodríguez-Granados MT, Carrascosa JM, Gárate T, Gómez-Díez S, Guimaraens-Juantorena D: Consensus document on bath-PUVA therapy. The Spanish Photobiology Group of the Spanish Academy of Dermatology and Venereology. Actas Dermosifiliogr. 2007; 98:164–170. PMID: 17504700

[55] Grundmann-Kollmann M, Ochsendorf F, Zollner TM, Spieth K, Sachsenberg-Studer E, Kaufmann R, Podda M: PUVA-cream photochemotherapy for the treatment of localized scleroderma. J Am Acad Dermatol. 2000; 43:675–678. PMID: 11004625. doi: 10.1067/mjd.2000.105503

[56] Engin B, Oguz O: Evaluation of time-dependent response to psoralen plus UVA (PUVA) treatment with topical 8-methoxypsoralen (8-MOP) gel in palmoplantar dermatoses. Int J Dermatol. 2005; 44:337–339. PMID: 15811091. doi: 10.1111/j.1365-4632.2004.02153.x

[57] Grundmann-Kollmann M, Ochsendorf FR, Zollner TM, Tegeder I, Kaufmann R, Podda M: Cream psoralen plus ultraviolet A therapy for granuloma annulare. Br J Dermatol. 2001; 144: 996–999. PMID: 11359387

[58] Pham CT, Koo JY: Plasma levels of 8-methoxypsoralen after topical paint PUVA. J Am Acad Dermatol. 1993; 28:460–466. PMID: 8445063

[59] Nimkulrat P, Leenutaphong V, Sudtim S: Phototoxicity of new psoralen-containing gels and creams versus bath PUVA. J Med Assoc Thai. 2005; 88:1406–1411. PMID: 16519387

[60] Archier E, Devaux S, Castela E, Gallini A, Aubin F, Le Maître M, Aractingi S, Bachelez H, Cribier B, Joly P, Jullien D, Misery L, Paul C, Ortonne JP, Richard MA: Carcinogenic risks of psoralen UV-A therapy and narrowband UV-B therapy in chronic plaque psoriasis: A systematic literature review. J Eur Acad Dermatol Venereol. 2012; 26:22–31. PMID: 22512677. doi: 10.1111/j.1468-3083.2012.04520.x

[61] Rácz E, Prens EP, Kurek D, Kant M, de Ridder D, Mourits S, Baerveldt EM, Ozgur Z, van IJcken WF, Laman JD, Staal FJ, van der Fits L: Effective treatment of psoriasis with narrow-band UVB phototherapy is linked to suppression of the IFN and Th17 pathways. J Invest Dermatol. 2011; 131:1547–1558. PMID: 21412260. doi: 10.1038/jid.2011.53

[62] Der-Petrossian M, Seeber A, Hönigsmann H, Tanew A: Half-side comparison study on the efficacy of 8-methoxypsoralen bath-PUVA versus narrow-band ultraviolet B phototherapy in patients with severe chronic atopic dermatitis. Br J Dermatol. 2000; 142:39–43. PMID: 10651692

[63] Lee E, Koo J, Berger T: UVB phototherapy and skin cancer risk: A review of the literature. Int J Dermatol. 2005; 44:355–360. PMID: 15869531. doi: 10.1111/j.1365-4632.2004.02186.x

[64] Kilinc Karaarslan I, Teban L, Dawid M, Tanew A, Kittler H: Changes in the dermoscopic appearance of melanocytic naevi after photochemotherapy or narrow-band ultraviolet B phototherapy. J Eur Acad Dermatol Venereol. 2007; 21:526–531. PMID: 17373982. doi: 10.1111/j.1468-3083.2006.02020.x

[65] Stern RS; PUVA Follow up Study: The risk of melanoma in association with long-term exposure to PUVA. J Am Acad Dermatol. 2001; 44:755–761. PMID: 11312420. doi: 10.1067/mjd.2001.114576

[66] Stern RS; PUVA follow-up study: The risk of squamous cell and basal cell cancer associated with psoralen and ultraviolet A therapy: A 30-year prospective study. J Am Acad Dermatol. 2012; 66:553–562. PMID: 22264671. doi: 10.1016/j.jaad.2011.04.004

[67] Kim YS, Park YL, Lee JS, Whang KU: Multiple actinic keratosis, squamous cell carcinoma and basal cell carcinoma occurred after PUVA therapy in a Korean patient. Photodermatol Photoimmunol Photomed. 2014; 305:277–279. PMID: 24456558. doi: 10.1111/phpp.12114

Chapter 9

The Use of Photomedicine in Musculoskeletal Pain

Abdullah M. Al-Shenqiti

Additional information is available at the end of the chapter

http://dx.doi.org/10.5772/65748

Abstract

Musculoskeletal pain is a major cause of disability. Myofascial trigger points (MTrPs) in particular are a common source of pain in a substantial number of patients presenting at a pain clinic. Many different invasive and non-invasive forms have been advocated to the treatment of MTrPs. However, favourable outcome rates are inconsistent and some of these treatment forms described are often painful and have potentially dangerous side effects. Photomedicine including the coherent light sources (lasers) and more recently, non-coherent light sources have been reported to be beneficial in soft tissue lesions including MTrPs. Their beneficial therapeutic effects can be obtained without undesired effects. The main intentions of this chapter are to bring the attention of the doctors and physical therapists to the scientific approach of photomedicine, in particular laser therapy for the relief of pain arising from MTrPs, and to demonstrate how this type of therapy can be utilized in a rational manner for the relief of musculoskeletal pain. In addition, it has been found necessary to include or to start with an overview of the recently recognized diagnostic and therapeutic importance of MTrPs. Attention will therefore first be drawn mainly to incidence, types, aetiology, clinical diagnostic criteria and conventional forms of MTrPs.

Keywords: photomedicine, myofascial pain, trigger points, laser therapy, phototherapy

1. Introduction

Skeletal muscle contractile tissues are subject to constant wear and tear, which makes them prone to development of myofascial trigger points (MTrPs) that result in referred pain and motor dysfunction [1]. MTrPs are extremely common and a major source of musculoskeletal pain and dysfunction that can affect anyone at one time or another [1–3].

MTrPs are one of the profound reasons of pain in clinical practice [4, 5]. They are the source of pain in 30% of patients seeking treatment or medical advices for pain in primary care and the greatly noticeable cause of pain in 85% of patients presenting at a pain centre [6, 7].

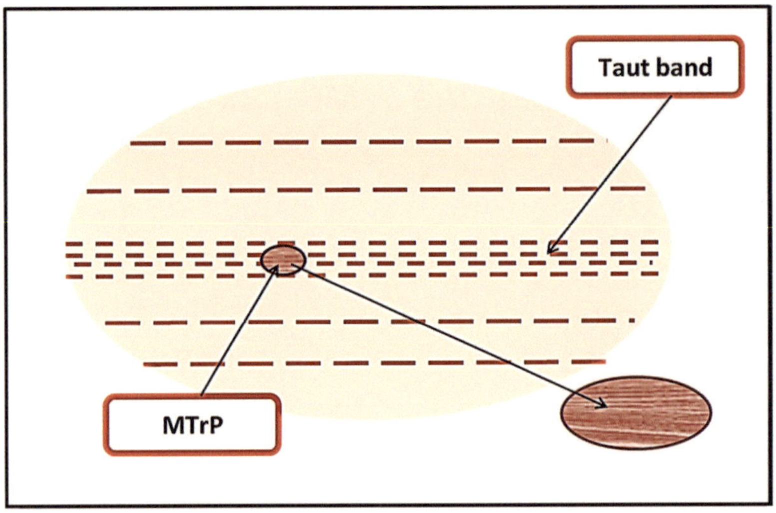

Figure 1. Simplified schematic of taut band and myofascial trigger point (MTrP).

Myofascial pain syndromes are common conditions that, by definition, result from trigger points (TrPs). Unfortunately, practitioners often do not recognise the myofascial pain syndrome [7, 8]. Unrecognised myofascial headaches, low back pain and shoulder pain have been considered to be one of the major causes of chronic pain, disability and industrial time lost, which plays a factor in most worker's compensation claims [1, 9].

Musculoskeletal pain originating from muscle has concerned the medical community for more than a century [10]. The subject has been appointed by multiple terms that emphasize various signs and symptoms representing basically the same phenomenon [11].

History has introduced terms such as fibrositis, myalgia, rheumatic myalgia and non-articular rheumatism. However, it should be noted that all of these terms and many others that are used for myofascial trigger points (primary cause of muscle pain) and fibromyalgia (central cause of muscle pain) are now no longer utilized [1, 10, 12].

The entity of MTrP has now been widely acknowledged on the basis of clinical observation and basic scientific research [13, 14]. A myofascial trigger point (MTrP) has been defined as a highly localised, sensitive, hyperirritable spot in a palpable taut band of skeletal muscle fibres [1, 15] (**Figure 1**). MTrPs are frequently found at or near to a muscle's origin and insertion, as well as along the belly of a muscle particularly at the motor points [2, 12].

2. Types of MTrPs

There are two main types of MTrPs active and latent. An active MTrP is one associated with spontaneous pain or occurring in response to movement [16–18]. It has also been defined as one whose nociceptors have undergone sufficient activation and sensitisation to cause pain to be referred to a site some distance from it (the zone of pain referral) [12].

A latent MTrP is a sensitive spot with pain or discomfort, which occurs in response to compression only [16, 17]. It may also be defined as one in which its nociceptors have undergone a limited amount of trauma-induced activation and sensitisation, but not sufficient to cause the development of pain [12].

Active TrPs might cause agonising incapacitating pain particularly when associated with active satellite TrPs in another muscles [1]. By contrast, despite the fact that, latent TrPs do not produce spontaneous pain, they can cause some increased muscle tension, limitation of passive range motion and may also cause some muscle shortening [1, 17]. Both active and latent TrPs can therefore cause motor dysfunction [1].

MTrPs may become activated either through a primary or through a secondary event [12, 18]. Primary activation of the TrPs usually takes place as a result of direct trauma to a muscle, sudden strain, or when there is excessive or unusual exercise. The activation might also be the result of cumulative effects due to long-standing repetitive minor trauma or overloading [1, 12, 17, 18].

Secondary activation of TrPs usually takes place in synergistic and antagonistic muscles. This may be due to compensatory actions or by counteracting tension in the primary muscles. Referral from visceral sources such as in a myocardial infarction or connective tissue disorder such as osteoarthritis, rheumatoid arthritis may also contribute to this secondary phenomenon [1, 19].

3. Clinical diagnostic criteria of MTrPs

There are certain clinical characteristics that should be looked for during the examination in order to confirm the presence of MTrPs. These include:

3.1. Taut band

Muscles sometimes contain taut cord-like bands. Palpable taut band is considered to be a basic diagnostic criterion of an MTrP [20].

3.2. Local twitch response

The local twitch response (LTR) is a transient contraction of the palpable taut band of muscles comprising MTrPs. It can be visualised, or palpated through the skin of the patient, or seen by ultrasound imaging [1, 15, 18].

The LTR is elicited mechanically, usually by a vigorous snapping palpation of the TrP in a direction opposite to the muscle fibres, or by needle penetration of the TrP [1, 18].

3.3. Spot tenderness or jump sign

Spot tenderness is an essential diagnostic criterion in the MTrP examination. However, spot tenderness alone has a limited value because it might be due to other reasons such as fibromyalgia.

The jump sign is a characteristic behavioural response to pressure on a MTrP. Patients often withdraw and sometimes complain of pain particularly with active MTrPs [1].

3.4. Pain recognition

Digital pressure on an MTrP can be used to elicit referred pain patterns characteristic of that muscle and the patient symptoms. This is considered as one of the most important diagnostic criteria particularly when accompanied by other signs [1, 20, 21].

3.5. Limited range of motion

Restricted range of motion is more severe in more active MTrPs and is a fundamental characteristic of MTrPs [1]. A muscle containing an MTrP restricts range of motion due to pain [1, 12, 22]. When MTrPs are treated, range of motion increases and often returns to normal [1].

3.6. Referred pain

Pain is often felt a considerable distance from the MTrPs and as a consequence, most patients are unaware of the presence of the TrP despite its exquisite tenderness. The referred pain either occurs spontaneously, particularly when the MTrP is very active [1, 2] or through palpation [15].

Referred pain by itself is not considered a diagnostic criterion of an MTrP unless accompanied by other findings [1, 20, 23]. However, the referred pain patterns play an important role in the initial examination as they direct the examiner to the muscle that harbours the MTrPs. In addition, knowledge of referral patterns minimises the chances of missing some TrPs [12] (**Figure 2**).

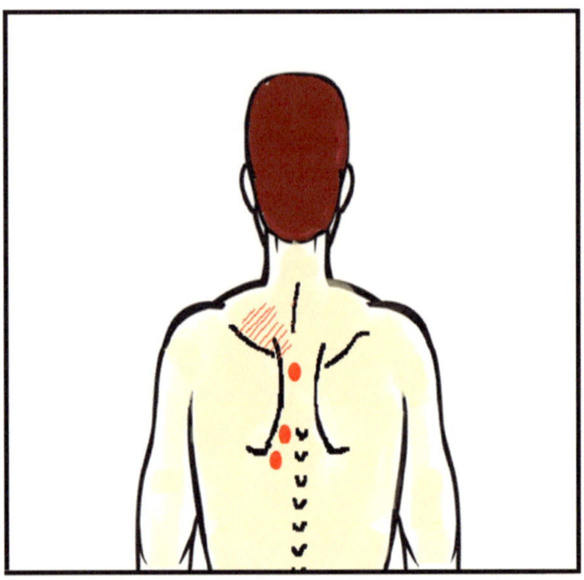

Figure 2. The pattern of pain referral from myofascial trigger points (•) in the rhomboid muscles.

4. Diagnosis of MTrPs

The diagnosis of MTrPs primarily relies on manual palpation and clinical judgment. However, manual palpation may be imprecise and not a reliable [24]. Therefore, specific training coupled with clinical experience is needed to obtain good reliability for the MTrP diagnosis. It has been showed that a combination of "spot tenderness," "taut band" and "pain recognition" are the basic clinical criteria to diagnose a MTrP, while "referred pain" and "local twitch response" are considered to be confirmatory signs [20, 21].

More recently, detection of biochemicals related to pain and inflammation in MTrP site [25], the sonographic methods of MTrPs [26] and the magnetic resonance elastography for taut band image [27] are potential objective outcome assessment tools in the MTrPs diagnosis.

5. Conventional forms of MTrPs treatment

There are several forms that are conventionally used to treat the MTrPs, which include:

5.1. Dry needling

The possibility of treating the MTrPs by dry needling techniques has been noted as early as 1952 [28], but Lewit [29] was the first investigator to employ dry needling techniques.

More recently, the effectiveness of dry needing in reducing the tenderness of MTrPs has been reported by a number of authors (e.g. [30–32]). However, dry needling is occasionally associated with adverse events such as post-needling soreness, bruising, dizziness and infection [32–34].

5.2. The injection of a local anaesthetic into an MTrP

The use of local anaesthetics such as Procaine Lidocaine has been reported to be an effective method for reducing post-injection soreness [1, 30, 32]. However, the use of them may occasionally give rise to toxic, allergic and anaphylactic reactions [15].

5.3. Botulinum toxin A injection

Botulinum toxin A injection (BTA) has been utilized in treatment for MTrPs [35–38]. However, it is rare clinically indicated, as it may be associated with possible local and systemic side effects such as muscle weakness and serious respiratory compromise [38, 39].

5.4. The injection of non-steroidal and steroidal anti-inflammatory drugs into MTrPs

The injection of non-steroidal anti-inflammatory drugs into the MTrPs has been used successfully to treat them [40, 41]. However, repeated injection of it into muscle might lead to skin necrosis [40]. The injection of steroids has also been used to treat the MTrP, and a good result has been reported [40, 42]. However, the use of steroids should be discouraged because of the risk of inducing local myopathy and the possible muscle fibre damage that is frequently associated with repeated injections [40].

5.5. Therapeutic ultrasound

The literature advocates therapeutic ultrasound as an effective modality for MTrP treatment in the clinical practice [1, 43]. In a study by Hong et al. [44] revealed that pain pressure threshold of MTrPs was increased immediately after ultrasound therapy with intensities of (1.2–1.5 W/cm^2) as compared to placebo therapy. However, Lee et al. [45] could not obtain similar finding at a lower intensity of ultrasound (0.5 W/cm^2).

More recently, two studies conducted by Srbely et al. [46] and Srbely and Dickey [47] revealed improvement in pressure pain threshold value (less tenderness). However, the study of Srbely and Dickey [47] was not blinded and did not address the long-term benefit.

5.6. Electric stimulation

Electrotherapy has been advocated as an effective therapeutic modality to alleviate pain emanating from MTrPs [43, 48, 49]. Graff-Radford et al. [50] showed that high frequency transcutaneous electrical nerve stimulation (TENS) could alleviate pain but they did not succeed to show any improvement in the MTrP sensitivity. More recently, Lee et al. [45] utilised electrical muscle stimulation and they concluded that pain was significantly decreased compared to the placebo group, but no significant improvement in pressure threshold or range of motion was found. The long-term influence of the electrical stimulation on MTrP was not addressed in the methodology of the above two trials.

6. Photomedicine

Photomedicine has progressed and come to be one of the most inspiring fields in the medical research in the past 50 years. The coherent light sources (lasers) and more recently, non-coherent light sources, e.g. light emitting diodes (LEDs) and superluminous diodes (SLDs) used in the musculoskeletal disorders are those with an athermic effect. Frequently used lasers include the helium-neon (HeNe gas) and infrared lasers with gallium arsenide (GaAs) or gallium aluminium arsenide (GaA1As) diodes [51–53].

Laser therapy (coherent sources) or low reactive-level laser therapy (LLLT) has been reported to be beneficial in soft tissue lesions including MTrPs [54–60]. Its beneficial therapeutic effect can be obtained without undesired effects. The below section of this chapter considers mainly the background of laser and characteristics of laser light, laser treatment parameters, treatment approaches and the possible mechanisms of action of laser in MTrPs.

7. Background and historical perspectives of laser

While laser is a relatively new form of treatment, the therapeutic benefits of light energy are not a new concept [51, 61, 62]. The sun was the first source of light that was employed in the treatment of several conditions.

http://dx.doi.org/10.5772/65748

Laser was not developed until 1960; however, the concept behind it was described at the beginning of the century by Albert Einstein in his 'quantum theory' [62, 63]. The development of LASER—Light Amplification by stimulated Emission of Radiation—then arose when Theodore Maiman in 1960 amplified light (using a ruby crystal as a lasing media) [51, 62].

In the 1960s, rapid development took place and variety of laser types appeared, based on different lasing media and resulting in different wavelengths. For example, Johnson in 1961 developed the neodymium YAG (Nd:YAG) laser followed by the Argon laser developed by Bennet in 1962. This was followed by the carbon dioxide (CO_2) laser 2 years later by Patel and colleagues [64]. These kinds of laser in their medical applications relied upon the photothermal and photoablative interactions with the tissues at relatively high power and energy densities [62, 63].

In contrast, other types of laser were developed by Professor Master's group in Budapest during the late 1960s and early 1970. These types of laser relied upon the non-thermal interactions of laser irradiation with tissues at low power and energy densities had a photobiostimulation effect on experimental wounds, which increased the rate of healing [62–65].

Another possible biological effect of low power laser was described in 1973 by Friedrich Plog in Canada, who presented his work on the use of HeNe laser as an alternative to metal needles for acupuncture treatments [51, 66, 67].

After these initial successful reports of Professor Mester's group at Budapest and Dr. Plog in Canada, low power laser treatment has become more frequently utilized by physicians and physical therapists for the alleviation of pain [68–70]. More recently, low power laser has got approval of Food and Drug Administration (FDA), as a pain reliever for soft tissue lesion in 2005 in the USA [71]. Furthermore, the appearance of a number of clinical research papers with very promising results particularly for MTrPs treatment have led to the popularity of laser therapy (e.g. [54–58]).

8. Principal components of a laser system

The laser device consists of three essential components.

8.1. Lasing medium

A lasing medium is a material that can absorb the energy generated by an external source. It can be gaseous, liquid, solid, crystal or a semiconductor [51, 62, 65, 72–74].

8.2. Energy source

Energy laser device must have an energy source to excite the lasing medium in order to emit laser radiation [51, 62, 65, 73, 74].

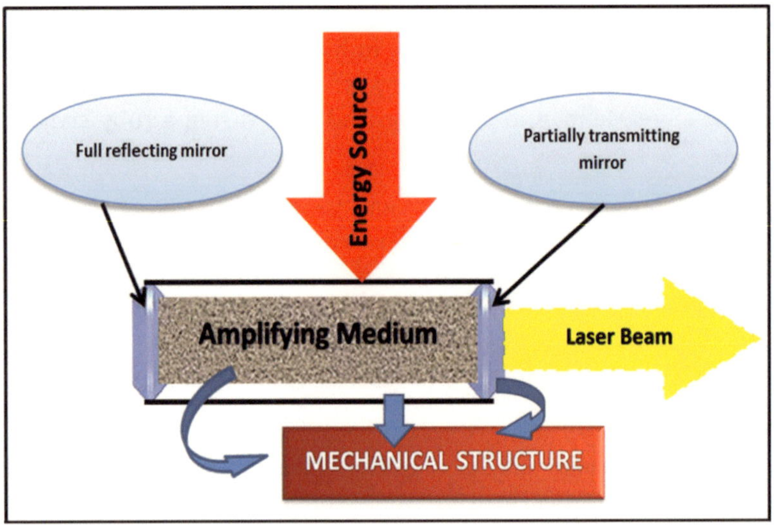

Figure 3. Simplified schematic of laser basic components.

8.3. Mechanical structure

The mechanical structure consists of the lasing medium within a central chamber located between two parallel mirrors. Reflection of photons of light back and forth between the two mirrors an across the chamber takes place, which lead to an intense photon production [51, 62, 72, 73].

The reflective extent of the two mirrors is not the same. While one of them is 100%, the other one is slightly less reflective to allow a small amount of the laser beam to pass through as irradiation output of the device [51, 62, 72, 73] (**Figure 3**). However, in the semiconductor devices, the ends of the diodes can be polished or coated with a highly reflective material to work as an alternative to the mirrors. Similarly, one end of the diode is slightly less reflective to allow a certain amount of the laser beam to pass as an output of irradiation [51, 73, 75].

9. Characteristics of laser light

Laser light differs from the ordinary light in terms of its monochromaticity, collimation and coherence. The biological and clinical significance of these characteristics is still relatively questionable and under investigations:

9.1. Monochromaticity

Monochromaticity indicates to single, defined wavelength, which consequently gives (mono) single colour [51, 73, 76–78]. Research evident showed that biological process possibly altered within a very narrow bandwidth, as distinct from the board spectrum of natural light [79].

9.2. Collimation

Collimation indicates to the minimal divergence of the laser beam. Compare to, the emitted radiation of non-laser light sources radiates in various directions [51, 72, 75].

9.3. Coherence

Coherence indicates to the inherent 'synchronicity' of the light emitted by laser devices, which means that all energy waves are in phase [51, 63, 75, 77, 78] (**Figure 4**).

Some in-vitro studies have found that it is substantially critical to use a coherent laser source to attain photobiological modulations (e.g. [80, 81]), whilst others have found that coherence is not necessary [79, 82, 83]. Therefore, some of manufacturers have presented a cheaper phototherapy units, e.g. superluminous diodes (SLDs) and light-emitting diodes (LEDs), which are non-coherent [51, 63].

Clinically, researchers have disputed over the possible loss of coherency when subjecting laser light to human tissues and recently have shown positive outcomes when using light-emitting diodes (LEDs) (non-coherent light sources) in experimental muscle injury [84, 85].

Conversely, it has been reported that the photon density of coherent laser beam ensures a greater and more efficient penetration [67, 86, 87]. Simunovic [88] has also shown that coherency possibly maintained when passing through tissue. The significance of coherency has been also stressed by Antipa [89], as one of the characteristics that are necessary to obtain a higher clinical efficacy of laser therapy [89].

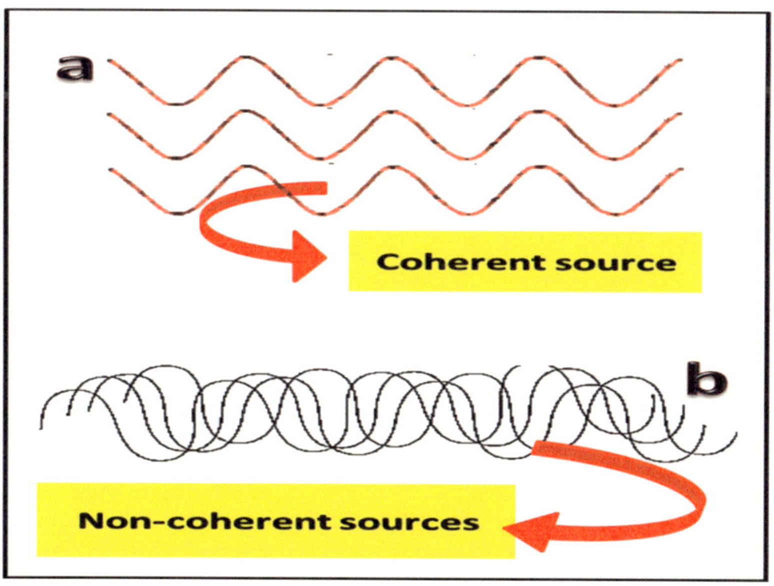

Figure 4. (a) Coherent light and (b) incoherent light.

9.4. Laser therapy treatment approaches

Laser therapy usually involves two main types of treatment approaches.

9.4.1. Contact approach

In the contact approach, the probe or the treatment head is applied perpendicular to the treated tissue. This technique greatly intensifies the irradiance on the tissue surface and consequently a greater proportion of laser energy can be directed to the target tissue [51, 63, 72, 75] (**Figure 5**).

The contact approach has been reported to be the most efficient treatment approach and must be used whenever it is possible [51, 62]. The treatment is also relatively safe as it reduces the potential hazard that comes from accidental intrabeam viewing [51, 62, 63].

A contact approach is commonly utilized in treating MTrPs. Beneficial effects have been shown in a number of clinical trials adopting this approach [54, 56, 90] while others failed to reveal any successful effects [91, 92]. However, in the latter two studies, no treatment parameters details and/or poor treatment parameters were evident.

9.4.2. Non-contact approach

In the non-contact approach, the probe or the treatment head is used out of contact with the tissue (**Figure 5**). This technique attenuates the irradiance on the irradiated tissue according to the 'inverse square law', thus more reflection of the incident photons will occur [51, 62, 63].

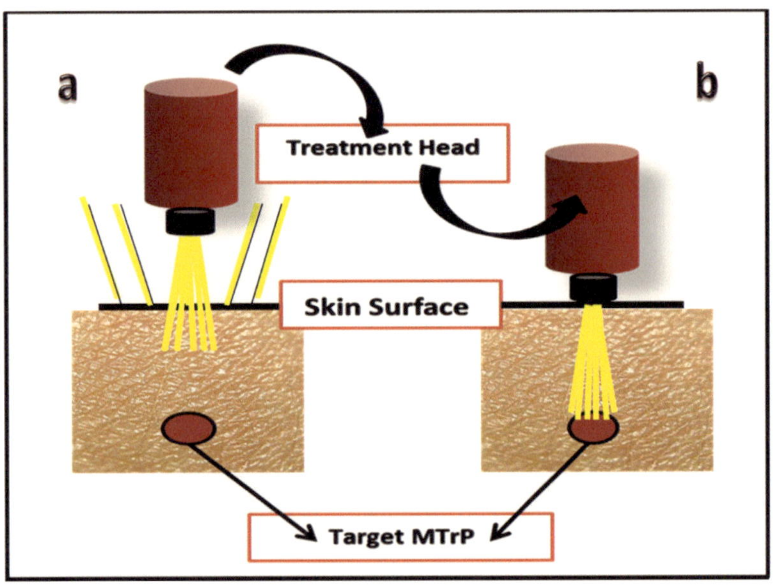

Figure 5. (a) Non-contact approach and (b) contact approach.

10. Treatment parameters

Treatment parameters are extremely important and their detailed specification can allow replication of experimental or clinical findings.

10.1. Wavelength

Wavelength is the most important treatment parameters that determine the depth of penetration of laser irradiation [93]. Laser therapy units are usually with single wavelength sources. However, more recently, laser therapy units with a broad spectrum of wavelengths are available.

Therapeutic lasers have commonly wavelengths of approximately 602–1064 nm and give visible (red) or invisible (near infra-red) radiation (HeNe laser) [51, 65, 94].

10.2. HeNe lasers (632.8 nm)

The insufficient of penetration of this visible short wavelength laser source (HeNe laser) [51, 65, 94] might be one the justifications for its ineffectiveness. However, positive outcomes were evident with this type of laser in some MTrP clinical studies (e.g. [54, 95]).

10.3. CO_2 Lasers (10,600 nm)

The CO_2 lasers produce infrared radiation at 10.600 nm and such devices have been used successfully as pain relief modalities by some researchers (e.g. [96–98]). However, this type of laser is almost totally absorbed by water, thus reducing great proportion of light penetration in biological tissue [67].

10.4. Diode lasers (820–950 nm)

Wavelengths that are in the range of 820–950 nm (diode lasers) are known as near infrared radiation in the electromagnetic spectrum [51]. Their tissue penetration ability is quite high compared to other sources with different wavelengths [67].

Most of myofascial trigger point clinical studies utilized lasers with longer wavelength, ranging from 780 to 904, because it can transmit light energy with greater penetration and, therefore, they are the most appropriate to treated trigger points that particularly located in deep muscles [99].

10.5. Radiant power output

The radiant power output of laser systems is generally measured in watts (W), but as a result of the relatively low power output employed in LLLT systems, it is more frequently measured in milliwatts (mW = thousands of a watt) [63, 65, 100].

It has also been reported that more penetration can be gained with greater average output power, as a greater number of photons will be presented at deeper depths [72]. However, radiant power output was greatly variable between studies with possible pain reduction when irradiating painful MTrPs with a range of radiant power outputs of 0.95–120 mW.

10.6. Irradiance

Irradiance is defined as the incident photon density of laser irradiation at the target tissue and utilized to express to the intensity of light [67]. The significance of irradiance has been stressed by a number of researchers as one of the most influential treatment parameters [101, 102]. However, unfortunately, quite few numbers of researchers reported this treatment parameter [99].

Some literature reported positive results for tissue repair and anti-inflammatory effects when the range of 5–55 mW/cm2 was employed [103–105], while higher irradiances of 300–1730 mW/cm2 was recommended for analgesic purposes [106].

The irradiance can be obtained from the following equation:

$$\text{Irradiance} = \frac{\text{Output power (W)}}{\text{Irradiated area (cm}^2\text{)}} \tag{1}$$

From the above equation, it can be seen that the value of the irradiance (measured in watts) will be profoundly affected by the spot size (measured in square centimetre) of the laser beam [67].

10.7. Radiant energy

The radiant energy delivered to a region of the target tissue over a period of time is commonly expressed in joules (J) and can be calculated by the following equation:

$$\text{Radiant Energy (J)} = \text{power output (W)} \times \text{time (s)} \tag{2}$$

From the above equation, if a certain energy is required in a treatment session, the time (in seconds) needed to obtain that energy can be obtained, by dividing the energy by the radiant power output [51, 63].

The total radiant energy is one of critical treatment parameters [107]. The energy employed in the MTrPs clinical trials ranged from 0.275 to 8 J/point [99].

10.8. Radiant exposure

Radiant exposure is a critical factor in ascertaining whether the laser light will influence photobiological modulation process [108, 109]. A recent study also revealed that the radiant exposure provided by laser therapy is one of the factors that can influence biochemicals related to pain in the treatment of MTrPs [60].

It is worth noting, energy density is not a fixed parameter as it is dependent on time and can be manipulated by the operator [110]. The radiant exposure can be obtained from the following equation:

$$\text{Energy density (J/cm}^2\text{)} = \frac{\text{Power (W)} \times \text{times (s)}}{\text{area (cm}^2\text{)}} \tag{3}$$

http://dx.doi.org/10.5772/65748

Treatment exposure is usually in a range between 1.44 and 12 J/cm^2 in the treatment of MTrPs. However, radiant exposures of up to 32 J/cm^2 have been employed also [75, 99].

10.9. Pulse repetition rate

Generally, the laser devices that are available in research or clinical applications deliver a continuous wave or allow some form of pulsing of their output [63, 65, 72, 73].

The pulse repetition rate in the pulsed devices is expressed in Hertz (Hz, pulses per second) and can vary from 2 to thousands of Hz [63]. However, the pulse rate is restricted in some laser devices.

It has been reported that pulsed light possibly more effective than continuous one, as it allow a potentially much higher peak power densities without causing a significant tissue heating and consequently greater treatment depth [93]. Additionally, different biological effects were obtained, when experiments were conducted to determine the effect of different pulsing frequencies (e.g. [111–115]).

10.10. Frequency of treatment and length of treatment course

Clinical practitioners and researchers advocate multiple treatment sessions for successful laser treatment [51, 65, 94] (**Figure 6**). In MTrPs studies, laser treatment were commonly

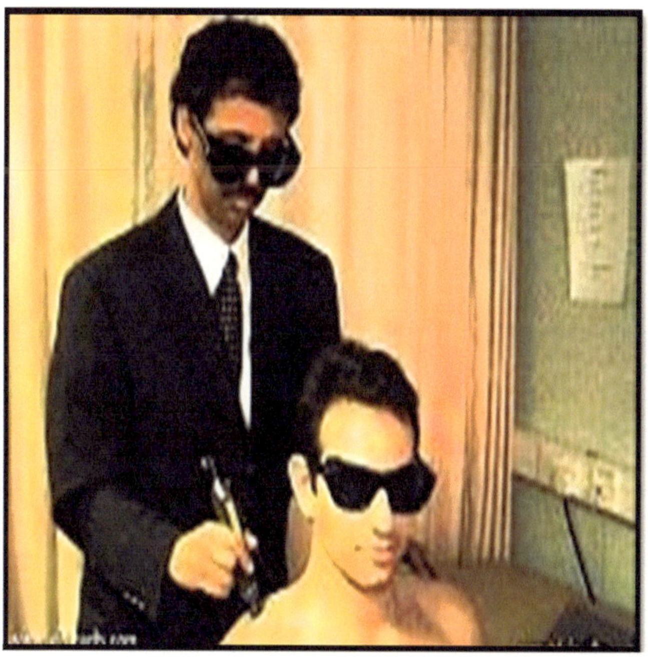

Figure 6. Clinical laser session.

utilized 2-3 times per week However, there is no consensus about the optimum frequency of treatment or length of treatment course [56, 99].

11. The possible mechanisms of action of laser in MTrPs

Three possible mechanisms of action were proposed included: stimulation of the local metabolism; modulation of neurotransmitter; anti-inflammatory effect and laser-induced neuronal suppression.

11.1. Stimulation of the local metabolism

In the mechanism of taut band formation, certain muscle fibres react to trauma or abnormal stress by excessive release of calcium ions. This would cause uncontrolled muscle fibres contracture with increase metabolic demands and consequently, MTrPs formation [1]. Laser therapy reported to have the potential to cause rotation and vibration on the membrane molecules that make up the calcium channels that may alter the function of these channels [116]. This might help in removing or minimizing the excessive amount of calcium that may causes uncontrolled shortening activity of the muscle fibres.

The characteristic shortening of muscle fibres associated with MTrPs results in deteriorated local circulation leading to loss of oxygen and nutrient supply. Laser therapy has the ability to enhance the local microcirculation and subsequently decrease the muscular tension and emanate pain in the area [88].

11.2. Modulation of neurotransmitter

Modulation of neurotransmitters has proposed as a mechanism for pain alleviation [117]. For instance, serotonin levels are relatively intensifying when the treatment of MTrPs with laser treatment are employed. A trial carried out by Walker [118] applied laser irradiation on MTrPs patients attributed the analgesic effects to changes in serotonin metabolism.

More recently, a double blind study conducted by Ceylan et al. [57] also found that laser irradiation is an effective method of treatment of MTrPs associated with the elevation of the serotonin. However, more studies may be required in this area.

11.3. Anti-inflammatory effect

The cause of pain in active MTrPs may be as a result of direct trauma to a muscle, sudden strain, or when there is excessive or unusual exercise, a study by Shah et al. [25] also documents a high concentration of nociceptive substances, e.g. protons, bradykinin, calcitonin gene-related peptide, substance p, serotonin and noradrenaline) in the active MTrPs.

As the rise of the above biochemical milieu of substances are usually associated with pain and inflammation and in accordance with the above findings, evidence from the literature reported that laser therapy inhibits peripheral nerves afferent terminals prohibits peripheral nerve sensitization and hinder further release of the nociceptive substances, thus possible mechanisms of pain relief and anti-inflammatory effect may occur [119, 120].

Research has also clearly revealed anti-inflammatory effects of laser irradiation particularly in acute injury [120]. The tissue repair is associated with the release of prostaglandins $E_{2.}$ Laser irradiation showed the ability to reduce the formation of the inflammatory markers including the prostaglandins E2 [119]. Therefore, laser might be able promote resolution of the inflammatory process vital for the tissue repair.

11.4. Laser-induced neuronal suppression

Laser-induced suppression of neuronal activity is another potential mechanism for pain relieving influences of laser irradiation. In advocate of laser-induced neuronal suppression mechanisms are a number of human trials that showed that laser relatively hinders nerve conduction velocity and augments latency in median [51], radial [121] and sural nerves [122]. However, light-emitting diodes (LEDs) and superluminous diodes (SLDs) more recently failed to act as a direct suppression of neuronal activity [123].

In consistent with the above findings, a number of electrophysiological experiments were carried out, to assess neuronal mediated inhibitory effects of laser irradiation [124–126]. Laser irradiations were able more specifically to influence the nerve conduction of small diameter, thinly myelinated A and unmyelinated C fibres. Therefore, in the light of these encouraging research reports using laser as an alternative to needle in acupuncture for MTrPs treatment might not be excluded.

Author details

Abdullah M. Al-Shenqiti

Address all correspondence to: monuhama@yahoo.co.uk

Faculty of Medical Rehabilitation Sciences, Taibah University, Al-Madinah Al-Munawarah, Saudi Arabia, Centre for Rehabilitation Science, University of Manchester, Manchester, UK

References

[1] Simons D, Travell J, Simons L. Travell & Simons's myofascial pain and dysfunction: the trigger point manual, vol. 1, second edition. William & Wilkins, Baltimore. 1999.

[2] Baldry P. Acupuncture, Trigger Points and Musculoskeletal Pain. Second Edition. Churchill Livingstone, Longman Group UK limited, Harcourt Publishers Limited, Edinburgh 1993.

[3] Fleckenstein J. Epidemiology. In: Irnish D (ed). Myofascial trigger points, comprehensive diagnosis and treatment. E-Book, 1st edition. Churchill Livingstone. 2013.

[4] Baldry P. Myfascial Pain and Fibromyalgia Syndromes. A clinical Guide to Diagnosis and Management. Churchill Livingstone, Harcourt Publishers Limited, London 2001.

[5] Cummings M, Baldry P. Regional myofascial pain: diagnosis and management. Best Pract Res Clin Rheumatol 2007; 21: 367–387.

[6] Fishbain D, Goldberg M, Meagher B, Steele R, Rosomoff H. Male and femal chronic pain patients categorized by DSM-III psychiatric diagnostic criteria. Pain 1986; 26: 181–197.

[7] Skootsky S, Jaeger B, Oye R. Prevalence of myofascial pain in general internal medicine practice. West J Med 1989; 151: 157–160.

[8] Sola A, Bonica J. Myofascial pain syndromes. In: Bonica J, Loeser J, Chapman C. (eds) The management of pain. Lea & Febiger, Philadelphia. 1990. pp. 352–367.

[9] Fricton J. Myofascial pain syndrome. Neurol Clin 1989; 7: 413–427.

[10] Simons D. Myofascial trigger points: the critical experiment. J Musculoskelet Pain 1997; 5: 113–118.

[11] Simons D, Stolov W. Microscpic features and transient contraction of palpable bands in canine muscle. Am J Phys Med 1976; 55: 65–88.

[12] Baldry P. Trigger point acupuncture. In: Filshie Jand white A. (eds) Medical acupuncture, a western scientific approach. Churchill Livingstone, London. 1998. pp. 33–60.

[13] Kuan T. Current studies on myofascial pain syndrome. Curr Pain Headache Rep 2009; 13: 365–369.

[14] Zhuang X, Tan S, Huang Q. Understanding of myofascial trigger points. Chin Med J 2014; 127(4): 4271–4277.

[15] Travell J, Simons D. Myofascial pain and dysfunction. The trigger point manual. Williams and Wilkins, Baltimore. 1983.

[16] Simons D. Myofascial pain syndrome due to trigger points. In: Goodgold J (ed). Rehabilitation medicine. St Louis, Mosby. 1988. pp. 686–723.

[17] Rachlin E. Trigger point. In: Rachlin E (ed) Myofascial pain and fibromyalgia: trigger point management. St. Louis, Mosby. 1994. pp. 145–157.

[18] Irnish D, Gautschi R, Behrens N. Terminology. In: Irnish D (ed) Myofascial trigger points, comprehensive diagnosis and treatment. E-Book, 1st edition. Churchill Livingstone. 2013.

[19] Renolds M. Myofascial trigger point syndromes in practice of rheumatology. Arch Phys Med Rehabil 1981; 62: 111–114.

[20] Gerwin R, Shannon S, Hong C, Hubbard D, Gevirtz R. Interrater reliability in myofascial trigger point examination. Pain 1997; 69: 65–73.

[21] Al-Shenqiti A, Oldham J. Test-retest reliability of myofascial trigger point detection in patients with rotator cuff tendonitis. Clin Rehabil 2005; 19: 482–487.

[22] Macdonald A. Abnormally tender muscle regions and associated painful movements. Pain 1980; 8: 197–205.

[23] Hong C. Pathophysiology of myofascial trigger point. J Formos Med Assoc 1996; 95: 93–104.

[24] Myburgh C, Larsen A, Hartvigsen J. A systematic, critical review of manual palpation for identifying myofascial trigger points: evidence and clinical significance. Arch Phys Med Rehabil. 2008; 89:1169–1176.

[25] Shah J, Phillips T, Danoff J, Gerber L. An in vivo microcanalytical technique for measuring the local biochemical milieu of human skeletal muscle. J Appl Physiol 2005; 99: 1977–1984.

[26] Sikdar S, Shah J, Gebreab T, et al. Novel applications of ultrasound technology to visualize and characterized myofascial trigger points and surrounding soft tissues. Arch Phys Med Rehabil 2009; 90: 1829–1838.

[27] Chen Q, Basford J, An K-N. Ability of magnetic resonance elastography to assess taut bands. Clin Biomech 2008; 23(5): 623–629.

[28] Travell J, Rinzler S. The myofascial genesis of pain. Postgrad Med 1952; 11: 425–435.

[29] Lewit K. The needle effect in the relief of myofascial pain. Pain 1979; 6: 83–90.

[30] Hong C. Trigger point injection: dry needling versus lidocaine injection. Am J Phys Med Rehabil 1994; 73: 256–263.

[31] Gunn C. The Gunn approach to the treatment of chronic pain. Intramuscular stimulation for myofascial pain of radiculopathic origin, 2nd edition. Churchill Livingstone, New York. 1996.

[32] Irnish D, Euler D, Gleditsch J, Banzer W, Bachmann J. Acupuncture and related procedures. In: Irnish D (ed) Myofascial trigger points, comprehensive diagnosis and treatment. E-Book, 1st edition. Churchill Livingstone. 2013.

[33] Ramps H. Adverse reactions to acupuncture. In: Filshie J, White A (eds) Medical acupuncture, a western scientific approach. Churchill Livingstone, London. 1998.

[34] Vickers A, Zollman C. ABC of complementary medicine: acupuncture. BMJ 1999; 319: 973–976.

[35] Ojala T, Arokoski J, Partanen J. The effect of small doses of Botulinum Toxin A on neck-shoulder myofascial pain syndrome: a double-blind randomized, and controlled cross-over trial. Clin J Pain 2006; 22: 90–96.

[36] Ho K, Tan, K. Botulinum toxin A for myofascial trigger point injection: a qualitative systematic review. Eur J Pain 2007; 11: 519–527.

[37] Jeynes L, Gauci C. Evidence for the use of Botulinum Toxin in the chronic pain setting—a review of the literature. Pain Pract 2008; 8: 269–279.

[38] Schmitt H, Irnish D. Triger point infiltration. In: Irnish D. Myofascial trigger points, comprehensive diagnosis and treatment. E-Book, 1st edition. Churchill Livingstone. 2013.

[39] Borodic J, Joseph M, Fay L. Botulinum A toxin for the treatment of spasmodic torticollis: dyphagia and regional toxin spread. Head Neck 1990; 12: 392–398.

[40] Drewes A, Andreason A, Poulsen L. Injection therapy for treatment of chronic myofascial pain: a double-blind study comparing corticosteroid versus diclofenac injections. J Musculoskelet Pain 1993; 1: 289–294.

[41] Frost A. Diclofenac versus lidocaine as an injection therapy in myofascial pain. Scand J Rheumatol 1986; 15: 153–156.

[42] Lang P, Irnish D. Systemic pharmacotherapy. In: Irnish D (ed) Myofascial trigger points, comprehensive diagnosis and treatment. E-Book, 1st edition. Churchill Livingstone. 2013.

[43] Schmitt H, Pothmann R, Banzer W, Hübscher M, Maier M, Kosub M. Physical procedures. In: Irnish D (ed) Myofascial trigger points, comprehensive diagnosis and treatment. E-Book, 1st edition. Churchill Livingstone. 2013.

[44] Hong, C.Z., Chen, Y.C., Pon, C.H., Yu, J. Immediate effects of various physical medicine modalities on pain threshold of an active myofascial trigger point. J Musculoskelet Pain 1993; 1: 37–53.

[45] Lee J, Lin D, Hong C. The effectiveness of simultaneous thermotherapy with ultrasound and electrotherapy with combined AC and DC current on the immediate pain relief of myofascialtrigger point. J Musculoskelet Pain 1997; 5: 81–90.

[46] Srbely J, Dickey J, Lowerison M, Edwards A, Nolet P, Wong L. Stimulation of myofascial trigger points with ultrasound induces asegmental antinociceptive effects: a randomized controlled study. Pain 2008; 139: 260–266.

[47] Srbely J, Dickey J. Randomized controlled study of the antinociceptive effect of ultrasound on trigger point sensitivity: novel applications in myofascial therapy? Clin Rehabil 2007; 21: 411–417.

[48] Khan J. Electrical modalities in the treatment of myofascial conditions. In: Rachlin E (ed) Myofascial pain and frbromyalgia. Trigger point management. St. Louis, Mosby. 1994.

[49] Hsueh T, Cheng P, Kuan T, Hong C. The immediate effectiveness of electrical nerve stimulation and electrical muscle stimulation on myofascial trigger points. Am J Phys Med Rehabil 1997; 76: 471–476.

[50] Graff-Radford S, Reeves J, Baker R, Chiu D. Effects oftranscutaneous electrical nerve stimulation on myofascial pain and trigger point sensitivity. Pain 1989; 37: 1–3.

[51] Baxter GD. Therapeutic laser. Theory and practice. Churchill Livingstone, London. 1994.

[52] Basford J. Low intensity laser therapy: still not an established clinical tool. Laser Surg Med 1995; 16: 331–342.

[53] Borges L, Cerqueira M, dos Santos Rocha J, Conrado L, Machado M, Pereira R, Net O. Light-emitting diode phototherapy improves muscle recovery after a damaging exercise. Lasers Med Sci 2014; 29: 1139–1144.

[54] Snyder-Mackler L, Barry A, Perkins A, Soucek M. Effects of helium-neon laser irradiation on skin resistance and pain in patients with trigger points in the neck or back. Phys Therapy 1989; 69: 336–341.

[55] Olavi A, Pekka R, Pertti K J. Effects of the infrared laser therapy at treated and non-treated trigger points. Acupunct Electrother Res Int J 1989; 14: 9–14.

[56] Al-Shenqiti A, Oldham J. The use of low level laser therapy (LLLT) in the treatment of trigger points that are associated with rotator cuff tendonitis. In: Longo L, Hofstetter AG, Pascu M-L, Waidelich WRA (eds) Proceedings of SPIE vol. 5287 Laser Florence 2002: a window on the Laser Medicine World, Bellingham, WA: SPIE. 2003. pp. 91–101.

[57] Ceylan Y, Hizmetli S, Silig Y. The effects of infrared laser and medical treatments on pain and serotonin degradation products in patients with myofascial pain syndrome. A Controlled Trial Rheumatol Int 2004; 24: 260–263.

[58] Lam L, Cheing G. Effects of 904 nm low-level laser therapy in the management of lateral epicondylitis: a randomized controlled trial. Photomed Laser Surg 2007; 25: 65–71.

[59] Demirkol N, Sari F, Bulbul M, Demirkol M, Simsek I, Usumez A. Effectiveness of occlusal splints and low-level laser therapy on myofascial pain. Lasers Med Sci 2015; 30: 1007–1012.

[60] Hsieh Y, Hong C, Chou L, Yang S, Yang C. Fluence-dependent effects of low-level laser therapy in myofascial trigger spots on modulation of biochemicals associated with pain in a rabbit model. Lasers Med Sci 2015; 30: 209–216.

[61] Castel J, Abergel R, Willner R, Baumann J. low energy laser biostimulation: new prospects for medical applications. Lasers Med 1986; 712: 242–247.

[62] Ohshiro T, Calderhead R. Low level laser therapy: a practical introduction. John Wiley and Sons, Chichester. 1988.

[63] Baxter D. Low intensity laser therapy. In: Kitchen S, Bazin S (eds) Clayton's electrotherapy. 10th edition. W. B. Saunders Company Limited, London. 1996. pp. 197–217.

[64] Patel C. CW high-power N_2-CO_2 laser. Applied Physics Letters 1965; 7: 15–17

[65] Turner J, Hode L. Low level laser therapy, clinical practice and scientific background, a guide for research scientists, doctors, dentists, veterinarians, and other interested parties within the medical field. Gra¨ngesberg: Prima Books in Sweden AB. 1999.

[66] Kitchen S, Patridge C. A review of low level laser therapy. Physiotherapy 1991; 77: 161–168.

[67] Ohshiro T. Light and life: a review of low reactive-level laser therapy, following 13 years' experience in over 12000 patients. Laser Ther 1993; 1: 5–22.

[68] Bischko J. Use of the laser beam in acupuncture. Acupunct Electrother Res 1980; 5: 29–40.

[69] Waylonis G, Wilke S, O'Tool D, Waylonis D, Waylonis D. Chronic myofascial pain: management by low-output helium-neon laser therapy. Arch Phys Med Rehabil 1988; 69: 1017–1020.

[70] Ceccherelli F, Altafini L, Lo Castro G, Avila A, Ambrosio F, Giron G. Diode laser in cervical myofascial pain: a double-blind study versus placebo. Clin J Pain 1989;5: 301–204.

[71] FDA report, (File 510 'K' Number: K043353) 1st July 2005. Department of health & human services. Public Health Service. Food and Drug Administration, Rockville MD 20850. Low level laser therapy (LLLT) Omega XP Laser System. Class II, Performance Standards.

[72] Kert J, Rose L. Clinical laser therapy: low level laser therapy. Scandinavian Medical Laser Technology, Copenhagen. 1989.

[73] Pontinen P. Low level laser therapy as a medical treatment modality. A manual for physician, dentists, physiotherapists and veterinary surgeons. Tampere. 1992.

[74] Pascu M. Laser physics. In: Simunovic Z (ed) Lasers in medicine and dentistry. Basic scientific and up-to-date clinical application of low energy-level laser therapy LLLT. European Medical Laser Association. Vitagraf d.o.o. 2000. pp. 24–74.

[75] Low J, Reed A. Electrotherapy explained. Principals and practice, 3rd edition. Butterworth-Heinemann, Oxford. 2000.

[76] England S. Introduction to mid laser therapy. Physiotherapy 1988; 74: 100–102.

[77] Snyder-Mackler L, Seitz L. Therapeutic uses of light in rehabilitation. In: Michlovitz S. Thermal agents in rehabilitation, 2nd edition. F A Davis Company, Philadelphia. 1990.

[78] Weisberg J. Ultraviolet irradiation. In: Hecox B, Mehreteab T, Weisberg J (eds). Physical agents. A comprehensive text for physical therapists. Appleton and Lange, Norwalk, Connecticut. 1994.

[79] Karu T. Photobiological fundamentals of low-power laser therapy. IEEE J Quantum Electron 1987; 23: 1703–1717.

[80] Boulton M, Marshall J. He-Ne laser stimulation of human fibroblast proliferation and attachment in vitro. Lasers Life Sci 1986; 1: 125–134.

[81] Berki T, Nemeth P, Hegedus J. Biological effect of low power Helium-Neon (HeNe) laser irradiation. Lasers Med Sci 1988; 3: 35–39.

[82] Karu T. Photochemical effects upon the cornea, skin and other tissues. Photobiology of low-power laser effects. Health Phys 1989; 56: 691–704.

[83] Young S, Bolton P, Dyson M, Harvey W, Diamantopoulos C. Macrophage responsiveness to light therapy. Lasers Surg Med 1989; 9: 497–505.

[84] Kelencz C, Muñoz I, Amorim C, Nicolau R. Effect of low-power gallium-aluminum-arsenium noncoherent light (640 nm) on muscle activity: a clinical study. Photomed Laser Surg 2010; 28: 647–52.

[85] Leal Junior E, de Godoi V, Mancalossi J, Rossi R, De Marchi T, Parente M, Grosselli D, Generosi R, Basso M, Frigo L, Tomazoni S, Bjordal J, Lopes-Martins R. Comparison between cold water immersion therapy (CWIT) and light emitting diode therapy (LEDT) in short-term skeletal muscle recovery after high-intensity exercise in athletes—preliminary results. Lasers Med Sci 2011; 26: 493–501.

[86] Kubota J, Ohshiro T. The effects of diode laser low-reactive-level laser therapy (LLLT) on flab survival in a rat model. Laser Ther 1989; 127–133.

[87] Ohshiro T. Low reactive level laser therapy. Practical applications. John Wiley and Sons, Chichester. 1991.

[88] Simunovic Z. Lasers in medicine and dentistry. Basic science and up-to-date clinical application of low energy-level laser therapy LLLT, part one, European Medical Laser Association. Vitagraf d.o.o. 2000.

[89] Antipa C. Contributions to LLL clinical therapy. In: Simunovic Z (ed) Lasers in medicine and dentistry. Basic science, and up-to-date clinical application of low energy-level laser therapy LLLT, part 1, European Medical Laser Association. Vitagraf d.o.d. 2000.

[90] Simunovic Z. Low level laser therapy with trigger points technique: a clinical study on 243 patients. J Clin Laser Med Surg 1996;14:163–167.

[91] Altan L, Bingol U, Aykac M, Yurtkuran M. Investigation of the effect of GaAs laser therapy on cervical myofascial pain syndrome. Rheumatol Int 2005; 25: 23–27.

[92] Dundar U, Evcik D, Samli F, Pusak H, Kavuncu V. The effect of gallium arsenide aluminium laser therapy in the management of cervical myofascial pain syndrome: a double blind, placebocontrolled study. Clin Rheumatol 2007; 26: 930–934.

[93] Hashmi J, Huang Y, Sharma S, Kurup D, MSEE L, Carroll J, Hamblin M. Effect of pulsing in low-level light therapy. Lasers Surg Med 2010; 42: 450–466.

[94] Laakso L, Richardson C, Cramond T. Factors affecting low level laser therapy. Australian Physiotherapy 1993; 39: 94–98.

[95] Simunovic Z, Trobonjaca T, Trobonjaca Z. Treatment of medial and lateral epicondylitis-tennis and golfer's elbow-with low level laser therapy: a multicenter double blind, placebo-controlled clinical study on 324 patients. J Clin Laser Med Surg 1998;16:145–151.

[96] Morselli M, Soragni O, Anselmi C, Farinelli F. Very low energy-density treatments by CO_2 laser in sport medicine. Laser Surg Med 1985; 5: 150

[97] Morselli M, Soragni O, Lupia P et al: Effects of very low energy-density treatment of joint pain by CO_2 laser, Laser Surg Med 1985; 5: 149

[98] Martino G, Fava G, Galperti G. CO_2 laser therapy for women with mastalgia. Lasers Surg Med 1987; 7: 78–82.

[99] Al-Shenqiti A, Oldham J. The use of low intensity laser therapy in the treatment of myofascial trigger points: an updated critical review. Phys Ther Rev 2009; 14: 115–123.

[100] Diamentopoulos C. Bioenergetics and tissues optics. In: Baxter GD (ed) Therapeutic lasers. Theory and practice. Churchill Livingstone, Edinburgh. 1994.

[101] Trelles M, Mayayo E, Miro L, Rigau J, Baudin G, Calderhead R. The action of low reactive level laser therapy (LLLT) on mast cells: a possible pain relief mechanism examined. Laser Ther 1989; 1: 27–30.

[102] Nussbaum E, Baxter GD, Lilge L. A review of laser technology and light-tissue interactions as a background to therapeutic applications of low intensity lasers and other light sources. Phys Ther Rev 2003; 8: 31–44.

[103] Castano A, Dai T, Yaroslavsky I et al. Low-level laser therapy for zymosan-induced arthritis in rats: Importance of illumination time. Laser Surg Med 2007; 39: 543–550.

[104] Lanzafame R, Stadler I, Kurtz A et al. Reciprocity of exposure time and irradiance on energy density during photoradiation on wound healing in a murine pressure ulcer model. Laser Surg Med 2007; 39: 534–542.

[105] Oron, U, Yaakobi T, Oronet A et al. Attenuation of infarct size in rats and dogs after myocardial infarction by lowenergy laser irradiation. Laser Surg Med 2001; 28: 204–211.

[106] Chow R, Armati P, Laakso E, Bjordal J, Baxter G D. Inhibitory effects of laser irradiation on peripheral mammalian nerves and relevance to analgesic effects: a systematic review. Photomed Laser Surg 2011; 29: 365–381.

[107] Enwemeka C. Intricacies of dose in laser phototherapy for tissue repair and pain relief. Photomed Laser Surg 2009; 27: 387–393.

[108] Karu T, Tiphlova O, Samokhina M, Diamontopoulos C, Sarantsev V, Shveikin V. Effects of infra-red laser and superluminous diode irradiation on Escherichia coli division rate. IEEE J Quantum Electron 1990; 26; 2163–2165.

[109] Karu T, Pyatibrat L, Kalendo G, Esenaliev R. Effects of monochromatic low-intensity light and laser irradiation on adhesion of HeLa cells in vitro. Lasers Surg Med 1996; 18: 171–177.

[110] Nussbaum E, Van Zuylen J, Baxter D. Specifications of treatment dosage in laser therapy: Unreliable equipment and radiant power determination as confounding factors. Physiother Can 1999; 51: 159–167.

[111] Dyson M, Young S. Effect of laser therapy on wound contraction and cellularity in mice. Lasers Med Sci 1986; 1: 125–130.

[112] Longo I, Evangelista S, Tinnaci G, Sesti A. Effects of diodes-laser-silver-aluminium (Ga-Al-As) 904 nm on healing of experimental wounds. Lasers Surg Med 1987; 7: 444–447.

[113] Rajaratnam S, Bolton P, Dyson M. Macrophage responsiveness to laser therapy with varying pulsing frequencies. Laser Ther 1994; 6: 107–112.

[114] El-Sayed S, Dyson M. Effect of laser pulse repetition rate and pulse duration on mast cell number and degranulation. Lasers Surg Med 1996; 19: 433–437.

[115] Sushko B, Lymans'kyi I, Huliar S. Action of the red and infrared electromagnetic waves of light-emitting diodes on the behavioral manifestation of somatic pain. Fiziol Zh. 2007; 53: 51–60.

[116] Smith K. The photobiological basis of low level laser radiation. Laser Ther 1991; 3: 19–24.

[117] Navratil L, Dyleysky I. Mechanisms of the analgesic effect of therapeutic lasers in vivo. Laser Ther 1997; 9: 33–39.

[118] Walker J. Relief from chronic pain by low power laser irradiation. Neurosci Lett 1983; 43: 339–344.

[119] Siddall P, Cousins M. Neural blockade in clinical anesthesia. In: Cousins M, Bridenbaugh P (eds) Introduction to pain mechanisms—implications for neural blockade. Lippincott-Raven, Philadelphia. 1998. pp. 675–713.

[120] Bjordal J, Johnson M, Iverson V, Aimbire F, Lopes-Martins R. Photoradiation in acute pain: a systematic review of possible mechanisms of action and clinical effects in randomized placebo-controlled trials. Photomed Laser Surg 2006; 24: 158–168.

[121] Kramer J, Sandrin M. Effect of low-power laser and white light on sensory conduction rate of the superficial radial nerve. Physiother Can 1993; 45:165–170.

[122] Cambier D, K. Blom, E. Witvrouw E, Ollevier G, De Muynck M, Vanderstraeten G. The influence of low intensity infrared laser irradiation on conduction characteristics of peripheral nerve: a randomised, controlled, double blind study on the sural nerve. Laser Med Sci 2000; 15:195–200.

[123] Telemeco T, Schrank E. The effect of light therapy on superficial radial nerve conduction using a clustered array of infrared superluminous diodes and red light emitting diodes. J Lasers Med Sci 2013; 4:17–24.

[124] Mezawa S, Iwata K, Naito K, Kamogawa H. 1988. The possible analgesic effect of soft-laser irradiation on heat nociceptors in the cat tongue. Archs Oral Biol 1988; 33: 693–694.

[125] Tsuchiya K, Kawatani M, Takeshige C, Sato T, Matsumoto I. Diode laser irradiation selectively diminishes slow component of axonal volleys to dorsal roots from the saphenous nerve in the rat. Neurosci Lett. 1993; 161: 65–68.

[126] Tsuchiya D, Kawatani M, Takeshige C. Laser irradiation abates neuronal responses to nociceptive stimulation of rat-paw skin. Brain Res Bull 1994; 34: 369–374.

Chapter 10

Intense Pulsed Light Therapy

Gu Weijie, Liu Hongmei and Liu Wei

Additional information is available at the end of the chapter

http://dx.doi.org/10.5772/65345

Abstract

Intense pulsed light (IPL) is one of the most effective nonablative approaches to treat skin photoaging. The broad range of wavelengths (500–1200 nm) emitted from IPL devices effectively target both melanin and hemoglobin in the skin. Numerous trials show the effectiveness and compatibility of IPL devices in a variety of skin conditions, especially in cosmetic indications such as hypertrichosis and telangiectasias. Compared with the wide clinical use of IPL, the biochemical and molecular mechanism is not clear. Both *in vivo* and *in vitro* studies demonstrate that IPL could increase the production of extracellular matrix, promote the proliferation of fibroblasts, and increase the secretion of TGF-β and matrix metalloproteinases, which play important roles in the photorejuvenation effects of IPL. However, investigations regarding the detailed underlying mechanism are necessary.

Keywords: intense pulsed light, photorejuvenation, fibroblast, collagen, matrix metalloprotease

1. Introduction

Intense pulse light (IPL) treatment currently represents one of the most popular nonablative photodamage skin treatments [1]. Initially, it was promoted as an approach for leg telangiectasias treatment. In continued use, this device was found to be of far greater utility for indications other than leg telangiectasias. IPL technology had its birthplace in San Diego in 1992, with the first commercial IPL system introduced in 1994, and cleared by the U.S. FDA in late 1995. In the last 22 years (1994–2016), more than 20 different laser companies have developed a wide variety of IPL devices, which testified the acceptance of IPL as a valid, efficacious technological breakthrough. First-generation IPL devices (Photoderm, ESC) emit light of the infrared part of the spectrum, which prevalently leads to epithelial damage and a high incidence of side effects. In second- (Vasculight VL, ESC) and third-generation IPL devices (Quantum SR, Lumenis), water filters out the infrared portion, significantly reducing the risk of side effects. The fourth-generation IPL devices (Lumenis one, Lumenis) have improved the defects of the existing IPL. They maximize the effectiveness and minimize the side effects by fairly transferring energy to the entire face. Their proportionate distribution of energy allows to treat not only the skin surface but also inside the dermis where discoloration originates.

IPL is now considered the gold standard for treatment of many signs of photoaging, including facial telangiectasias, hyperpigmentation, and fine wrinkling. The main advantages of IPL are the lower risk of postinflammatory hyperpigmentation, minimal recovery downtime, long-term improvement, etc. [1].

2. Main body

2.1. Biophysical interactions

IPL is situated in the visible light and infrared radiation of the electromagnetic spectrum (**Figure 1**). The broad range of wavelengths (500–1200 nm) emitted from IPL devices effectively target all the three main chromophores (hemoglobin, water, and melanin) in human skin [2]. The wavelength determines not only the absorption behavior but also the penetration depth of the light, which increases with the wavelength (**Figure 2**). Cut-off filters are used to eliminate the shorter than desired wavelengths from a particular treatment to focus the residual emissions on the feature to be treated. The patient's skin type and the skin condition determine the choice of suitable cut-off filters and therefore the spectrum of wavelengths to be emitted. In addition, to avoid the burning of the epidermis, the skin can be cooled by applying a thick layer of cold gel or, with newer models, by integrated cooling on the IPL crystal [3, 4]. Compared with lasers devices, an important advantage of the IPL system is its relatively large spot size, which can increase the speed of treatment given that large areas can be treated quickly with fewer pulses. However, the hand pieces are larger and have a flat surface, hindering treatment of irregular surfaces.

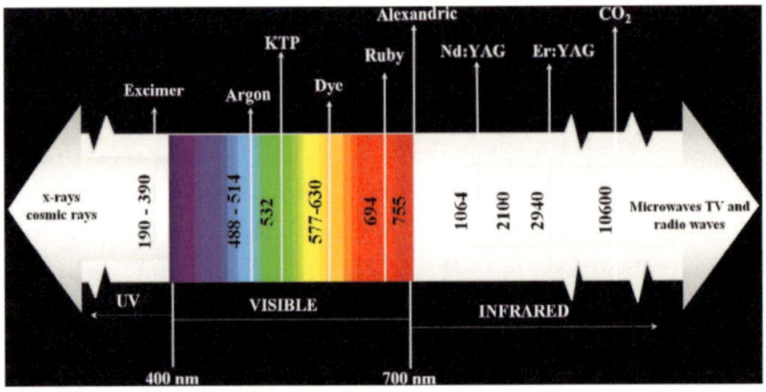

Figure 1. IPL is situated in the visible light and infrared radiation of the electromagnetic spectrum (reprinted with permission of Lumenis company, Yokneam, Israel).

http://dx.doi.org/10.5772/65345

Pulses can be delivered singly, doubly, or triply, with variable delay between the pulses. Pulse duration can range widely from 0.5 to over 20 ms. Selective photothermolysis is the basic principle of IPL treatment. This often leads to cell necrosis, blood coagulation, and structure alterations, which contribute to the clinical and side effects of IPL. To prevent unselective damage to the surrounding tissue, pulse duration should be lower than the thermal relaxation time of the target structure. The particular wavelengths combined with pulse durations, pulse intervals, and fluences facilitates the treatment of a wide spectrum of skin conditions, such as vascular lesions, pigmented lesions, fine wrinkling, and unwanted hair growth.

The incidence of acute side effects has been markedly reduced with the newest progressive set of parameters. Most side effects associated to IPL photodepilation are transient and minimal, including stinging pain, swelling, and erythema. Blistering and scattered crusting are permanent side effects of overfluenced treatment. Before IPL treatment, a signed informed consent is mandatory. Therapy sequelae and potential side effects have to be mentioned.

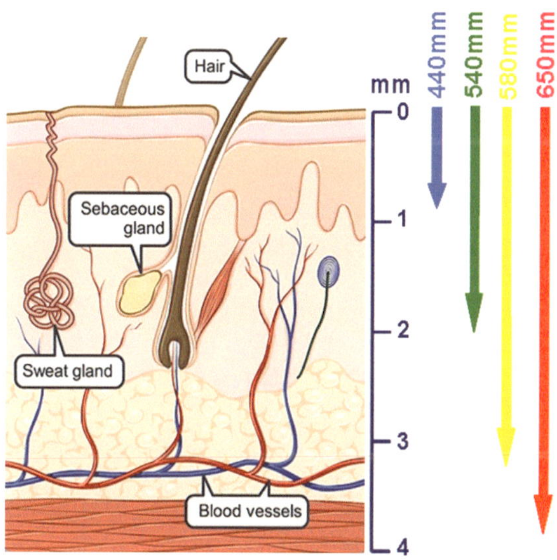

Figure 2. Depth of light penetration into the skin, at various wavelengths.

2.2. Indications of IPL therapy

2.2.1. Facial telangiectasias

Pulsed dye laser (PDL) is considered the gold standard for vascular lesions. However, this technique is limited by the need to achieve postoperative purpura that lasts 10–14 days. In contrast, the absence of postoperative purpura and minimized postprocedure downtime are main advantages of IPL technology. IPL is able to raise the blood vessel temperature high enough to cause its coagulation, leading to its destruction and replacement by fibrous granulation tissue. The successful treatment of vascular lesions with IPL depends on the type and size of vessels targeted, with cherry angiomas and superficial telangiectatic veins typically demonstrating the best response. A study analyzed the effect of IPL on facial telangiectasias and found that 79.2% of patients achieved greater than 50% reduction of vessels after one to four treatments [5]. In the largest study to date, Clementoni analyzed 1000 patients with telangiectasias treated using IPL and found that 89.7% experienced 75–100% improvement. These telangiectasias included leg veins that had no associated feeding reticular veins [6]. In our clinical experience, facial telangiectasias achieved marked improvement after IPL treatment (**Figure 3a** and **b**).

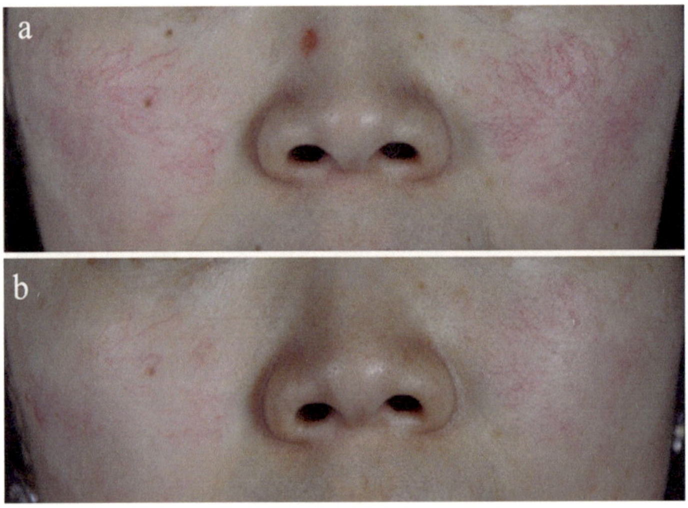

Figure 3. (a) Facial telangiectasias before treatment and (b) after a single IPL treatment. (reprinted with the permission of Liu Hongmei Laser Center, Huangsi Aesthetic Surgery Hospital, Beijing, China).

2.2.2. Pigmented lesions

Pigmented lesions are frequent targets of laser and IPL treatment. Deep (dermal) pigmented lesions such as melanocytic nevi, nevi of Ota and Ito, drug-induced hyperpigmentation, Becker's nevi, nevus spilus, and tattoos may be preferred to Q-switched lasers [7, 8]. Superficial pigments include solar lentigines, ephelides, café-au-lait macules, and epidermal melasma, which respond well to IPL. Moreno Arias published a study in which 20 patients with pigmented lesions were treated with IPL. They concluded that greater efficacy (76–100%) was attained with superficial lesions (ephelides, epidermal melasma, café-au-lait spots) compared with efficacy of less than 25% for deep lesions (Becker's nevus, epidermal nevus, and mixed melasma) [9–11]. It is important to carefully assess each patient's skin type preoperatively and adjust the IPL settings appropriately to avoid complications. In darker skin types, there is a risk of inducing hyperpigmentation. The immediate endpoint from IPL treatment of dyschromia should be visible darkening of the treated brown spots. These typically crust over 24–48 h and peel off within 7 days. Satisfied results were achieved in café-au-lait macules (**Figure 4a** and **b**) and ephelides (**Figure 5a** and **b**) treatment by IPL.

http://dx.doi.org/10.5772/65345

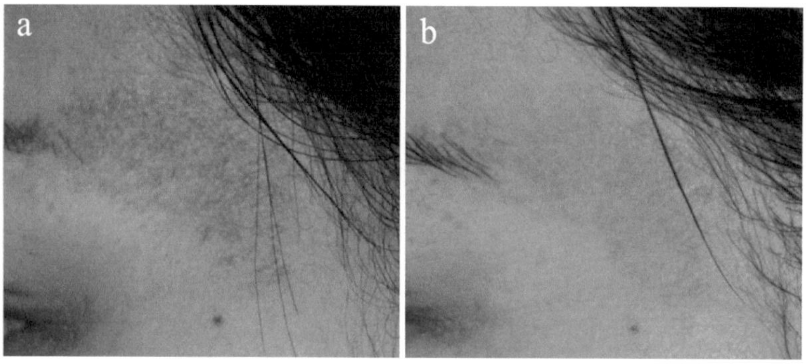

Figure 4. Café-au-lait macules (a) before treatment and (b) after a single IPL treatment (reprinted with the permission of Liu Hongmei).

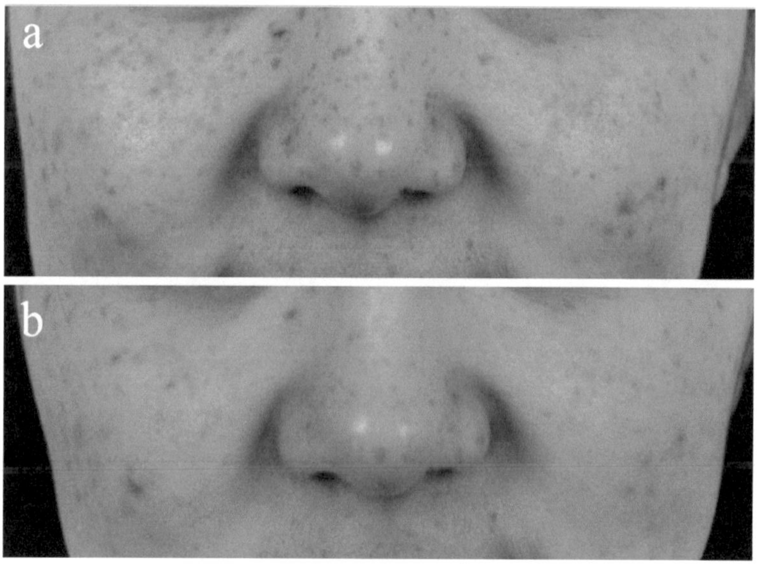

Figure 5. Ephelides (a) before treatment and (b) after a single IPL treatment.

Melasma is commonly seen in the Asian population. Traditional therapies including depigmenting agents, chemical peels, and Chinese medicine have some therapeutic effects but are often unsuccessful for refractory melasma. IPL technology provided an effective approach for melasma treatment. Over the last decade, the demand for IPL therapy in treating melasma has risen steadily, although IPL was traditionally considered as a second-line treatment. Li reported that 69 of 89 Chinese patients (77.5%) being treated for melasma improved by more than 50% following a total of four IPL treatments at 3-week intervals [12]. Recently, low-fluence IPL and fractionated IPL were used in treating melasma. The latter IPL system delivers more than 40 subpulses of 40 μs duration within milliseconds. In contrast to conventional IPL, fractionated IPL attenuates peak fluence and reduces nonselective heat diffusion, and is assumed to be safer than its conventional IPL. Bae demonstrated that low-fluence and short-pulse duration IPL at dose of 10 and 13 J significantly decreased the modified MASI score in 20 Korean melasma patients. Yun's study showed that fractionated IPL had modest effectiveness in female Asian melasma patients. With regard to safety, fractionated IPL is a good alternative to conventional IPL with no indication that it exacerbates melasma [13, 14]. They suggested that low-fluence IPL protocol could provide more effective treatment for melasma with minimal side effects in Asian skin.

2.2.3. Hair removal

Hair removal has become a key indication for IPL devices. Safe and long-lasting hair reduction in cosmetically undesirable locations can be achieved with IPL devices. These IPL systems emit red and infrared light with wavelengths ranging 600–1200 nm, which are capable of targeting melanin in the hair shaft, follicular epithelium, and hair matrix. During treatment, concomitant epidermal cooling sources help to minimize unwanted thermal injury induced by epidermal melanin (particularly in patients with darker skin) [15]. To protect the epidermal melanin from thermal injury, IPL pulses can be divided in synchronized millisecond pulses separated by short thermal relaxation times. The hair follicle is most susceptible to IPL treatment during the anagen phase. In addition, the darker the skin and the brighter the hair, the less effective the treatment will be (**Figure 6**).

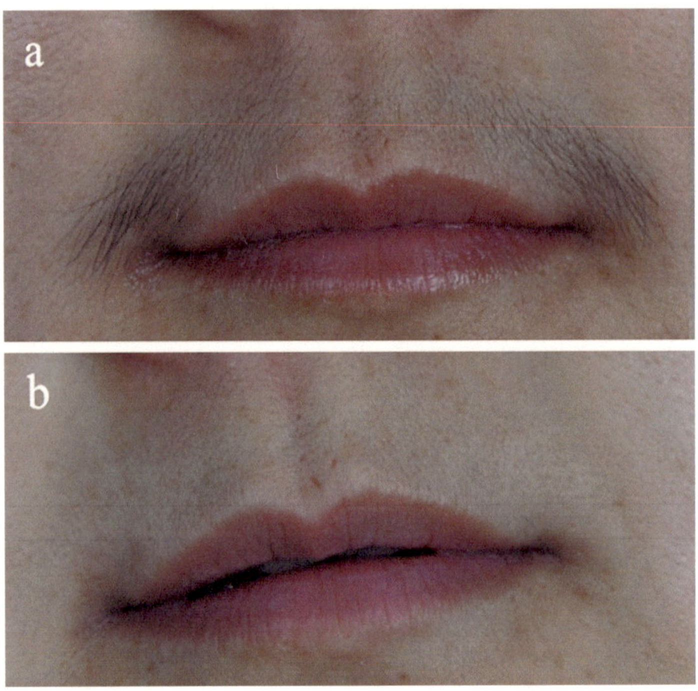

Figure 6. A woman with hypertrichosis (a) prior to treatment and (b) after five IPL treatments.

2.2.4. *Photorejuvenation*

Photorejuvenation has been described as a dynamic nonablative process involving the use of the IPL to reduce mottled pigmentation and telangiectasias and smooth the textural surface of the skin. There are two types of photorejuvenation: type I photorejuvenation refers to vascular anomalies, pigmentary changes, or pilosebaceous changes, while type II is related to dermal and subcutaneous senescence. Histologically, analysis showed that both type I and type III collagens increased after IPL treatment, whereas the elastin content decreased but elastin fibers were more neatly arranged. According to transmission electron microscope investigations, the amount of fibroblast activity increased, the fibroblasts were more active, and more collagen fibers were neatly rearranged within the stroma. Thus, morphological evidence exists for clinical improvement of the skin texture [16].

2.2.5. *Poikiloderma of Civatte*

Poikiloderma of Civatte consists of a reddish-brown reticolate pattern of pigmentation with associated telangiectasias and atrophic changes of the skin. There is no single effective treatment for poikiloderma of Civatte. Because of their ability to target vascular and pigment abnormalities simultaneously, IPL sources have been utilized in the treatment of poikiloderma of Civatte. Treatment of poikiloderma is one of the most effective uses of IPL technology [17]. In a previous study, 135 randomly selected patients with typical changes of poikiloderma of Civatte on the neck and/or upper chest underwent one to five IPL treatments [17]. Parameters included the 515- and 550-nm filters with pulse durations of 2–4 ms, either single or double with a 10-ms delay. Fluences were between 20 and 40 J/cm^2. Clearance over 75% of hyperpigmentation was reported.

2.2.6. *Rosacea*

Rosacea affects the appearance and can have important psychosocial effects.

Erythematotelangiectatic rosacea is the most common and may have the strongest vascular component among the four subtypes. Studies showed that IPL significantly reduces erythema and telangiectasia of rosacea and this is sustained for at least 6 months.

2.2.7. *Acne*

Acne vulgaris is a common disease in adolescents and young adults. Effective conventional therapies include oral and topical antibiotics and occasionally with oral and topical vitamin A. But these therapies were limited for adverse effects such as antibiotic resistance, teratogenicity, and skin dryness and irritation. IPL has been demonstrated to be an effective treatment for acne in Caucasians and Asian [18, 19]. Proposed mechanisms for the effects of our IPL therapy include photoinactivation of P. acnes and photothermolysis of the sebaceous glands, as well as anti-inflammatory action.

In our experience, significant improvement was observed in patients after two IPL treatments (**Figure 7a** and **b**).

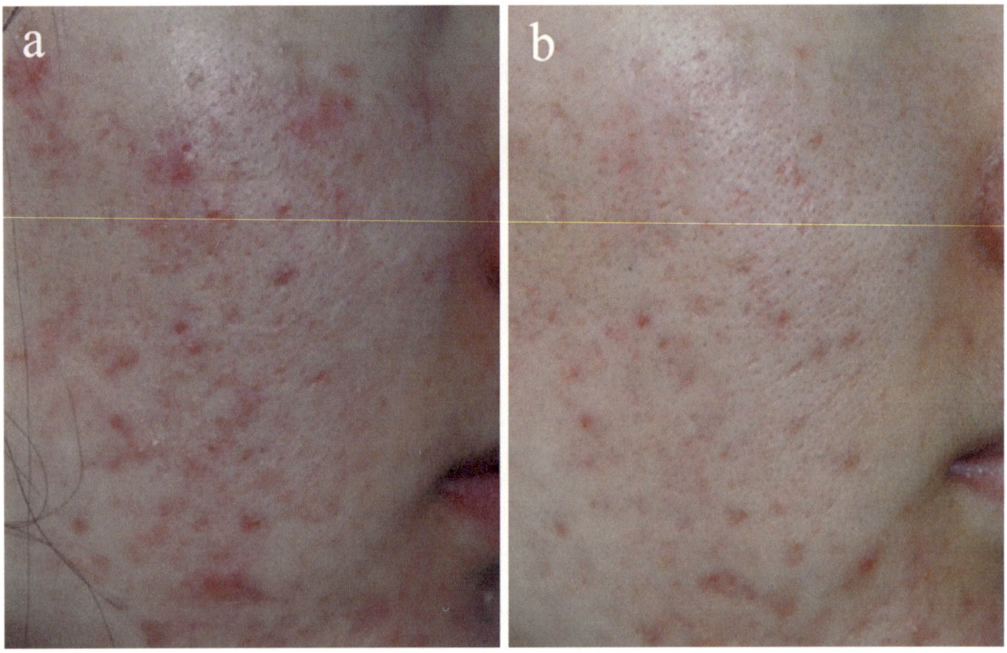

Figure 7. Acne vulgaris (a) before treatment and (b) after two IPL treatment.

2.2.8. Unconventional use of IPL

It is well known that UV irradiation resulted in DNA damage in microorganism. A study by Takeshita revealed that DNA damage, such as formation of single-strand breaks and pyrimidine dimers, was induced in IPL irradiated yeast cells. A new sterilization technique/technology based on the use of pulsed light, which has been developed by PurePulse Technologies (San Diego, CA, USA), is suggested to have great potential in the development of a new method of sterilization [20].

2.3. Mechanisms involved in IPL therapy

The efficacy of IPL in photorejuvenation of aged skin had been proven by numerous clinical trials. However, information regarding the precise mechanisms of IPL's actions is currently still far from complete, despite some achievements in recent years. The basic principle of IPL treatment is heating and selective photothermolysis, which can lead to cell necrosis (melanin damage), blood coagulation, and structure alterations. It has been proved that pigmented and vascular lesions treatment is based on the cell necrosis (melanin damage) and blood coagulation effects. The elimination of superficial wrinkles results from the structure alterations and collagen remodeling. However, the detailed mechanism involved in collagen remodeling, which many studies focus on, is not clear. Two aspects were included in the mechanism of IPL treatment, *in vivo* effects of IPL on the skin and *in vitro* effects of IPL on fibroblasts, cytokines, etc.

http://dx.doi.org/10.5772/65345

2.3.1. *In vivo effects of IPL on the skin*

Accumulation of procollagen I and procollagen III in porcine and human skin after IPL treatment has been documented by several studies [21, 22]. Enrique investigated the gross and microscopic changes after nonablative IPL facial resurfacing. All the patients showed clinical and microscopic improvement after IPL treatment. Microscopic improvement includes increased epidermal thickness, elimination of horny plugs, appearance of new rete ridges, and increase in the number of melanocytes and melanophages. Thickness of the epidermis showed a statistically significant increase after treatment ($p < 0.01$; 0.24 vs. 0.36) [23]. Elastosis and collagen damage showed improvement after treatment, the elastotic masses disappeared and showed a more orderly and fibrillar pattern, parallel to the basal cell layer. In Gu's study, similar increase in epidermal thickness was found in IPL irradiated human buttock skin (17 J/cm^2, four irradiations at 2-week intervals). Compared with the untreated control skin, IPL irradiated skin showed thicker stratum corneum and epidermis. Collagen fibers showed a more orderly pattern, parallel to the basal cell layer (**Figure 8a** and **b**). Immunohistochemistry showed more compactly arranged collagen I fibers and smaller interspaces in IPL-treated skin (**Figure 9a** and **b**).

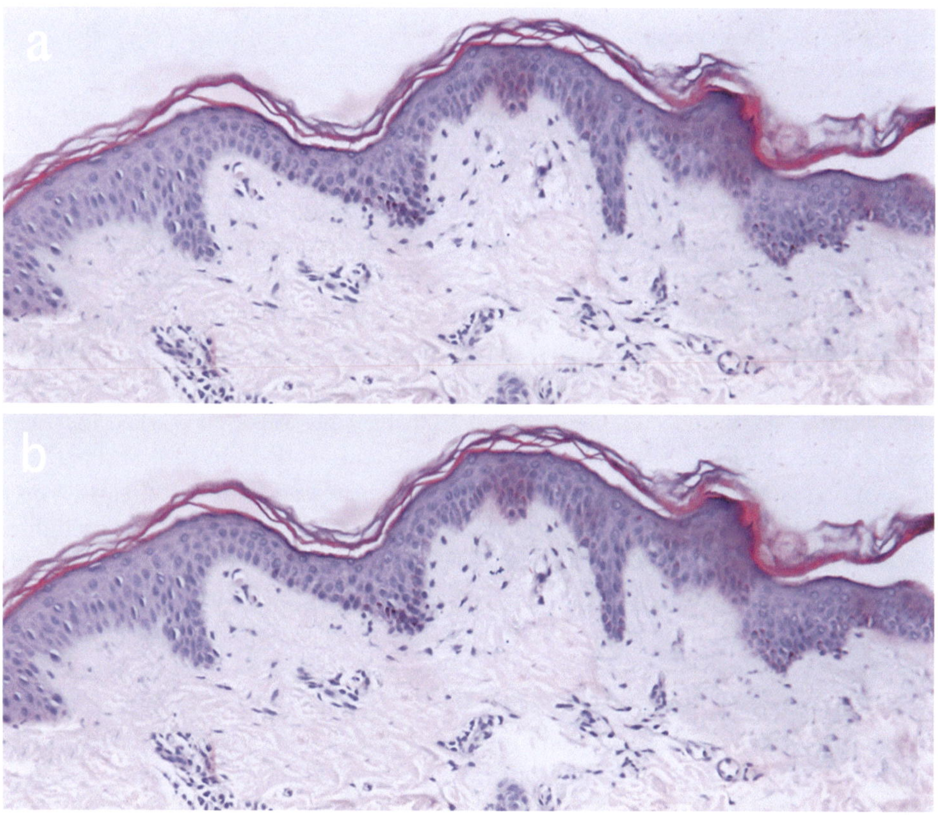

Figure 8. Histological manifestation in (a) untreated human buttock skin and (b) human buttock skin after four IPL irradiations (hematoxylin and eosin staining, magnification 10×).

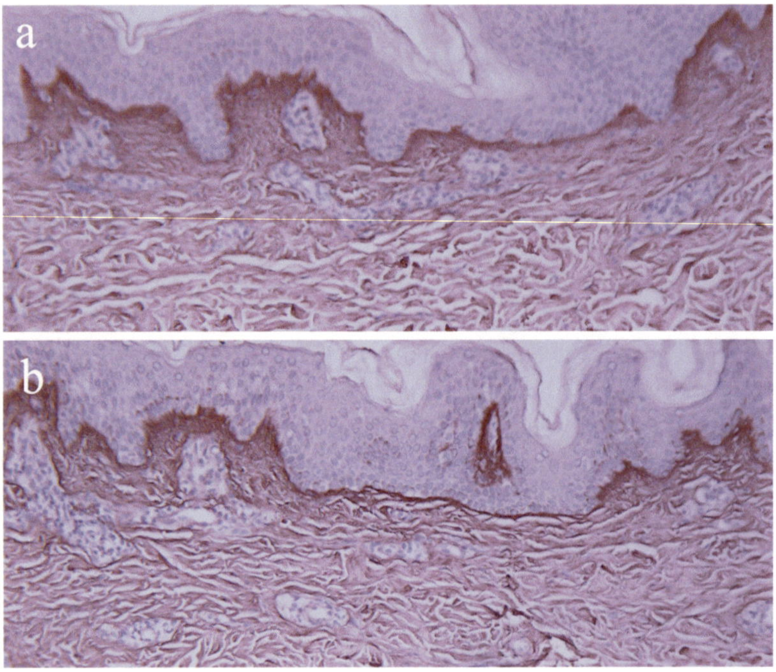

Figure 9. Collagen I fibers in (a) untreated human buttock skin and (b) human buttock skin after four IPL irradiations (immunohistochemistry, magnification 10×).

Matrix metalloproteases (MMPs) play important roles in many physiological and pathological processes, such as skin ageing, wound healing, and even in tumor invasion. In the process of IPL photorejuvenation, MMPs are thought to be responsible for the turnover and degradation of extracellular matrix (ECM) [24, 25]. MMPs are composed of 23 family members, the main target molecules being connective tissue and basement membrane proteins (e.g., all types of collagens [both native and denatured ones, i.e., gelatins], laminins, integrins, elastin, proteoglycans, fibronectin, vitronectin, tenascins, etc.) Orringer has revealed marked increases in messenger RNA levels of MMP-1, MMP-3, MMP-9, and MMP-13 in carbon dioxide laser resurfaced photodamaged human skin. Wang detected increased MMP-1 and TIMP-1 protein levels in IPL-irradiated rat skin, which concord with Orringer's study. They proposed that the increased matrix metalloproteinase may play a constructive role in collagen synthesis in the IPL-activated wound healing process [26, 27]. On the contrary, Luo found increased procollagens but decreased matrix metalloproteinase mRNA levels in BALB/C mouse skin, suggesting IPL irradiation can not only enhance new collagen production, but also decrease collagen degradation though downregulation of MMP [28]. So far, few studies documented decreased matrix metalloproteinase mRNA levels in IPL-irradiated skin *in vivo*. Gu confirmed the elevation of MMP protein levels in IPL-treated human buttock skin. In addition, by comparing with the UVA-induced MMP expression patterns, they found that IPL induced a different MMP expression pattern (remarkable increase of MMP-1, MMP-3, and MMP-12 in UVA-exposed skin, while lower MMP-1, MMP-3, and MMP-12 but higher MMP-9 levels in IPL-irradiated skin). They proposed MMP-1, MMP-3, and MMP-12 could play a destructive role, whereas MMP-9 may play a constructive one in ECM metabolism (**Figures 10a** and **b**, **11a** and **b**, and **12a** and **b**).

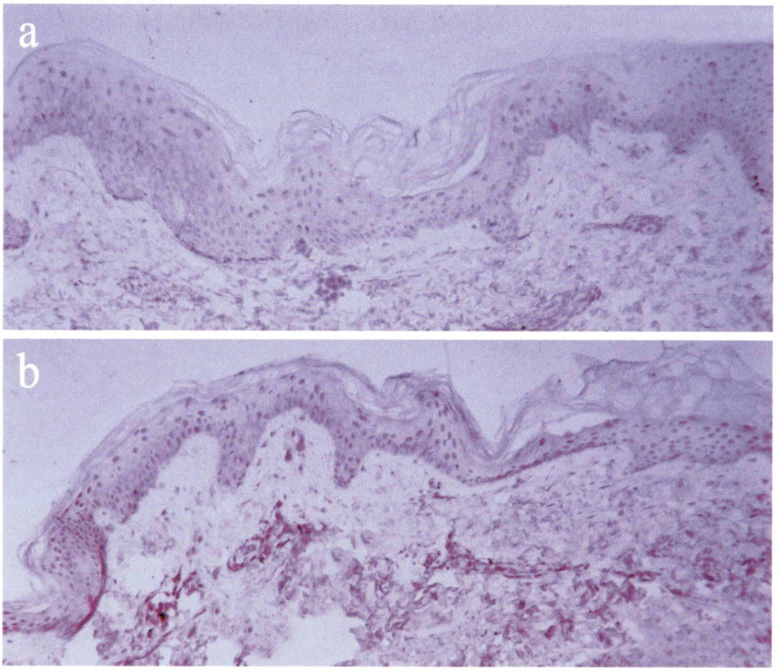

Figure 10. Protein expression of MMP-1 before (a) and after (b) IPL irradiation (immunohistochemistry, magnification 10×).

Transforming growth factor-β (TGF-β) is a major regulator of the synthesis of ECM proteins in human skin as it stimulate fibroblast proliferation and collagen production. A study by Wang showed that TGF-β may be involved in the IPL photorejuvenation process. *In situ* hybridization showed strong positive TGF-β1 mRNA expression levels in rat skin 7 days after IPL exposure, as compared with the negative TGF-β1 mRNA expression in the nonexposed skin. Thus, they suggest TGF-β1 plays an important role in photorejuvenation [29]. Ali's study confirmed that IPL elicits a statistically significant increase in epidermal TGF-β1 expression 48 h following the first treatment session, and this increase was maintained 1 week following the last treatment session. The induction of TGF-β1 was epidermal and limited to the upper differentiated layers of the epidermis [30]. However, another study by El-Domyati showed no significant differences ($p < 0.05$) in TGF-β1 protein expression levels among the IPL-treated and the control groups (baseline [before treatment]; end of treatment [after 3 months]; posttreatment [6 months after the start of treatment]) [31], which did not concord with Ali's study. This may be due to the different time points to obtain skin biopsies (the former detected the TGF-β1 7 days after IPL irradiation, whereas the latter obtained the biopsies 3 and 6 months after IPL irradiation) and different IPL devices and parameters.

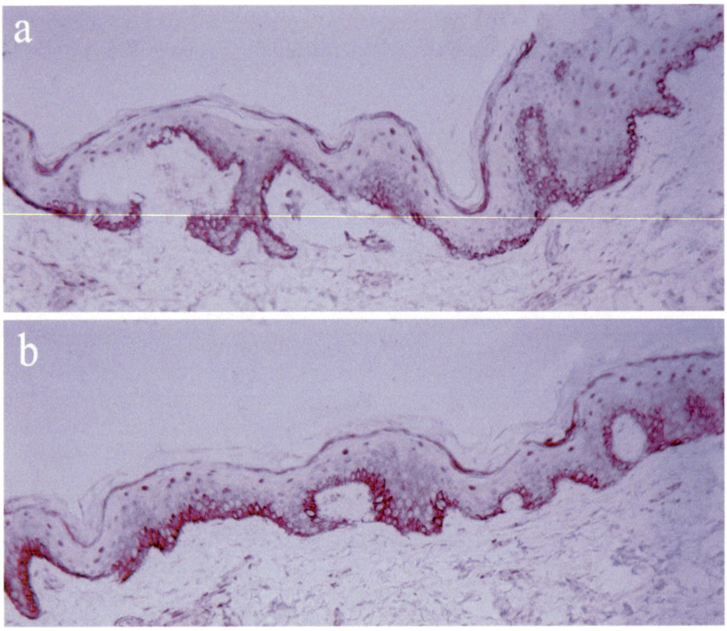

Figure 11. Protein expression of MMP-3 before (a) and after (b) IPL irradiation (immunohistochemistry, magnification 10×).

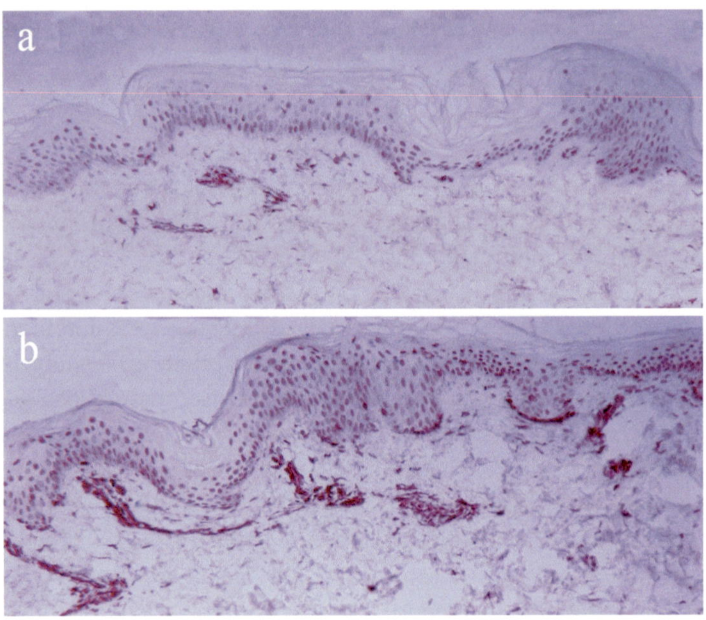

Figure 12. Protein expression of MMP-9 before (a) and after (b) IPL irradiation (immunohistochemistry, magnification 10×).

http://dx.doi.org/10.5772/65345

Some results indicated that IPL activates a wound healing process and leads to vascular formation, which may play roles in IPL photorejuvenation. Recently, a study with mouse island skin flap model revealed that IPL at lower dose could improve wound healing through the dilation of tissue vasculature and heat-shock protein production [32]. An investigation by Wu demonstrated that IPL irradiation significantly enhanced aquaporin 3 protein levels in rat skin, which is responsible for substratum corneum hydration, biosynthesis of the substratum corneum, and wound healing process [33].

2.3.2. *In vitro effects of IPL on fibroblasts, cytokines, etc*

IPL treatment has been shown to be highly effective for skin rejuvenation but the biochemical and molecular mechanism are not well known. Fibroblasts secrete procollagen and then covert it to collagen, which is an important component of ECM. Effects of IPL on fibroblasts were focused by many *in vitro* studies.

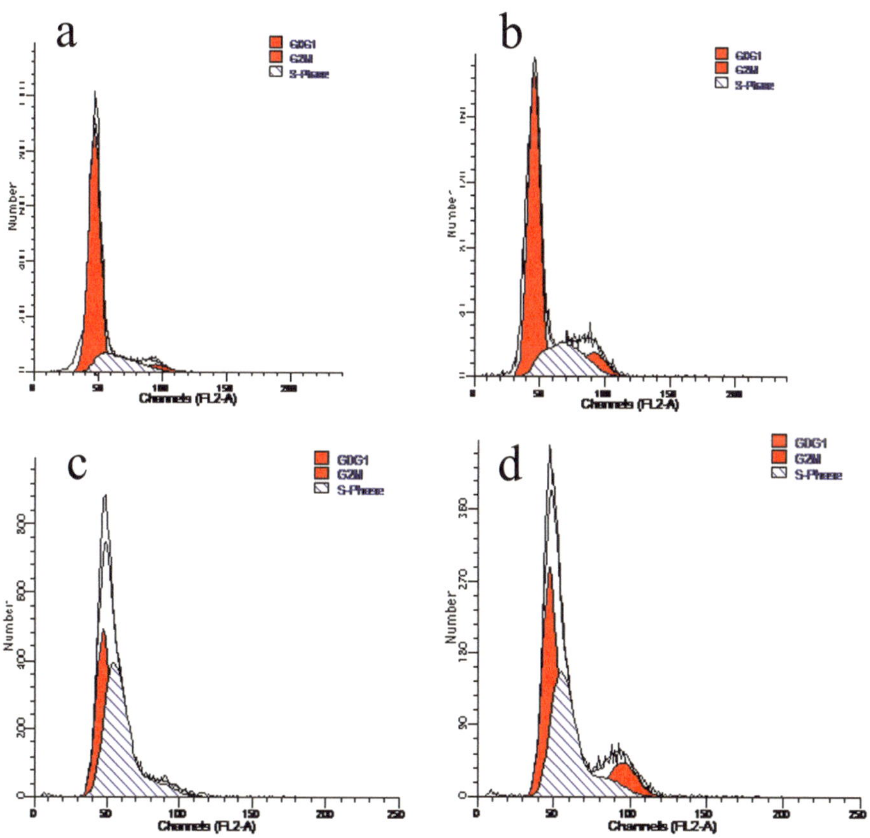

Figure 13. Cell cycle in fibroblasts was assessed by flow cytometry after cells were stained with PI. (a) Control group, (b) UVA I irradiated group, (c) IPL irradiated group, and (d) IPL irradiation after PUVA exposure. Cells were stained by PI before flow cytometry. IPL irradiation, wavelength 570–960 nm, pulse duration 12 ms, energy intensity 15 J/cm^2, irradiated once a day, for 2 days.

Liu investigated the effects of IPL and UVA on fibroblasts proliferation. In untreated control group, most cells were in cell cycle phase G1, while minor cells were in cell cycle phase S. UVA I irradiated group was designed to construct a cell injury model and compare the effects of IPL and UVA on human skin fibroblasts. Compared with the control, UVA induced no significant changes in proportion of cells in cycle phase S, as well as cell cycle phase G2. As compared with the UVA I irradiated group and the control group, the UVA+IPL group (fibroblasts irradiated with IPL after PUVA exposure) proliferate at a faster rate ($p < 0.05$) [34] (**Figure 13a–d**).

Cells were also stained by CCK-8 and assessed by flow cytometry to detect the proliferation ability. Note that 72 h after therapeutic dose of IPL irradiation, results showed an increase of cell proliferating index than the control ($p < 0.01$). As compared with the UVA I irradiated group, the UVA+IPL group increased in cell proliferating index ($p < 0.05$). Cell cycle protein cyclin D1 and CDK2 expression levels were also upregulated after IPL irradiation (**Figure 14**).

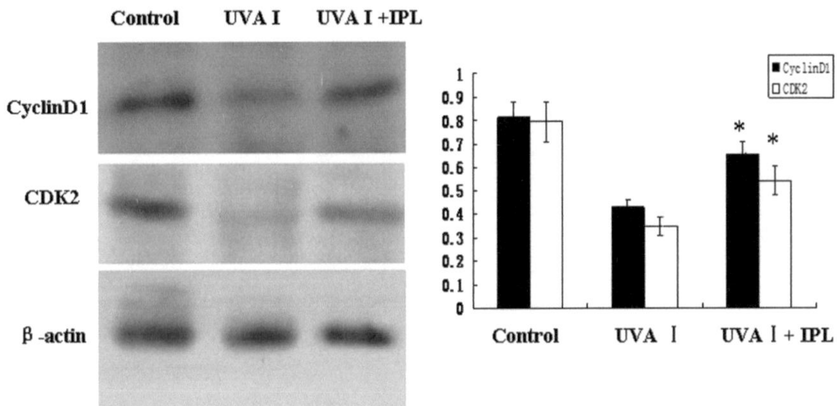

Figure 14. Cyclin D1 and CDK2 protein expression levels were detected by Western blot.

Cuerda-Galindo did a series of studies regarding the effects of IPL on fibroblasts. Their study showed that SA Filter 800–1200 nm using a 60.1 J/cm^2 energy density double-pulse induces a significant skin fibroblast proliferation. Note that 48 h after IPL irradiation, 1BR3G human skin fibroblasts were observed to proliferate at a faster rate, showing a significant increase of cells in S and G2/M cell cycle phases (S cell cycle phase, 8.23 vs. 10; G2/M cell cycle phase, 8.63 vs. 17.5), which is consistent with the results of Liu [34].

Further studies show IPL could reverse or rejuvenate the cell senescence in fibroblasts. Wang evaluated the influence of IPL irradiation on 8-methoxypsoralen plus ultraviolet-A irradiation (PUVA)-induced senescence of fibroblasts. In their study, PUVA treatment increased the number of SA-β-gal-positive fibroblasts, increased the level of ROS, and shortened the telomere length. However, irradiation with IPL after PUVA exposure decreased the number of SA-β-gal-positive cells, decreased the ROS level, and prevented telomere shortening, in comparison with PUVA treatment only ($p < 0.05$) (**Figure 15a–c**). They proposed that irradiation with IPL after PUVA exposure partially rejuvenated the cells, demonstrating a protective effect against PUVA-induced fibroblast senescence [36].

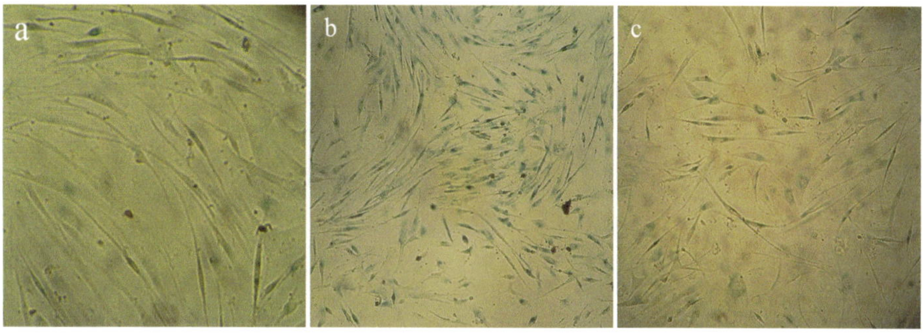

Figure 15. The staining of SA-β-gal in (a) control (untreated) human fibroblasts, (b) PUVA-induced senescence of fibroblasts, and (c) fibroblasts irradiated with IPL after PUVA exposure (reprinted with the permission of Wang Ruiyan).

It is well known that collagen in the dermis is mainly composed of type I (80%) and III (10%) collagens, which are responsible for the elasticity and integrity of the skin. Fibroblasts secrete procollagens and then convert them into collagens, which decreased in photoaged skin. More and more studies have proved that IPL irradiation could promote the production of collagens in fibroblasts [21, 22]. Besides collagen, other molecular components are present and contribute to the overall mechanical properties of skin. Among the noncollagenous components of the dermis, there are proteoglycans (PG), glycosaminoglycan conjugated proteins (GAG), hyaluronic acid, and versican, which are important constituents of human skin connective tissue and essential for maintaining mechanical strength of the skin. A study by Cuerda-Galindo detected an increase in the amount of collagens, accompanied by an elevation in protein production of hyaluronic acid and versican, which can be a possible mechanism of action for IPL devices in aging skin treatment [35, 37].

When referred to the biochemical and molecular mechanism of IPL treatment, three aspects should be mentioned: fibroblasts proliferation, ECM production, and ECM degrading enzymes. MMPs are endopeptidases that perform a degradative function, generally targeting the extracellular matrix. MMP1 is called collagenase and its main substrate are collagen type III, I, II, VII, and X. Although it is well established that MMP expression was increased in damaged or photoaged skin [38, 39], Cuerda-Galindo observed MMP-1 increased following IPL irradiation, consistent with the previous findings induced by laser treatment [40, 41]. Based on the above theories, these authors speculate that increased MMP could be an overlooked mechanism of skin rejuvenation, in which it will be implicated, contributing to the degradation of senescent collagens and then the turnover of the ECM [35]. So, it is reasonable that upregulation of MMPs levels following IPL irradiation did not contradict with the photorejuvenation effects and upregulation of collagen levels.

According to the effects of IPL on MMPs levels, there was another tendency, the downregulation of MMPs levels following IPL irradiation. Wong demonstrated reduced protein levels of MMP-2, MMP-14, and TIMP-2 in primary human skin fibroblasts following IPL irradiation [28]. Other authors reported that the IPL management had no impact on MMP secretion levels in fibroblasts [42]. More than the stimulation of ECM proteins production observed by many studies, they postulate that photorejuvenation effect of IPL also involves the inhibition of

MMPs and therefore the decrease of ECM protein destruction [43]. Recent studies demonstrated that significant differences in the expression of MMP (down- and upregulation) may be related to the laser parameters such as wavelength and fluence [44, 45].

TGF-β acts as a multifunctional cytokine in regulating cell growth and differentiation and the biosynthesis of ECM proteins. Previous studies confirmed that TGF-β substantially increases elastin and type I collagen expression, via a Smads signaling pathway [46, 47]. Wong's study verified upregulated expression of collagen III and TGF-β in dermal fibroblasts cultured within contracted collagen lattices, provided a potential mechanistic explanation for the mechanism of clinical photorejuvenation effects of IPL. This was verified by Byun, who observed slight increases in TGF-β1 mRNA and protein levels after IPL treatment.

Other cytokines involved in IPL treatment include interleukin 10 (IL-10), one of the regulatory cytokines that inhibit cytokine production in activated T lymphocytes and antigen-presenting cells. In Byun's study, IL-10 protein increased up to 5.95-fold in IPL-irradiated cultured keratinocytes (HaCaT cells), which may contribute to the anti-inflammatory effect and the therapeutic benefit of IPL for inflammatory dermatoses such as acne vulgaris [48].

To determine the principal mechanism that is involved in IPL hair removal treatment, the hair structures targeted by IPL were observed. Human scalp specimens were exposed *ex vivo* to IPL pulses and were then processed for histological analysis, immunofluorescence labeling of keratin 19, and endogenous alkaline phosphatase activity. Histological analysis confirmed that the melanin-rich matrix cells of the bulb in anagen follicles and the hair shaft are principally targeted by IPL treatment, while white hairs and epidermis remained unaffected. Damage caused by heat sometimes extended over the dermal papilla cells, while stem cells were mostly spared [49]. Collateral damage does not deplete stem cells. Damage at the dermal papilla was observed only with high-energy treatment modalities. These observations histologically verified the mechanism of IPL hair removal technology, explained why some hairs grow back after a single IPL treatment.

3. Summary

IPL systems are a successful and a noninvasive means of treatment, providing a viable alternative to laser systems and conventional therapeutic options when it comes to treating a series of indications, such as telangiectasias, skin photoaging, dyspigmentation, and unwanted hair. Compared with the wide clinical use, molecular mechanism involved in IPL therapy has not been thoroughly investigated. However, there are enough data to show that various biological effects have been shown to be exerted via IPL including fibroblasts proliferation, collagen production, and MMP secretion. It has also been shown that IPL protect PUVA induced senesce of fibroblasts. Advances have been made with respect to mechanism of IPL therapy, but a great deal is still unknown.

http://dx.doi.org/10.5772/65345

Author details

Gu Weijie[1], Liu Hongmei[2] and Liu Wei[1*]

*Address all correspondence to: lwei5811@126.com

1 Department of Dermatology, The General Hospital of Air Force, Beijing, China

2 Laser Center, Huangsi Aesthetic Surgery Hospital, Beijing, China

References

[1] Goldman MP, Weiss RA, Weiss MA. Intense pulsed light as a nonablative approach to photoaging. Dermatol Surg. 2005 Sep;31(9 Pt 2):1179–87; discussion 87.

[2] Steiner R. Laser-Tissue Interactions [A]. In: Raulin C GB(ed). Laser and IPL Technology in Dermatologic and Aesthetic Medicine[M]. 1st ed. Springer, Heidelberg, Germany; 2011.1:23.

[3] Goldman MP. Treatment of benign vascular lesions with the photoderm VL high-intensity pulsed light source. Adv Dermatol. 1997;13:503–21.

[4] Sadick NS, Weiss R. Intense pulsed-light photorejuvenation. Semin Cutan Med Surg. 2002 Dec;21(4):280–7.

[5] Bjerring P, Christiansen K, Troilius A. Intense pulsed light source for treatment of facial telangiectasias. J Cosmet Laser Ther. 2001 Dec;3(4):169–73.

[6] Clementoni MT, Gilardino P, Muti GF, Signorini M, Pistorale A, Morselli PG, et al. Intense pulsed light treatment of 1,000 consecutive patients with facial vascular marks. Aesthetic Plast Surg. 2006 Mar–Apr;30(2):226–32.

[7] Tanzi EL, Lupton JR, Alster TS. Lasers in dermatology: four decades of progress. J Am Acad Dermatol. 2003 Jul;49(1):1–31; quiz-4.

[8] Kilmer SL, Garden JM. Laser treatment of pigmented lesions and tattoos. Semin Cutan Med Surg. 2000 Dec;19(4):232–44.

[9] Kawada A, Shiraishi H, Asai M, Kameyama H, Sangen Y, Aragane Y, et al. Clinical improvement of solar lentigines and ephelides with an intense pulsed light source. Dermatol Surg. 2002 Jun;28(6):504–8.

[10] Sasaya H, Kawada A, Wada T, Hirao A, Oiso N. Clinical effectiveness of intense pulsed light therapy for solar lentigines of the hands. Dermatol Ther. 2012 Nov–Dec;24(6):584–6.

[11] Moreno Arias GA, Ferrando J. Intense pulsed light for melanocytic lesions. Dermatol Surg. 2001 Apr;27(4):397–400.

[12] Li YH, Chen JZ, Wei HC, Wu Y, Liu M, Xu YY, et al. Efficacy and safety of intense pulsed light in treatment of melasma in Chinese patients. Dermatol Surg. 2008 May;34(5):693–700; discussion 1.

[13] Bae MI, Park JM, Jeong KH, Lee MH, Shin MK. Effectiveness of low-fluence and short-pulse intense pulsed light in the treatment of melasma: a randomized study. J Cosmet Laser Ther. 2015;17(6):292–5.

[14] Yun WJ, Lee SM, Han JS, Lee SH, Chang SY, Haw S, et al. A prospective, split-face, randomized study of the efficacy and safety of a novel fractionated intense pulsed light treatment for melasma in Asians. J Cosmet Laser Ther. 2015;17(5):259–66.

[15] Dierickx CC. Hair removal by lasers and intense pulsed light sources. Dermatol Clin. 2002 Jan;20(1):135–46.

[16] Feng Y, Zhao J, Gold MH. Skin rejuvenation in Asian skin: the analysis of clinical effects and basic mechanisms of intense pulsed light. J Drugs Dermatol. 2008 Mar;7(3):273–9.

[17] Weiss RA, Goldman MP, Weiss MA. Treatment of poikiloderma of Civatte with an intense pulsed light source. Dermatol Surg. 2000 Sep;26(9):823–7; discussion 8.

[18] Kawana S, Tachihara R, Kato T, Omi T. Effect of smooth pulsed light at 400 to 700 and 870 to 1,200 nm for acne vulgaris in Asian skin. Dermatol Surg. 2009;36(1):52–7.

[19] Choi YS, Suh HS, Yoon MY, Min SU, Lee DH, Suh DH. Intense pulsed light vs. pulsed-dye laser in the treatment of facial acne: a randomized split-face trial. J Eur Acad Dermatol Venereol. 2009 Jul;24(7):773–80.

[20] Takeshita K, Shibato J, Sameshima T, Fukunaga S, Isobe S, Arihara K, et al. Damage of yeast cells induced by pulsed light irradiation. Int J Food Microbiol. 2003 Aug;85(1–2): 151–8.

[21] Goldberg DJ. New collagen formation after dermal remodeling with an intense pulsed light source. J Cutan Laser Ther. 2000 Jun;2(2):59–61.

[22] Iyer S, Carranza D, Kolodney M, Macgregor D, Chipps L, Soriano T. Evaluation of procollagen I deposition after intense pulsed light treatments at varying parameters in a porcine model. J Cosmet Laser Ther. 2007 Jun;9(2):75–8.

[23] Hernandez-Perez E, Ibiett EV. Gross and microscopic findings in patients submitted to nonablative full-face resurfacing using intense pulsed light: a preliminary study. Dermatol Surg. 2002 Aug;28(8):651–5.

[24] Bruckner-Tuderman L. Biology of the extracellular matrix. In: Bolognia JL, Jorizzo, JL, Rapini, RP, editors. Dermatology. 2nd ed. London: Elsevier; 2007. pp. 1447–54.

[25] Sardy M. Role of matrix metalloproteinases in skin ageing. Connect Tissue Res. 2009;50(2):132–8.

[26] Wang ML, Liu DL, Yuan Q, Du, B.J. Study of effect of intense pulsed light on TIMP-1 expression in rat skin. Chin J Aesth Med. 2006;15:122–5.

[27] Wang ML, Liu DL, Yuan Q. Effect of intense pulsed light on MMP-1 expression in rat skin. Chin J Aesth Plast Surg. 2006;17:392–4.

[28] Luo D, Cao Y, Wu D, Xu Y, Chen B, Xue Z. Impact of intense pulse light irradiation on BALB/c mouse skin-in vivo study on collagens, matrix metalloproteinases and vascular endothelial growth factor. Lasers Med Sci. 2009 Jan;24(1):101–8.

[29] Wang ML, Liu DL, Yuan Q, Du BJ. Effect of intense pulsed light on transforming growth factor-β1 mRNA expression in rat skin. J South Med Univ. 2009;29(1):92–6.

[30] Ali MM, Porter RM, Gonzalez ML. Intense pulsed light enhances transforming growth factor beta1/Smad3 signaling in acne-prone skin. J Cosmet Dermatol. 2013 Sep;12(3): 195–203.

[31] El-Domyati M, El-Ammawi TS, Medhat W, Moawad O, Mahoney MG, Uitto J. Expression of transforming growth factor-beta after different non-invasive facial rejuvenation modalities. Int J Dermatol. 2015 Apr;54(4):396–404.

[32] Cao MT, Xuan HD, Thi NP. Effects of intense pulsed light on tissue vascularity and wound healing: a study with mouse island skin flap model. Plast Surg Int. 2015;2015:429367.

[33] Wu CJ, Chen CC, Shih HS, Chang LR, Liu CH, Liu YT, et al. Effect of intense pulsed light on the expression of aquaporin 3 in rat skin. Lasers Med Sci. 2015 Sep;30(7):1959–65.

[34] Liu HM, Liu W, Zhao XZ, Tian Y, Yuan XY, Wang RY. Protective effect of intense pulsed light on fibroblast injury induced by UVA I. Chinese J Med Aest Cosmetol. 2011;17(2): 117–20.

[35] Cuerda-Galindo E, Diaz-Gil G, Palomar-Gallego MA, Linares-GarciaValdecasas R. Increased fibroblast proliferation and activity after applying intense pulsed light 800–1200 nm. Ann Anat. 2015 Mar;198:66–72.

[36] Wang R, Liu W, Gu W, Zhang P. Intense pulsed light protects fibroblasts against the senescence induced by 8-methoxypsoralen plus ultraviolet-A irradiation. Photomed Laser Surg. 2011 Oct;29(10):685–90.

[37] Cuerda-Galindo E, Diaz-Gil G, Palomar-Gallego MA, Linares-GarciaValdecasas R. Intense pulsed light induces synthesis of dermal extracellular proteins in vitro. Lasers Med Sci. 2015 Sep;30(7):1931–9.

[38] Jansen PL, Rosch R, Jansen M, Binnebosel M, Junge K, Alfonso-Jaume A, et al. Regulation of MMP-2 gene transcription in dermal wounds. J Invest Dermatol. 2007 Jul;127(7):1762–7.

[39] Ohnishi Y, Tajima S, Akiyama M, Ishibashi A, Kobayashi R, Horii I. Expression of elastin-related proteins and matrix metalloproteinases in actinic elastosis of sun-damaged skin. Arch Dermatol Res. 2000 Jan;292(1):27–31.

[40] Kuo YR, Wu WS, Jeng SF, Wang FS, Huang HC, Lin CZ, et al. Suppressed TGF-beta1 expression is correlated with up-regulation of matrix metalloproteinase-13 in keloid regression after flashlamp pulsed-dye laser treatment. Lasers Surg Med. 2005 Jan;36(1):38–42.

[41] Orringer JS, Kang S, Johnson TM, Karimipour DJ, Hamilton T, Hammerberg C, et al. Connective tissue remodeling induced by carbon dioxide laser resurfacing of photo-damaged human skin. Arch Dermatol. 2004 Nov;140(11):1326–32.

[42] Wu D, Zhou B, Xu Y, Yin Z, Luo D. Impact of intense pulsed light irradiation on cultured primary fibroblasts and a vascular endothelial cell line. Exp Ther Med. 2009 Oct;4(4):669–74.

[43] Wong WR, Shyu WL, Tsai JW, Hsu KH, Lee HY, Pang JH. Intense pulsed light modulates the expressions of MMP-2, MMP-14 and TIMP-2 in skin dermal fibroblasts cultured within contracted collagen lattices. J Dermatol Sci. 2008 Jul;51(1):70–3.

[44] Dang Y, Ye X, Weng Y, Tong Z, Ren Q. Effects of the 532-nm and 1,064-nm Q-switched Nd:YAG lasers on collagen turnover of cultured human skin fibroblasts: a comparative study. Lasers Med Sci. 2010 Sep;25(5):719–26.

[45] Huang J, Luo X, Lu J, Chen J, Zuo C, Xiang Y, et al. IPL irradiation rejuvenates skin collagen via the bidirectional regulation of MMP-1 and TGF-beta1 mediated by MAPKs in fibroblasts. Lasers Med Sci. 2011 May;26(3):381–7.

[46] Kucich U, Rosenbloom JC, Abrams WR, Rosenbloom J. Transforming growth factor-beta stabilizes elastin mRNA by a pathway requiring active Smads, protein kinase C-delta, and p38. Am J Respir Cell Mol Biol. 2002 Feb;26(2):183–8.

[47] Ghosh AK, Yuan W, Mori Y, Varga J. Smad-dependent stimulation of type I collagen gene expression in human skin fibroblasts by TGF-beta involves functional cooperation with p300/CBP transcriptional coactivators. Oncogene. 2000 Jul;19(31):3546–55.

[48] Byun JY, Choi HY, Myung KB, Choi YW. Expression of IL-10, TGF-beta(1) and TNF-alpha in cultured keratinocytes (HaCaT Cells) after IPL treatment or ALA-IPL photodynamic treatment. Ann Dermatol. 2009 Feb;21(1):12–7.

[49] Larouche D, Kim DH, Ratte G, Beaumont C, Germain L. Effect of intense pulsed light treatment on human skin in vitro: analysis of immediate effects on dermal papillae and hair follicle stem cells. Br J Dermatol. 2013 Oct;169(4):859–68.

Chapter 11

Biological Function of Low Reactive Level Laser Therapy (LLLT)

Toshihiro Kushibiki and Miya Ishihara

Additional information is available at the end of the chapter

http://dx.doi.org/10.5772/65747

Abstract

Low reactive level laser therapy (LLLT) and photobiomodulation are mainly focused on the activation of intracellular or extracellular photoabsorbable molecule (chromophore) and the initiation of cellular signaling using low power lasers and lights. Over the past 40 decades, a number of basic and clinical researches were reported that the laser therapy had the potential to improve wound healing and reduce pain and inflammation. In recent years, the term "LLLT" has become widely recognized. In this review, the mechanisms of action of LLLT at a cellular level are described. Finally, our recent research results that LLLT enhanced the cells differentiation are also described.

Keywords: low reactive level laser therapy (LLLT), intracellular chromophore, regulation of gene expression

1. Introduction

Low reactive level laser therapy (LLLT) is a form of medical treatment in which human tissue is irradiated with a low-powered laser (on the order of several 100 mW) to induce therapeutic changes. In an attempt to explore the carcinogenic potential of laser light, Mester et al. applied a low-powered ruby laser with a 694-nm wavelength to the shaved dorsal skin of mice [1]. Contrary to their expectations, the laser irradiation did not cause cancer, but instead improved hair growth. As the first study to document the biological effect of lasers, their findings became a springboard for subsequent LLLT research. Although light-based therapies had been used for a long time, and ultraviolet therapy has a history longer than a century [2], the work of Mester et al. was significant in demonstrating the effects of laser light, which has the unique characteristics of monochromaticity and coherence. Following subsequent experiments, Mester and colleagues reported in 1971 that low-level laser rays accelerated wound healing [3]. From this time onward, experimental and clinical studies demonstrated many therapeutic effects of LLLT, including improvements in wound healing, collagen synthesis, cell proliferation, fracture repair, and local blood circulation, as well as suppression of inflammation and pain. These effects will be explained in more details in the sections to follow. The accumulated volume of clinical research suggests that LLLT has the potential to gain wide acceptance in clinical practice as a modality with few adverse effects. Today, however, that potential remains incompletely developed. What are the roadblocks to the clinical application of LLLT?

In their 1971 articles [3, 4], Mester et al. proposed irradiation of wounds with 5–25 mW helium-neon laser at an energy density (fluence) of 1–1.5 J/cm^2. Although many subsequent studies reported positive effects under these irradiation conditions, several studies did not demonstrate reproducibility. In addition, some scientists claimed that these positive effects were merely the result of laser-induced temperature increases, and others argued that outcomes differed significantly by study site and operator. These conflicting results and interpretations underscore the need to investigate and elucidate the therapeutic mechanisms of LLLT using an interdisciplinary approach involving molecular biology and other advanced sciences. To this end, we believe it is important to scrutinize published clinical studies of low-energy laser effects and to translate the clinical observations into molecular, cellular, and biological mechanisms. Although large volumes of *in vitro, in vivo,* and clinical articles on LLLT are published every year, this 50-year-old technique has not gained wide acceptance as a first-line option for treatment in clinical settings. A common problem described in review articles about the therapeutic use of lasers is that laser irradiation parameters vary considerably among operators, sites, and manufacturers. However, it is not technically feasible to apply particular uniform irradiation conditions to different types of patients or experimental animal species, because one must consider differences in the biological and physical conditions of the target organisms (cells) to which these lasers are administered.

In the following paragraphs, the typical biologic effects of LLLT are described, and then the cellular effects of LLLT that underlie its biological actions are discussed. Through our research, we have discovered (i) the presence of intracellular photoreceptors and physiological changes resulting from photoreception, (ii) postirradiation modifications in cellular signal transduction cascades, and (iii) postirradiation alterations in gene expression. These various effects do not occur in an isolated manner. Here, we focus on how these effects interact with each other to induce modifications in cellular functions. We also describe the typical results of several of our experiments involving different laser wavelengths, output levels, pulse lengths, irradiation times, and a variety of species and cell types.

2. Biologic effects of LLLT

2.1. Wound healing

A large number of studies have shown that LLLT accelerates wound healing, and we present some typical results here. Irradiation of cultured human keratinocytes with a 632-nm helium-neon laser elevated the interleukin-1α and interleukin-8 mRNA levels, promoted keratinocyte migration and proliferation, and accelerated would repair [5]. In addition, *in vitro* studies of laser-irradiated cells revealed elevated levels of vascular endothelial growth factor (VEGF) [6] and transforming growth factor β(TGF β)expression [7]. These findings illustrate the laser-enhanced expression of many cytokines and growth factors in keratinocytes and fibroblasts, the key cellular mediators of the wound-healing process.

2.2. Antiinflammatory action

When mice with lipopolysaccharide-induced peritonitis were irradiated with a 904-nm gallium arsenide laser, inflammatory cell migration was inhibited [8]. In a rat model of carrageenan-induced pleuritis, a 660-nm indium-gallium-aluminum-phosphate laser suppressed the production of inflammatory cytokines and the migration of inflammatory cells [9]. A group of researchers led by Albertini are actively pursuing research on LLLT's antiinflammatory effects [10–30].

2.3. Bone growth and repair

LLLT accelerates osteoblast proliferation, bone formation [31], and bone repair [32]. Various groups have suggested the involvement of insulin-like growth factor 1 (IGF-1) [33], mitogen-activated protein kinase (MAPK)/extracellular signal-regulated kinase (ERK) [34], and bone morphogenetic protein (BMP)/Smad signaling cascades [35].

2.4. Neurologic effect

In addition to regeneration of damaged neurons [36–39], LLLT is effective in reducing pain. A rapidly growing body of literature has described the pain-relieving effect of LLLT. For more details, refer to the review article on this topic in those special journal issues.

2.5. Other effects

LLLT confers physiological effects on the articular cartilage [40] and muscle tissue [41–43]. In addition, LLLT confers aesthetic benefits, including its effects on hair growth/regrowth [44–48], acne treatment, [49, 50] and skin rejuvenation [51, 52].

3. Laser-induced cellular responses

In order to elucidate the biological mechanisms underlying effects of low-level lasers documented in experimental and clinical studies, one must consider the cellular responses to laser irradiation. In this section, we describe the intracellular photoreceptors and the cellular responses to laser light.

3.1. Intracellular photoreceptor

In photobiology, photoreception refers to the intracellular process whereby wavelength-specific photoreceptors absorb photon energy [53]. Photoreceptors are biomolecules that are capable of absorbing photoenergy, either intrinsically or through a molecular component. The mitochondrial respiratory chain includes multiple photoreceptors, as described below.

3.1.1. *Cytochrome c oxidase*

The enzyme cytochrome *c* oxidase receives electrons from respiratory-chain substrates through the cytochrome pathway and transfers them to oxygen molecules. The photoabsorption spectra of cytochrome *c* oxidase in its various oxidation states are very close to the action spectra for various biological responses. Cytochrome *c* oxidase has been proposed as the endogenous photoreceptor in the visible to near-infrared region (above 600 nm) [54]. Scientists have conducted extensive research on the photobiomodulation by cytochrome *c* oxidase, particularly in neuronal cells. In a study of neurons functionally inactivated by tetrodotoxin, a voltage-dependent sodium channel blocker [55], near-infrared irradiation restored the activity of intoxicated cytochrome *c* oxidase by altering its redox state. In another study, laser irradiation of mitochondria increased cytochrome *c* oxidase activity, polarographically measured levels of oxygen uptake, and subsequent ATP production [56]. Many other *in vitro* and *in vivo* studies of laser-induced cell growth have reported changes in cytochrome *c* oxidase activity and ATP production following irradiation [57–65].

3.1.2. *Porphyrin*

Porphyrins are a group of macrocyclic organic compounds that contain four pyrrole subunits joined by methine bridges. These mostly green- or red-colored compounds have specific absorption spectra and emit red fluorescence. Naturally occurring porphyrins, including those found in the human body, often form complexes with an iron or magnesium ion coordinated to the four pyrrole nitrogen atoms. For example, iron protoporphyrin IX (PPIX) complexes (i.e., heme *b*) form the prosthetic groups of hemoglobin, catalase, and peroxidase. Mitochondrial cytochromes also contain iron-porphyrin groups (nonheme *b*). The PPIX absorption spectrum has five major peaks in the range of 400–650 nm, with peak height decreasing as the absorption wavelength increases. The excited triplet state of PPIX, formed by absorption of laser photons, generates reactive oxygen species by transferring energy to ground-state oxygen atoms. A mode of photodynamic therapy that exploits this feature has been developed for anticancer treatment. In this technique, patients are administered PPIX or its precursor, 5-aminolevulinic acid (ALA), and reactive oxygen species are generated with local laser irradiation to kill malignant cells or epithelial cells of vascular neoplasms. In addition to the tumoricidal effects of reactive oxygen species, photodynamic therapy also induces energy-demanding apoptotic process by maintaining intracellular ATP levels [66]. Furthermore, my colleagues and we also discovered changes in the functions of cells irradiated with lasers in the presence of low doses of PPIX [67]. As the intracellular photoacceptors, porphyrins mediate a wide variety of biochemical reactions through the production of reactive oxygen species following photoreception. We refer to the roles of reactive oxygen species in more details below.

3.1.3. Flavoproteins (flavin proteins)

Flavoproteins are a group of protein complexes containing a riboflavin prosthetic group (e.g., flavin adenine dinucleotide [FAD] or flavin mononucleotide [FMN]). Most flavoproteins function as flavin enzymes, which use iron, molybdenum, copper, manganese, and other heavy metal ions as cofactors. These proteins have major absorption peaks in the range of 350–500 nm. Flavoproteins mediate a wide array of biological processes, such as bioluminescence, quenching of oxidative stress–induced radicals, DNA repair, and apoptosis [68]. A large number of researchers, including the present author, have reported the roles of flavoproteins as intracellular photoacceptors [69–71].

3.1.4. Other groups of photoreceptors

In addition to the three major groups of photoreceptors explained above, there are other types of photoreceptors, including rhodopsin, bilirubin, melanin, pterin, vitamin B6, vitamin K, nicotinamide adenine dinucleotide (phosphate) hydrogen [NAD(P)H], urocanic acid, and tryptophan.

3.2. Laser-induced changes in signaling cascades

Many researchers believe that the photon energy captured by intracellular receptors leads to alterations in gene and protein expression through a series of processes that modify signaling cascades. However, little is known regarding how light-stimulated receptors transduce their signals to the nucleus, or how these signals mediate the expression of particular genes. We have studied the mechanisms underlying the promotion and suppression of stem-cell differentiation, with a focus on FAD-containing cryptochromes as cellular photoreceptors [70, 71]. Our research suggested that light-activated cryptochromes migrate into the nucleus, where they regulate the expression of proteins located downstream of the E-box sequence. As a matter of course, cell functions are regulated by an array of other factors, including reactive oxygen species. Therefore, We now describe the biochemical changes LLLT induces beyond the photoreceptor absorption of light energy, as reported in the literature.

3.2.1. Redox pathways

Several oxygen and nitrogen radicals have been proposed to transduce mitochondrial signals to the nucleus. Those species react with NAD, NADH, NADP, NADPH, glutathione, glutathione sulfide, thioredoxin, and thioredoxin sulphide [72]. The cell contains several endogenous sensors for these species (typically, superoxide dismutase [SOD]) [73]. Upon detection of reactive oxygen species, the cell activates self-defense pathways by altering its gene expression patterns [74]. If these self-defense mechanisms fail, the cell will undergo apoptosis. The levels of reactive oxygen species strictly determine the expression of proteins regulating cell proliferation, suggesting that oxygen radicals act as second messengers [75, 76]. Reactive oxygen species are considered to play key roles in the control of cellular functions [77]. Low-level laser beams with wavelengths around 630 nm generate oxygen radicals in exposed cells [78, 79]. We have also discovered significant increases in the levels of oxygen radicals in cells exposed to 405-nm laser light [80]. Although the specific mechanism remains unknown, laser-induced intracellular generation of reactive oxygen species probably involves energy transfer from PPIX and other photoacceptors present in the cell. In addition, several groups have described cellular functions mediated by nitric oxide (NO), which is upregulated by laser irradiation, as well as by inducible nitric oxide synthase (iNOS) [79, 81–84]. The mechanism of laser-induced control of cellular functions is believed to hinge on the regulation of photoacceptor activity and the intracellular levels of reactive oxygen species.

3.2.2. Transcription factors

Several researchers have reported that the aforementioned redox pathways trigger changes in the expression of many transcription factors. Here, We do not go beyond a brief description of one of the best-characterized transcription factors, nuclear factor (NF)-κB [85, 86]. Published articles on other transcription factors mediating a multitude of cell functions have made it clear that their expression levels are also modified upon exposure to laser irradiation. As a transcription factor, NF-κB can simultaneously induce the expression of interleukin (IL)-1, IL-2, IL-6, IL-8, IL-12, tumor necrosis factor (TNF)-α, and other proinflammatory cytokines. It also controls the expression of apoptosis-related proteins, which play a critical role in tumor cell growth and immortalization. Several studies have shown that the aforementioned redox pathways trigger increases in NF-κB levels. [85, 86] This mechanism is considered to account, at least in part, for the observation that low-level laser irradiation induces the expression of various cytokines.

3.2.3. Circadian rhythm

The circadian rhythm, a roughly 24-h cycle of cellular events, was probably acquired during the early stages of evolution, and is ubiquitous from unicellular organisms to mammals. Several mammalian clock genes work together to establish a stable oscillation of approximately 24 h. Circadian clock proteins, such as brain-muscle Arnt-like protein 2 (Bmal2), CLOCK (Clk), cryptochrome (Cry), and Period (Per), set the pace of the clock in almost all cell types (e.g., the timing of cell division and other cellular activities). Cry, a blue-light receptor in higher plants and Drosophilidae [87], utilizes as its chromophore the FAD coenzyme, which undergoes blue-light excitation. The intramolecular changes that occur in Cry upon photoreception remain unclear. Most photoreceptors identified so far undergo a conformational change to their apo state when their chromophore is photoisomerized, and the resultant structural change in the protein molecule triggers photoreceptor signaling. In the case of Cry, however, no photoisomerization takes place, because FAD is the chromophore. This observation led to the idea that light-excited FAD transfers electrons to a certain substrate. However, the validity of this theory has not been tested.

Bone metabolism (remodeling) is a continuous homeostatic process involving resorption of existing bone by osteoclasts and formation of new bone by osteoblasts. Fu et al. showed that circadian rhythms mediate bone formation [88], and Kawasaki et al. reported that the E-box motif, a circadian regulatory sequence, is involved in the osteoblast expression of MBP-4 [89]; these findings indicate that Cry proteins regulate various homeostatic and physiological events through E-box elements. We conducted research on the effects of lasers on endocellular distribution and expression of Cry using 405-nm laser beams, which correspond to the absorption band of the Cry coenzyme FAD [70]. **Figure 1** presents the beam profile of the 405-nm laser used in the study (Panel A) and the changes in mouse marrow mesenchymal

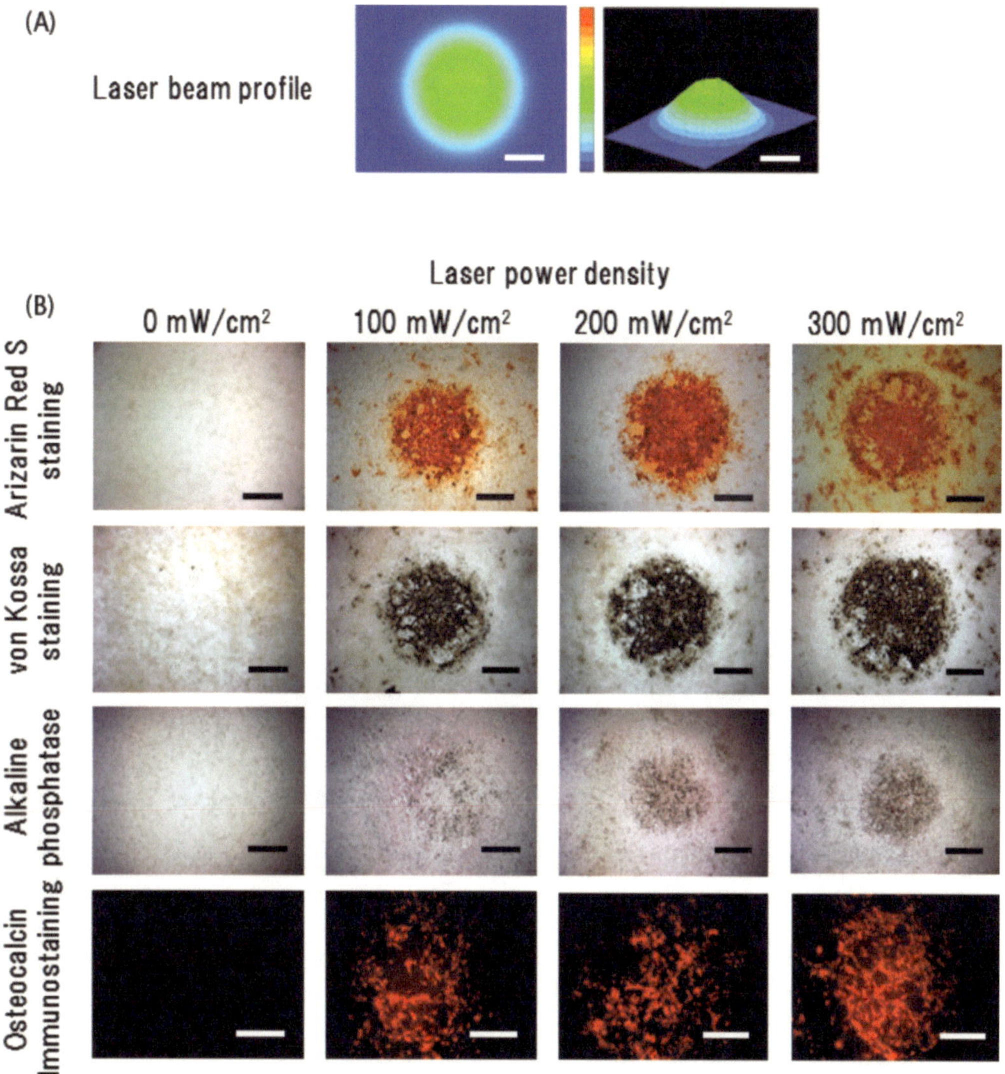

Figure 1. (A) The beam profile of the blue laser (wavelength; 405 nm, continuous wave). Mouse mesenchymal stromal cells were irradiated for 180 s at various laser power densities. Scale bars = 200. (B) Histochemical analysis of laser-irradiated mouse mesenchymal stromal cells. Calcium deposition of laser-irradiated mouse mesenchymal stromal cells was stained by Alizarin red-S (magnification: ×50). At 5 days postirradiation, calcium deposition had increased around the cells in a dose-dependent manner. Calcium phosphate deposition was evaluated by von Kossa staining (magnification: ×50). The area expressing alkaline phosphatase (ALP) activity was stained (magnification: ×50). Laser-irradiated samples displayed immunopositive staining for osteocalcin, a marker of osteoblast differentiation (magnification: ×100). Scale bars = 200 (for Alizarin red-S, von Kossa, and ALA staining) and 100 μm (for osteocalcin immunostaining). Adapted with permission from [70], copyright (2008).

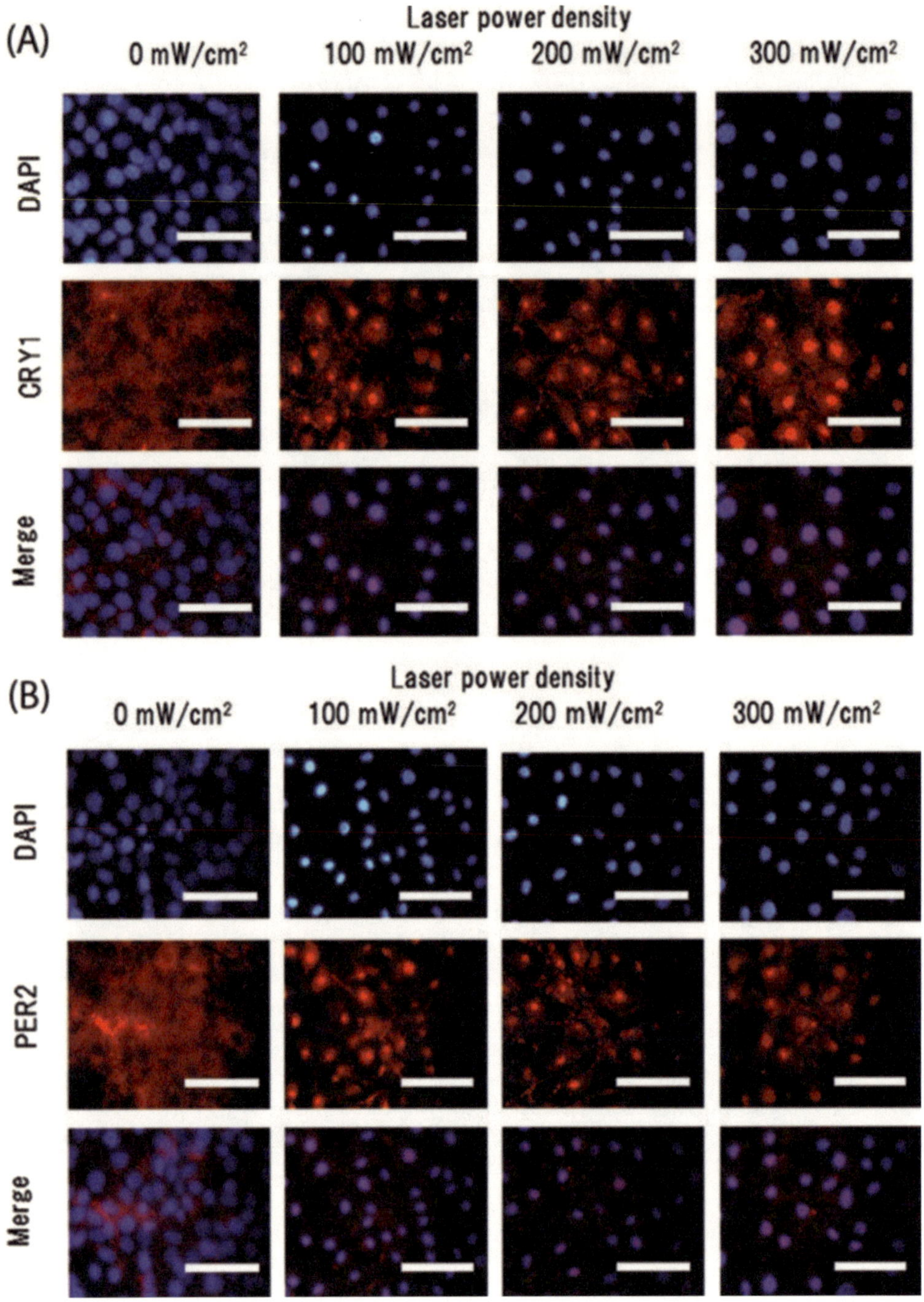

Figure 2. Intracellular location of mCRY1 (A) and mPER2 (B) proteins in mouse mesenchymal stromal cells 24 h after laser irradiation. Cells were double-labeled with DAPI (blue and upper panel) and mCRY1 or mPER2 (red and center panel). The lower panel provides a merged image. mCRY1 and mPER2 localized to the cytoplasm prior to laser irradiation. After laser irradiation, proteins translocated to the nucleus. Scale bars = 30 μm. Adapted with permission from [70], copyright (2008).

stromal cells irradiated for 3 min and then cultured for 5 days in osteoblast differentiation medium (Panel B). Alizarin red and von Kassa treatments, performed to detect calcium phosphate deposits, revealed that the stained cells were distributed in a circular area with a diameter similar to that of the laser beam. **Figure 1** also shows positive immunostaining results for alkaline phosphatase and osteocalcin, markers for osteoblast differentiation. These results confirmed that 405-nm laser irradiation accelerated osteoblast differentiation from mesenchymal stromal cells. In addition, the results of immunostaining for Cry1 and Per2 proteins are represented in **Figure 2**. Although Cry1 and Per2 were distributed across the cytosol in control cells, they were localized to the nucleus in cells exposed to 405-nm laser irradiation. Our results show that 405-nm laser beams promote the nuclear localization of Cry1 and mediate the expression of Cry1 and other proteins downstream of the E-box. We also reported that low-level laser irradiation suppressed the adipocyte differentiation of mesenchymal stromal cells [70], and accelerated their differentiation into chondrocytes [90].

4. Conclusions

Since the inception of life on earth, light has been one of the fundamental sources of biological energy. Today, researchers are conducting intensive basic and clinical research in the arena of laser medicine and photobiology, with the goal of developing new diagnostic and therapeutic modalities. Here, We described some of the latest advances in research on the cellular effects of irradiation with lasers and other forms of light. A great deal of future work will be required in order to broaden the applications of LLLT and achieve technical breakthroughs. In my past research, We found that living organisms and cells always respond to lasers and other forms of light in one way or another. The biological mechanisms underlying such responses significantly differ by the type of laser, target, and other experimental conditions. We must accumulate a systematic knowledge base by carefully analyzing the vast amount of experimental data currently available, as well as data collected in the future. We believe that light-based biomedical research will open new horizons for photodiagnosis, LLLT, and photodynamic therapy.

Acknowledgements

This paper was supported by KAKENHI Grant Numbers 16K15176 from Japan Society for the Promotion of Science (JSPS).

Author details

Toshihiro Kushibiki* and Miya Ishihara

*Address all correspondence to: toshi@ndmc.ac.jp

Department of Medical Engineering, National Defense Medical College, Namiki, Tokorozawa, Saitama, Japan

References

[1] E. Mester, B. Szende, P. Gartner: The effect of laser beams on the growth of hair in mice. Radiobiol Radiother (Berl), 9: 621–626, 1968.

[2] R. Roelandts: The history of phototherapy: something new under the sun? J Am Acad Dermatol, 46: 926–930, 2002.

[3] E. Mester, T. Spiry, B. Szende, J.G. Tota: Effect of laser rays on wound healing. Am J Surg, 122: 532–535, 1971.

[4] E. Mester, E. Jaszsagi-Nagy: Biological effects of laser radiation. Radiobiol Radiother (Berl), 12: 377–385, 1971.

[5] H.S. Yu, K.L. Chang, C.L. Yu, J.W. Chen, G.S. Chen: Low-energy helium-neon laser irradiation stimulates interleukin-1 alpha and interleukin-8 release from cultured human keratinocytes. J Invest Dermatol, 107: 593–596, 1996.

[6] N. Kipshidze, V. Nikolaychik, M.H. Keelan, L.R. Shankar, A. Khanna, R. Kornowski, M. Leon, J. Moses: Low-power helium: neon laser irradiation enhances production of vascular endothelial growth factor and promotes growth of endothelial cells in vitro. Lasers Surg Med, 28: 355–364, 2001.

[7] A. Khanna, L.R. Shankar, M.H. Keelan, R. Kornowski, M. Leon, J. Moses, N. Kipshidze: Augmentation of the expression of proangiogenic genes in cardiomyocytes with low dose laser irradiation in vitro. Cardiovasc Radiat Med, 1: 265–269, 1999.

[8] F. Correa, R.A. Lopes Martins, J.C. Correa, V.V. Iversen, J. Joenson, J.M. Bjordal: Low-level laser therapy (GaAs lambda = 904 nm) reduces inflammatory cell migration in mice with lipopolysaccharide-induced peritonitis. Photomed Laser Surg, 25: 245–249, 2007.

[9] E.S. Boschi, C.E. Leite, V.C. Saciura, E. Caberlon, A. Lunardelli, S. Bitencourt, D.A. Melo, J.R. Oliveira: Anti-Inflammatory effects of low-level laser therapy (660 nm) in the early phase in carrageenan-induced pleurisy in rat. Lasers Surg Med, 40: 500–508, 2008.

[10] F. Aimbire, R. Albertini, M.T. Pacheco, H.C. Castro-Faria-Neto, P.S. Leonardo, V.V. Iversen, R.A. Lopes-Martins, J.M. Bjordal: Low-level laser therapy induces dose-dependent reduction of TNFalpha levels in acute inflammation. Photomed Laser Surg, 24: 33–37, 2006.

[11] F. Aimbire, A.P. Ligeiro de Oliveira, R. Albertini, J.C. Correa, C.B. Ladeira de Campos, J.P. Lyon, J.A. Silva, Jr., M.S. Costa: Low level laser therapy (LLLT) decreases pulmonary microvascular leakage, neutrophil influx and IL-1beta levels in airway and lung from rat subjected to LPS-induced inflammation. Inflammation, 31: 189–197, 2008.

[12] F. Aimbire, F.V. Santos, R. Albertini, H.C. Castro-Faria-Neto, J. Mittmann, C. Pacheco-Soares: Low-level laser therapy decreases levels of lung neutrophils anti-apoptotic factors by a NF-kappaB dependent mechanism. Int Immunopharmacol, 8: 603–605, 2008.

[13] R. Albertini, F. Aimbire, A.B. Villaverde, J.A. Silva, Jr., M.S. Costa: COX-2 mRNA expression decreases in the subplantar muscle of rat paw subjected to carrageenan-induced inflammation after low level laser therapy. Inflamm Res, 56: 228–229, 2007.

[14] R. Albertini, F.S. Aimbire, F.I. Correa, W. Ribeiro, J.C. Cogo, E. Antunes, S.A. Teixeira, G. De Nucci, H.C. Castro-Faria-Neto, R.A. Zangaro, R.A. Lopes-Martins: Effects of different protocol doses of low power gallium-aluminum-arsenate (Ga-Al-As) laser radiation (650 nm) on carrageenan induced rat paw ooedema. J Photochem Photobiol B, 74: 101–107, 2004.

[15] R. Albertini, A.B. Villaverde, F. Aimbire, J. Bjordal, A. Brugnera, J. Mittmann, J.A. Silva, M. Costa: Cytokine mRNA expression is decreased in the subplantar muscle of rat paw subjected to carrageenan-induced inflammation after low-level laser therapy. Photomed Laser Surg, 26: 19–24, 2008.

[16] R. Albertini, A.B. Villaverde, F. Aimbire, M.A. Salgado, J.M. Bjordal, L.P. Alves, E. Munin, M.S. Costa: Anti-inflammatory effects of low-level laser therapy (LLLT) with two different red wavelengths (660 nm and 684 nm) in carrageenan-induced rat paw edema. J Photochem Photobiol B, 89: 50–55, 2007.

[17] A.C. Alves, R.D. Vieira, E.C. Leal-Junior, S.A. Dos Santos, A.P. Ligeiro, R. Albertini, J.A. Junior, P.D. de Carvalho: Effect of low-level laser therapy on the expression of inflammatory mediators and on neutrophils and macrophages in acute joint inflammation. Arthritis Res Ther, 15: R116, 2013.

[18] F. Bortone, H.A. Santos, R. Albertini, J.B. Pesquero, M.S. Costa, J.A. Silva, Jr.: Low level laser therapy modulates kinin receptors mRNA expression in the subplantar muscle of rat paw subjected to carrageenan-induced inflammation. Int Immunopharmacol, 8: 206–210, 2008.

[19] H.L. Casalechi, E.C. Leal-Junior, M. Xavier, J.A. Silva, Jr., T. de Carvalho Pde, F. Aimbire, R. Albertini: Low-level laser therapy in experimental model of collagenase-induced tendinitis in rats: effects in acute and chronic inflammatory phases. Lasers Med Sci, 28: 989–995, 2013.

[20] P. de Almeida, R.A. Lopes-Martins, S.S. Tomazoni, G.M. Albuquerque-Pontes, L.A. Santos, A.A. Vanin, L. Frigo, R.P. Vieira, R. Albertini, T. de Carvalho Pde, E.C. Leal-Junior: Low-level laser therapy and sodium diclofenac in acute inflammatory response induced by skeletal muscle trauma: effects in muscle morphology and mRNA gene expression of inflammatory markers. Photochem Photobiol, 89: 501–507, 2013.

[21] F.M. de Lima, R. Albertini, Y. Dantas, A.L. Maia-Filho, L. Santana Cde, H.C. Castro-Faria-Neto, C. Franca, A.B. Villaverde, F. Aimbire: Low-level laser therapy restores the oxidative stress balance in acute lung injury induced by gut ischemia and reperfusion. Photochem Photobiol, 89: 179–188, 2013.

[22] F.M. de Lima, A.B. Villaverde, R. Albertini, J.C. Correa, R.L. Carvalho, E. Munin, T. Araujo, J.A. Silva, F. Aimbire: Dual Effect of low-level laser therapy (LLLT) on the acute

lung inflammation induced by intestinal ischemia and reperfusion: action on anti- and pro-inflammatory cytokines. Lasers Surg Med, 43: 410–420, 2011.

[23] F.M. de Lima, A.B. Villaverde, R. Albertini, A.P. de Oliveira, H.C. Faria Neto, F. Aimbire: Low-level laser therapy associated to N-acetylcysteine lowers macrophage inflammatory protein-2 (MIP-2) mRNA expression and generation of intracellular reactive oxygen species in alveolar macrophages. Photomed Laser Surg, 28: 763–771, 2010.

[24] E.M. Laraia, I.S. Silva, D.M. Pereira, F.A. dos Reis, R. Albertini, P. de Almeida, E.C. Leal Junior, P. de Tarso Camillo de Carvalho: Effect of low-level laser therapy (660 nm) on acute inflammation induced by tenotomy of Achilles tendon in rats. Photochem Photobiol, 88: 1546–1550, 2012.

[25] R.A. Lopes-Martins, R. Albertini, P.S. Martins, J.M. Bjordal, H.C. Faria Neto: Spontaneous effects of low-level laser therapy (650 nm) in acute inflammatory mouse pleurisy induced by carrageenan. Photomed Laser Surg, 23: 377–381, 2005.

[26] F. Mafra de Lima, M.S. Costa, R. Albertini, J.A. Silva, Jr., F. Aimbire: Low level laser therapy (LLLT): attenuation of cholinergic hyperreactivity, beta(2)-adrenergic hyporesponsiveness and TNF-alpha mRNA expression in rat bronchi segments in E. coli lipopolysaccharide-induced airway inflammation by a NF-kappaB dependent mechanism. Lasers Surg Med, 41: 68–74, 2009.

[27] F. Mafra de Lima, K.T. Naves, A.H. Machado, R. Albertini, A.B. Villaverde, F. Aimbire: Lung inflammation and endothelial cell damage are decreased after treatment with phototherapy (PhT) in a model of acute lung injury induced by Escherichia coli lipopolysaccharide in the rat. Cell Biol Int, 33: 1212–1221, 2009.

[28] F. Mafra de Lima, A.B. Villaverde, M.A. Salgado, H.C. Castro-Faria-Neto, E. Munin, R. Albertini, F. Aimbire: Low intensity laser therapy (LILT) in vivo acts on the neutrophils recruitment and chemokines/cytokines levels in a model of acute pulmonary inflammation induced by aerosol of lipopolysaccharide from Escherichia coli in rat. J Photochem Photobiol B, 101: 271–278, 2010.

[29] D. Pires, M. Xavier, T. Araujo, J.A. Silva, Jr., F. Aimbire, R. Albertini: Low-level laser therapy (LLLT; 780 nm) acts differently on mRNA expression of anti- and pro-inflammatory mediators in an experimental model of collagenase-induced tendinitis in rat. Lasers Med Sci, 26: 85–94, 2011.

[30] M. Xavier, D.R. David, R.A. de Souza, A.N. Arrieiro, H. Miranda, E.T. Santana, J.A. Silva, Jr., M.A. Salgado, F. Aimbire, R. Albertini: Anti-inflammatory effects of low-level light emitting diode therapy on Achilles tendinitis in rats. Lasers Surg Med, 42: 553–558, 2010.

[31] Y. Ozawa, N. Shimizu, G. Kariya, Y. Abiko: Low-energy laser irradiation stimulates bone nodule formation at early stages of cell culture in rat calvarial cells. Bone, 22: 347–354, 1998.

[32] A.N. Silva Junior, A.L. Pinheiro, M.G. Oliveira, R. Weismann, L.M. Ramalho, R.A. Nicolau: Computerized morphometric assessment of the effect of low-level laser therapy on bone repair: an experimental animal study. J Clin Laser Med Surg, 20: 83–87, 2002.

[33] N. Shimizu, K. Mayahara, T. Kiyosaki, A. Yamaguchi, Y. Ozawa, Y. Abiko: Low-intensity laser irradiation stimulates bone nodule formation via insulin-like growth factor-I expression in rat calvarial cells. Lasers Surg Med, 39: 551–559, 2007.

[34] V. Aleksic, A. Aoki, K. Iwasaki, A.A. Takasaki, C.Y. Wang, Y. Abiko, I. Ishikawa, Y. Izumi: Low-level Er:YAG laser irradiation enhances osteoblast proliferation through activation of MAPK/ERK. Lasers Med Sci, 25: 559–569, 2010.

[35] S. Hirata, C. Kitamura, H. Fukushima, I. Nakamichi, Y. Abiko, M. Terashita, E. Jimi: Low-level laser irradiation enhances BMP-induced osteoblast differentiation by stimulating the BMP/Smad signaling pathway. J Cell Biochem, 111: 1445–1452, 2010.

[36] D. Gigo-Benato, T.L. Russo, E.H. Tanaka, L. Assis, T.F. Salvini, N.A. Parizotto: Effects of 660 and 780 nm low-level laser therapy on neuromuscular recovery after crush injury in rat sciatic nerve. Lasers Surg Med, 42: 673–682, 2010.

[37] C.C. Shen, Y.C. Yang, T.B. Huang, S.C. Chan, B.S. Liu: Neural regeneration in a novel nerve conduit across a large gap of the transected sciatic nerve in rats with low-level laser phototherapy. J Biomed Mater Res A, 101: 2763–2777, 2013.

[38] D. Gigo-Benato, S. Geuna, S. Rochkind: Phototherapy for enhancing peripheral nerve repair: a review of the literature. Muscle Nerve, 31: 694–701, 2005.

[39] J.J. Anders, S. Geuna, S. Rochkind: Phototherapy promotes regeneration and functional recovery of injured peripheral nerve. Neurol Res, 26: 233–239, 2004.

[40] M. Bayat, E. Ansari, N. Gholami, A. Bayat: Effect of low-level helium-neon laser therapy on histological and ultrastructural features of immobilized rabbit articular cartilage. J Photochem Photobiol B, 87: 81–87, 2007.

[41] D. Avni, S. Levkovitz, L. Maltz, U. Oron: Protection of skeletal muscles from ischemic injury: low-level laser therapy increases antioxidant activity. Photomed Laser Surg, 23: 273–277, 2005.

[42] R.A. Lopes-Martins, R.L. Marcos, P.S. Leonardo, A.C. Prianti, Jr., M.N. Muscara, F. Aimbire, L. Frigo, V.V. Iversen, J.M. Bjordal: Effect of low-level laser (Ga-Al-As 655 nm) on skeletal muscle fatigue induced by electrical stimulation in rats. J Appl Physiol (1985), 101: 283–288, 2006.

[43] E.C. Leal Junior, R.A. Lopes-Martins, F. Dalan, M. Ferrari, F.M. Sbabo, R.A. Generosi, B.M. Baroni, S.C. Penna, V.V. Iversen, J.M. Bjordal: Effect of 655-nm low-level laser therapy on exercise-induced skeletal muscle fatigue in humans. Photomed Laser Surg, 26: 419–424, 2008.

[44] P. Avci, G.K. Gupta, J. Clark, N. Wikonkal, M.R. Hamblin: Low-level laser (light) therapy (LLLT) for treatment of hair loss. Lasers Surg Med, 2013.

[45] E.F. Bernstein: Hair growth induced by diode laser treatment. Dermatol Surg, 31: 584–586, 2005.

[46] N. Bouzari, A.R. Firooz: Lasers may induce terminal hair growth. Dermatol Surg, 32: 460, 2006.

[47] T.C. Wikramanayake, R. Rodriguez, S. Choudhary, L.M. Mauro, K. Nouri, L.A. Schachner, J.J. Jimenez: Effects of the Lexington LaserComb on hair regrowth in the C3H/HeJ mouse model of alopecia areata. Lasers Med Sci, 27: 431–436, 2012.

[48] T.C. Wikramanayake, A.C. Villasante, L.M. Mauro, K. Nouri, L.A. Schachner, C.I. Perez, J.J. Jimenez: Low-level laser treatment accelerated hair regrowth in a rat model of chemotherapy-induced alopecia (CIA). Lasers Med Sci, 28: 701–706, 2013.

[49] T. Omi, P. Bjerring, S. Sato, S. Kawana, R.W. Hankins, M. Honda: 420 nm intense continuous light therapy for acne. J Cosmet Laser Ther, 6: 156–162, 2004.

[50] P. Papageorgiou, A. Katsambas, A. Chu: Phototherapy with blue (415 nm) and red (660 nm) light in the treatment of acne vulgaris. Br J Dermatol, 142: 973–978, 2000.

[51] M.A. Trelles, I. Allones, J.L. Levy, R.G. Calderhead, G.A. Moreno-Arias: Combined nonablative skin rejuvenation with the 595- and 1450-nm lasers. Dermatol Surg, 30: 1292–1298, 2004.

[52] S.Y. Lee, K.H. Park, J.W. Choi, J.K. Kwon, D.R. Lee, M.S. Shin, J.S. Lee, C.E. You, M.Y. Park: A prospective, randomized, placebo-controlled, double-blinded, and split-face clinical study on LED phototherapy for skin rejuvenation: clinical, profilometric, histologic, ultrastructural, and biochemical evaluations and comparison of three different treatment settings. J Photochem Photobiol B, 88: 51–67, 2007.

[53] J.C. Sutherland: Biological effects of polychromatic light. Photochem Photobiol, 76: 164–170, 2002.

[54] T.I. Karu, S.F. Kolyakov: Exact action spectra for cellular responses relevant to phototherapy. Photomed Laser Surg, 23: 355–361, 2005.

[55] M.T. Wong-Riley, H.L. Liang, J.T. Eells, B. Chance, M.M. Henry, E. Buchmann, M. Kane, H.T. Whelan: Photobiomodulation directly benefits primary neurons functionally inactivated by toxins: role of cytochrome c oxidase. J Biol Chem, 280: 4761–4771, 2005.

[56] D. Pastore, M. Greco, V.A. Petragallo, S. Passarella: Increase in <--H+/e- ratio of the cytochrome c oxidase reaction in mitochondria irradiated with helium-neon laser. Biochem Mol Biol Int, 34: 817–826, 1994.

[57] D. Barolet, P. Duplay, H. Jacomy, M. Auclair: Importance of pulsing illumination parameters in low-level-light therapy. J Biomed Opt, 15: 048005, 2010.

[58] J. Chu, S. Wu, D. Xing: Survivin mediates self-protection through ROS/cdc25c/CDK1 signaling pathway during tumor cell apoptosis induced by high fluence low-power laser irradiation. Cancer Lett, 297: 207–219, 2010.

[59] T.I. Karu, L.V. Pyatibrat, N.I. Afanasyeva: Cellular effects of low power laser therapy can be mediated by nitric oxide. Lasers Surg Med, 36: 307–314, 2005.

[60] C.C. Lan, S.B. Wu, C.S. Wu, Y.C. Shen, T.Y. Chiang, Y.H. Wei, H.S. Yu: Induction of primitive pigment cell differentiation by visible light (helium-neon laser): a photoacceptor-specific response not replicable by UVB irradiation. J Mol Med (Berl), 90: 321–330, 2012.

[61] J. Lim, R.A. Sanders, A.C. Snyder, J.T. Eells, D.S. Henshel, J.B. Watkins, 3rd: Effects of low-level light therapy on streptozotocin-induced diabetic kidney. J Photochem Photobiol B, 99: 105–110, 2010.

[62] L. Santana-Blank, E. Rodriguez-Santana, K. Santana-Rodriguez: Theoretic, experimental, clinical bases of the water oscillator hypothesis in near-infrared photobiomodulation. Photomed Laser Surg, 28 Suppl 1: S41–52, 2010.

[63] P.C. Silveira, E.L. Streck, R.A. Pinho: Evaluation of mitochondrial respiratory chain activity in wound healing by low-level laser therapy. J Photochem Photobiol B, 86: 279–282, 2007.

[64] S. Wu, D. Xing, X. Gao, W.R. Chen: High fluence low-power laser irradiation induces mitochondrial permeability transition mediated by reactive oxygen species. J Cell Physiol, 218: 603–611, 2009.

[65] Z.H. Wu, Y. Zhou, J.Y. Chen, L.W. Zhou: Mitochondrial signaling for histamine releases in laser-irradiated RBL-2H3 mast cells. Lasers Surg Med, 42: 503–509, 2010.

[66] K. Plaetzer, T. Kiesslich, B. Krammer, P. Hammerl: Characterization of the cell death modes and the associated changes in cellular energy supply in response to AlPcS4-PDT. Photochem Photobiol Sci, 1: 172–177, 2002.

[67] T. Kushibiki, Y. Tu, A. Abu-Yousif, T. Hasan: Photodynamic activation as a molecular switch to promote osteoblast cell differentiation via AP-1 activation. Sci Rep, 5: 13114, 2015.

[68] V. Massey: The chemical and biological versatility of riboflavin. Biochem Soc Trans, 28: 283–296, 2000.

[69] M. Eichler, R. Lavi, A. Shainberg, R. Lubart: Flavins are source of visible-light-induced free radical formation in cells. Lasers Surg Med, 37: 314–319, 2005.

[70] T. Kushibiki, K. Awazu: Controlling osteogenesis and adipogenesis of mesenchymal stromal cells by regulating a circadian clock protein with laser irradiation. Int J Med Sci, 5: 319–326, 2008.

[71] T. Kushibiki, K. Awazu: Blue laser irradiation enhances extracellular calcification of primary mesenchymal stem cells. Photomed Laser Surg, 27: 493–498, 2009.

[72] F.Q. Schafer, G.R. Buettner: Redox environment of the cell as viewed through the redox state of the glutathione disulfide/glutathione couple. Free Radic Biol Med, 30: 1191–1212, 2001.

[73] P. Storz: Mitochondrial ROS--radical detoxification, mediated by protein kinase D. Trends Cell Biol, 17: 13–18, 2007.

[74] H. Liu, R. Colavitti, Rovira, II, T. Finkel: Redox-dependent transcriptional regulation. Circ Res, 97: 967–974, 2005.

[75] K. Irani, Y. Xia, J.L. Zweier, S.J. Sollott, C.J. Der, E.R. Fearon, M. Sundaresan, T. Finkel, P.J. Goldschmidt-Clermont: Mitogenic signaling mediated by oxidants in Ras-transformed fibroblasts. Science, 275: 1649–1652, 1997.

[76] R. Schreck, P.A. Baeuerle: A role for oxygen radicals as second messengers. Trends Cell Biol, 1: 39–42, 1991.

[77] W. Droge: Free radicals in the physiological control of cell function. Physiol Rev, 82: 47–95, 2002.

[78] R. Lavi, A. Shainberg, H. Friedmann, V. Shneyvays, O. Rickover, M. Eichler, D. Kaplan, R. Lubart: Low energy visible light induces reactive oxygen species generation and stimulates an increase of intracellular calcium concentration in cardiac cells. J Biol Chem, 278: 40917–40922, 2003.

[79] V. Borutaite, A. Budriunaite, G.C. Brown: Reversal of nitric oxide-, peroxynitrite- and S-nitrosothiol-induced inhibition of mitochondrial respiration or complex I activity by light and thiols. Biochim Biophys Acta, 1459: 405–412, 2000.

[80] T. Kushibiki, T. Hirasawa, S. Okawa, M. Ishihara: Blue laser irradiation generates intracellular reactive oxygen species in various types of cells. Photomed Laser Surg, 31: 95–104, 2013.

[81] G.A. Guzzardella, M. Fini, P. Torricelli, G. Giavaresi, R. Giardino: Laser stimulation on bone defect healing: an in vitro study. Lasers Med Sci, 17: 216–220, 2002.

[82] M.C. Leung, S.C. Lo, F.K. Siu, K.F. So: Treatment of experimentally induced transient cerebral ischemia with low energy laser inhibits nitric oxide synthase activity and up-regulates the expression of transforming growth factor-beta 1. Lasers Surg Med, 31: 283–288, 2002.

[83] Y. Moriyama, E.H. Moriyama, K. Blackmore, M.K. Akens, L. Lilge: In vivo study of the inflammatory modulating effects of low-level laser therapy on iNOS expression using bioluminescence imaging. Photochem Photobiol, 81: 1351–1355, 2005.

[84] H. Tuby, L. Maltz, U. Oron: Modulations of VEGF and iNOS in the rat heart by low level laser therapy are associated with cardioprotection and enhanced angiogenesis. Lasers Surg Med, 38: 682–688, 2006.

[85] M. Eichler, R. Lavi, H. Friedmann, A. Shainberg, R. Lubart: Red light-induced redox reactions in cells observed with TEMPO. Photomed Laser Surg, 25: 170–174, 2007.

[86] C.F. Rizzi, J.L. Mauriz, D.S. Freitas Correa, A.J. Moreira, C.G. Zettler, L.I. Filippin, N.P. Marroni, J. Gonzalez-Gallego: Effects of low-level laser therapy (LLLT) on the nuclear factor (NF)-kappaB signaling pathway in traumatized muscle. Lasers Surg Med, 38: 704–713, 2006.

[87] C. Lee, J.P. Etchegaray, F.R. Cagampang, A.S. Loudon, S.M. Reppert: Posttranslational mechanisms regulate the mammalian circadian clock. Cell, 107: 855–867, 2001.

[88] L. Fu, M.S. Patel, A. Bradley, E.F. Wagner, G. Karsenty: The molecular clock mediates leptin-regulated bone formation. Cell, 122: 803–815, 2005.

[89] S. Kawasaki, S. Ebara, K. Nakayama, K. Takaoka: The E-Box motif, recognized by tissue-specific nuclear factor(s), is important for BMP-4 gene expression in osteogenic cells. Biochem Biophys Res Commun, 263: 560–565, 1999.

[90] T. Kushibiki, T. Tajiri, Y. Ninomiya, K. Awazu: Chondrogenic mRNA expression in pre-chondrogenic cells after blue laser irradiation. J Photochem Photobiol B, 98: 211–215, 2010.

Chapter 12

Photobiological Basics and Clinical Indications of Phototherapy for Skin Rejuvenation

Robert Glen Calderhead and Yohei Tanaka

Additional information is available at the end of the chapter

http://dx.doi.org/10.5772/intechopen.68723

Abstract

Sunlight is essential to almost all forms of life for both light and heat. Plants need sunlight for photosynthesis, and man and animals alike need plants for many vital purposes. The sun featured many Millennia ago not only as a deity but also as a therapeutic source, so phototherapy is by no means a recent phenomenon. Niels Finsen's therapeutic arc lamp system in the early 1900s replaced the sun as a therapeutic source. Since then, many light sources have been successfully applied for phototherapy, with laser diodes and light-emitting diodes the most efficient. This chapter will explore what phototherapy is, and examine its important role in the fast-developing indication of skin rejuvenation. Systems used in phototherapy will be discussed and compared. Photobiological basics and light/tissue interaction underlying the process will be examined, together with the importance of treatment parameters. The wound healing process, on which skin rejuvenation rests, will be dissected with a discussion of the optimum wavelengths to photoactivate the skin cells, leading to the clinical indications in photorejuvenation.

Keywords: phototherapy, photobiomodulation, low level light therapy (LLLT), laser diodes (LDs), light-emitting diodes (LEDs), skin rejuvenation, wound healing, mitochondrion

1. Introduction

The authors believe that the first question we need to ask, and answer, is; what is 'phototherapy'? The word is a compound derived from *phos, photos*, Greek for 'light' and from modern Latin *therapia*, from Greek *therapeia* 'healing,' from *therapeuein* 'minister to, treat medically.' In its broadest meaning, it is therefore the use of light to treat someone or something. The modern accepted definition is 'the use of low incident levels of photon energy at a particular wavelength, targeting tissue to achieve a clinically useful local or systemic effect, but without the creation of heat (athermal) or damage (atraumatic).' We can compare that with 'photosurgery,' where heat and damage are deliberately created in tissue to achieve the desired clinical result.

Other terms have evolved which can be found in the literature. 'Photobiomodulation' was recently adopted as a MeSH (Medical Subject Headings) term, part of the US National Library of Medicine's controlled vocabulary thesaurus, which is used for indexing articles for MEDLINE, PubMed Central and so on. However, equally useful, and well-used in the literature, is the term 'low level light therapy,' with its acronym LLLT. This was born in 1988 with the publication by John Wiley and Sons of Chichester, UK, and authored by Ohshiro and Calderhead, of the pivotal and first volume on the clinical use of laser therapy, 'Low Level Laser Therapy; A Practical Introduction' [1]. The authors of the current chapter like to use both terms, with 'photobiomodulation' (PBM) being used to describe how low incident levels of photon intensity interact with the target at a cellular and subcellular level, and the term 'LLLT' being used to describe the therapeutic application and final result of PBM. Based on that, the reader will mostly see LLLT talked about in this chapter.

There are some other inaccurate terms which have been coined, mostly as marketing-driven language, which the reader may come across in the literature, including 'soft laser,' 'cold laser,' low power laser' and so on. One can see how a thermal reaction attracts the name 'cold laser,' but in actual fact, the lasers used for LLLT, either defocused surgical lasers or laser diodes, run very hot and require a lot of cooling, so they are not 'cold lasers.' 'Soft laser' is attractive as it gives the idea of a gently acting laser, but again, inappropriate scientifically speaking. It is true that many LLLT systems, laser- or LED-based, deliver output powers in milliwatts (mW), so it is tempting to call them 'low power' lasers. When we consider these misnomers, please realize that the most important consideration for both the scientist and the clinician is the **therapeutic reaction** in the tissue to the incident light that occurs at a level below the damage threshold of the target cells to give the PBM effect which delivers the LLLT-mediated therapeutic result: the system used to obtain this low level of reaction is, however, unimportant. A 50 W CO_2 laser is not a 'low power' laser, but if defocused to a 10 cm spot size, in the treatment of a nonresponsive leg ulcer, for example, the incident power density, or irradiance, is actually only 635 mW/cm^2, under 1 W/cm^2. On the other hand, an 830 nm 60 mW laser diode (LD)-LLLT system can be focused to a 50 μm spot on the retina by the human eye. The incident intensity in this case is in excess of 3000 W/cm^2. In the first example, the 'high level' laser, target tissue will not be heated at all: in other words, phototherapy. In the second example, the 'low level laser,' the retinal tissue will be severely damaged with ablation and vaporization: in other words, photosurgery. In short, the 'level' in LLLT has therefore got nothing to do with the device used to produce the incident light; it is, rather, the **level of reaction** in the target cells which must be below the cellular damage threshold. This is illustrated in **Figure 1** and the legend thereto.

In 1988, light-emitting diodes (LEDs) were available and were very bright, but they were drastically low-powered with an unstable and extremely divergent output. Furthermore, they emitted at a very broad waveband, so it was possible to source a 'red' LED, but it was very difficult to find a narrow-band 633 nm LED (**Figure 2**), essential when targeting wavelength-specific chromophores. 'Chromophore' is in general the term given to tissue, cellular or subcellular targets for incident light energy at specific wavelengths. The clinical efficacy of LEDs at that time was thus extremely limited. Ohshiro and Calderhead had to concentrate their research and clinical findings on laser sources, both to some extent defocused continuous wave (CW) surgical lasers, for example, 10,600 nm carbon dioxide (CO_2) and 1064 nm neodymium-yttrium aluminum garget (Nd:YAG) lasers, very low-output lasers such as the 632.8 nm helium neon (HeNe) laser, but especially on specific-use gallium aluminum arsenide (GaAlAs) laser diodes incorporated in laser therapy systems, developed by Ohshiro in conjunction with Matsushita Electronics, and emitting at

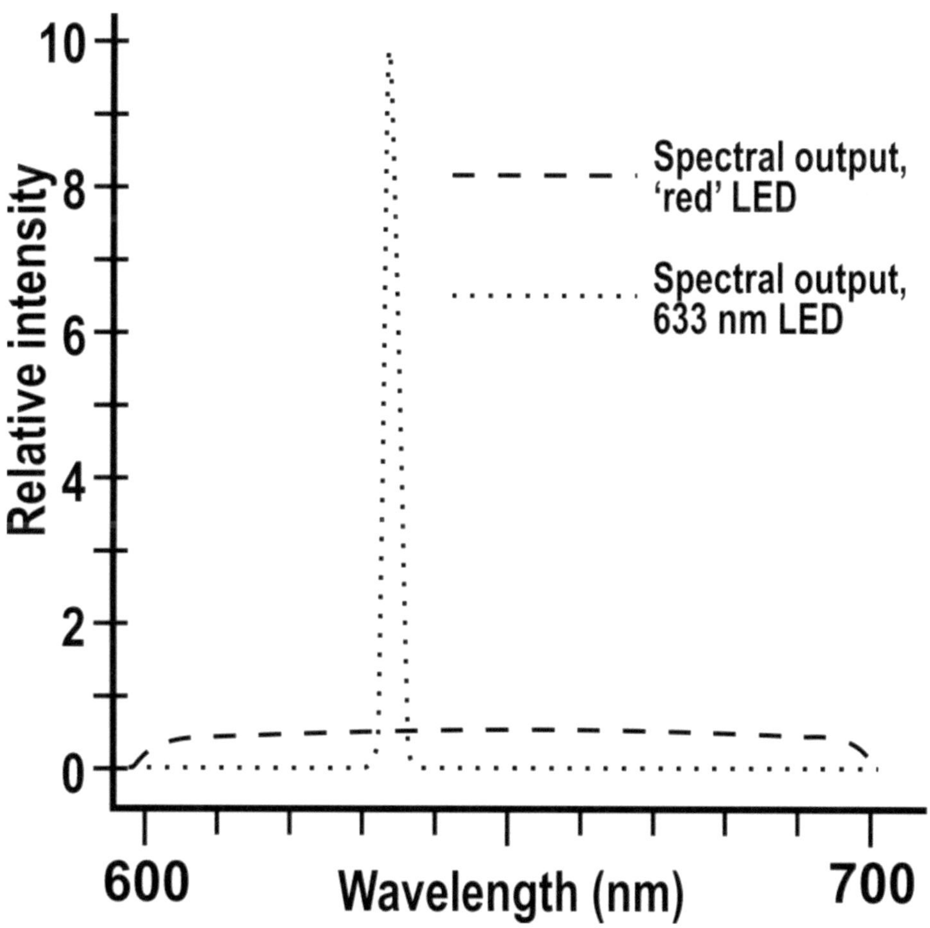

Figure 1. Difference in spectral distribution and relative output power (photon intensity) between an old-generation broad bandwidth red light-emitting diode (LED) and the new generation type, emitting in the example shown at 633 ± 5 nm. With the new generation LEDs, even though they are non-coherent, more than 90% of the photons are emitted at the rated wavelength with a very narrow bandwidth, conferring quasimonochromaticity on the beam.

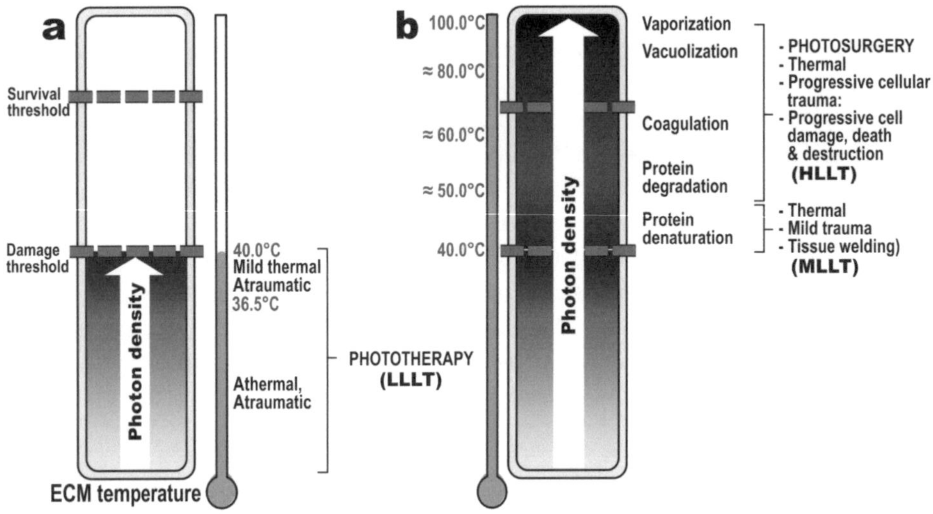

Figure 2. Schematic representation of a cell irradiated with two different irradiances, one low, one high, with the cell's arbitrary damage and survival thresholds indicated, showing changes in the extracellular matrix (ECM) temperature on the thermometer images. In (a), as the intensity of the absorbed incident photon energy increases, cellular activity is enhanced (photobiomodulated): the result of this is characterized as athermal and atraumatic LLLT. In (b), the continuing increase in incident photon intensity raises the level of reaction in the cell, and the internal temperature, beyond the damage threshold: although damaged, however, the cell is still alive. This is classed as mid level laser treatment (MLLT) following Ohshiro's classification system [Ohshiro T: A new effect-based classification of laser applications in surgery and medicine. Laser Ther, 1996; 8: 233–239]. As the temperatures in the target tissue rise to around 60°C, more intensive damage occurs as ECM collagen coagulation begins resulting in necrosis. Temperatures continue to rise with even higher intensities until tissue temperatures reach 100°C and the tissue is ablated with the vaporization of cellular and extracellular water. This is classed as high level laser treatment, HLLT, or photosurgery.

830 ± 3 nm. Low-level laser therapy thus became LLLT, but with the advent of clinically useful LEDs, as will be discussed in Section 3 below, low-level *laser* therapy became low level *light* therapy but with the acronym left as LLLT [2]. Please see Section 3 below for a detailed discussion of what lasers, laser diodes and light-emitting diodes are, and how they are used in LLLT.

2. Nothing new under the sun

LLLT is often thought of as 'new,' only some three decades old or so, and even the laser itself is not long over its half-century, having been first successfully demonstrated by Dr Theodore Maiman in 1960 [3]. The use of light in medicine dramatically precedes laser treatment by not just centuries, but by millennia. In Ancient Egyptian friezes from around 4000 BC, the sun is depicted as delivering rays to man, dogs and plants, with each ray ending in a little hand, 'patting' the target. In addition, in front of the face of the Pharaoh, the sun's ray ends in the ankh, the symbol for life (**Figure 3**). This illustrates the sun as the source of light and life. In addition, it is written in papyrus records that a herb similar to parsley was crushed and rubbed onto depigmented skin, probably a form of vitiligo,

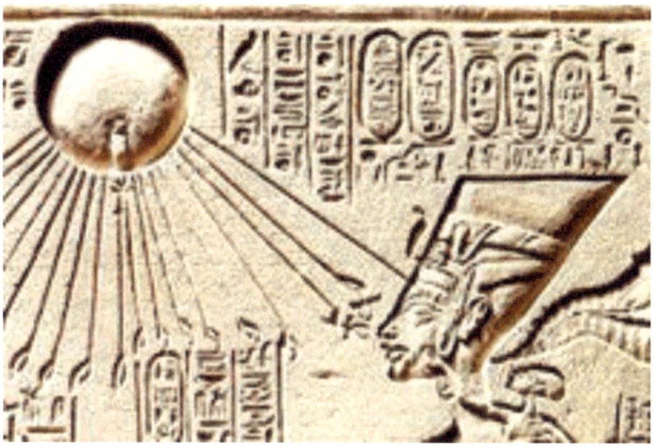

Figure 3. A portion of a frieze from Egypt's Tell el-Amarna, showing the Pharaoh Amenhotep IV in the rays of the sun (deified as Aten), where the 'patting' hands and the ankh symbol at the end of the rays can be clearly seen.

which in dark-skinned Ancient Egyptians must have been quite stigmatic. The area was then exposed to the full force of the sun, and the activation of the coumarins in the crushed parsley by the shortwave blue component of sunshine instigated a very strong photosensitive reaction resulting in severe sunburn. This was followed, at least partly, by postinflammatory hyperpigmentation, the much feared PIH following today's laser treatment, thus hopefully repigmenting the depigmented area.

Almost 2 millennia later, Hippocrates of Kos, the 'Father of Medicine,' was of the opinion that sunshine was one of the fuels of life, because his fellow Greeks, basking in Sunshine most of the year round, were of a much better and happier disposition than the barbarians to the north, which Hippocrates attributed to the fact that the northerners did not get enough sun.

Treatment using the sun is referred to as heliotherapy, from the Greek *Helios*, 'the sun.' However, the definition became a little broader, also involving exposure to specific wavebands, not necessarily from the sun. For many years, it was really only the sun that was powerful enough, and one of the treatments for 'melancholia' involved shutting the patient in a room with many windows to let in natural light, with red curtains to increase the ant-melancholic component of sunlight. One famous patient was King George III of the UK (1760–1820), who in his later years was believed to suffer from severe 'melancholia' and was shut in red-curtained rooms for treatment. It is now believed that he actually had a form of the blood disease porphyria, so this treatment probably exacerbated his condition and it is probably no wonder the poor monarch was known as 'Mad King George.'

At the turn of the twentieth century, man's dependence on the sun as a therapeutic light source was broken by the brilliant Danish scientist and clinician, Niels Finsen, who developed an artificial light source based on light energy emitted by an electric arc lamp, from which all heat had been filtered out. He was particularly successful for his work using this lamp on lupus vulgaris, for which he won the Nobel Prize for Medicine in 1903. Finsen did not enjoy good health, and died in 1904. However, his vast interest in phototherapy inspired by his own experiments into the use of sunshine and particular filtered wavelengths for treating his own Niemann-Pick disease [4], lived on, and the Finsen Medal is awarded to outstanding contributors to phototherapy up to this day.

More recently, blue light phototherapy (460–490 nm) has been routinely used in the treatment of neonate hyperbilirubinemia, that is, jaundice in newborns, in whom the bilirubin in the bloodstream has not been sufficiently filtered out by the mother's placenta.

However, one of the largest examples of a breakthrough for a unique medical light source came in 1960, with the successful oscillation of the first ruby laser by Dr Theodore Maiman. The major difference between laser energy and other filtered light sources is the coherent nature of laser energy, comprising monochromaticity (one single wavelength), temporal and spatial phase of the photons in the laser beam, and the ability to collimate a laser beam so it can travel large distances with minimal divergence.

Maiman's laser was based on a ruby crystal, and as the laser medium usually gives its name to the laser, it became known as a ruby laser. In the 5 short years from 1660 to 1965, almost all of the lasers used today in surgery and medicine were swiftly developed, including the 1046 nm neodymium:YAG (and other members of the YAG family), the argon laser (488 and 514.5 nm), the 10,600 nm carbon dioxide (CO_2) laser and the helium neon (HeNe) laser. Visible red and near-infrared (near-IR) semiconductor (diode) lasers were also developed. The clinical potential of this unique pure light source was quickly realized, as was of course the military implications. Ophthalmology was the first field to explore the use of the laser for retinal disorders in the mid-60s, followed quickly by dermatology for removal of cutaneous lesions. Both these specialities used the selective but destructive photocoagulative power of the visible light lasers, particularly the green 514.5 nm band of the argon laser, and the 694.3 nm band of the ruby laser. The CO_2 laser became a powerful 'light scalpel' for comparatively blood-free and precise incisional, excisional and ablative indications in a variety of specialities, including oto-rhino-laryngologists, neurosurgeons and gynecologists.

However, an interesting anomaly was quickly noted by those using the CO_2 laser in particular, in that patients complained of less postoperative pain, shorter-lasting erythema and almost equally good wound healing following laser surgery as compared with the cold scalpel. It was thought at first that it was the heat generated by the laser that brought about this serendipitous occurrence, but it was gradually realized it was the 'L' component of laser that was the causative element … the light, not the heat. In 1969, Professor Endrè Mester practicing in Semmelweis University, Budapest, Hungary, published a pivotal paper in Hungarian on the use of the athermal and atraumatic 5 mW HeNe laser to treat over 1000 cases of severely recalcitrant crural ulcers, followed by an English overview in 1971 [5]. Astonishingly, he achieved a cure rate of better than 80%, with less than 2% of the patients not responding at all [6]. This was the birth of modern-age phototherapy, so that Prof Endre Mester is regarded rightly as the Father of Phototherapy. Finally, something new had been found under the sun after all.

Smaller and for-purpose laser sources were developed enabling the delivery of low incident levels of photon energy at wavelengths found useful in cellular biomodulation, in particular laser diodes. More recently, a new generation of light-emitting diode was developed by the Space Medicine Laboratory in the National Aeronautics and Space Administration (NASA) in the USA, and LEDs are taking their place as useful and verified phototherapy light sources. All of these will be explored in the next section.

3. Phototherapy devices

The main devices used in modern state-of-the-art phototherapy have already been mentioned in the previous sections. These are filtered polychromatic non-laser light sources, such as xenon lamps and (more rarely) incandescent lamps; defocused continuous wave surgical laser systems, such as the CO_2 and Nd:YAG laser, although more rarely these days; dedicated low-irradiance laser diode-based systems; and made-for-purpose LED-based systems.

3.1. Filtered lamps

There are a number of filtered non-laser light sources available for phototherapy practice, based on high-intensity xenon or other continuous-output gas-based lamps. These offer greater photon intensities than incandescent lamps and also require much less in the way of cooling. The filters are typically in the blue, yellow, red and near-infrared (near-IR) range, with bandwidths in tens of nanometers or less. The spectral output from these systems is heavy in the near-IR waveband and then tends to trail off through the visible to the UV-A band. The pattern of a typical spectral output is seen in **Figure 4**. The entire output power is spread over the entire emitted spectrum. There are two possible methods to filter the light to obtain the desired 'color.' A narrow bandwidth cut-off/cut-on filter for example, used to obtain a small 10–20 nm band at the desired wavelength, for example, around 633 nm which is a popular wavelength for activating cellular activity, as will be explained later. The reader will however appreciate that this will dramatically reduce the available photon intensity to give an irradiance of a very few mW/cm^2, given that the output through the entire visible waveband from 400 to 700 nm is comparatively low in the first place. Another method is to cut-off the unwanted shorter wavelengths. A cut-off filter rated at 630 nm will allow light energy all the way from the near-IR components up to around 630 nm, but will cut off all wavelengths shorter than that. The emitted light is still a polychromatic waveband and therefore not really suitable for any indication requiring wavelength selectivity for the target chromophore. However, many of those who use these lamps find them effective, but very long exposure times are needed to achieve the desired final dose in even a few joules per square centimeter (J/cm^2).

3.2. Defocused surgical lasers

When Ohshiro and Calderhead started researching the field of phototherapeutic indications in the late 1970s, the only dedicated low output laser system available was the helium neon (HeNe), delivering milliwatt ranges at 632.8 nm. The HeNe laser was the system used by Mester in his early papers, and it was these data from Mester that first encouraged Ohshiro

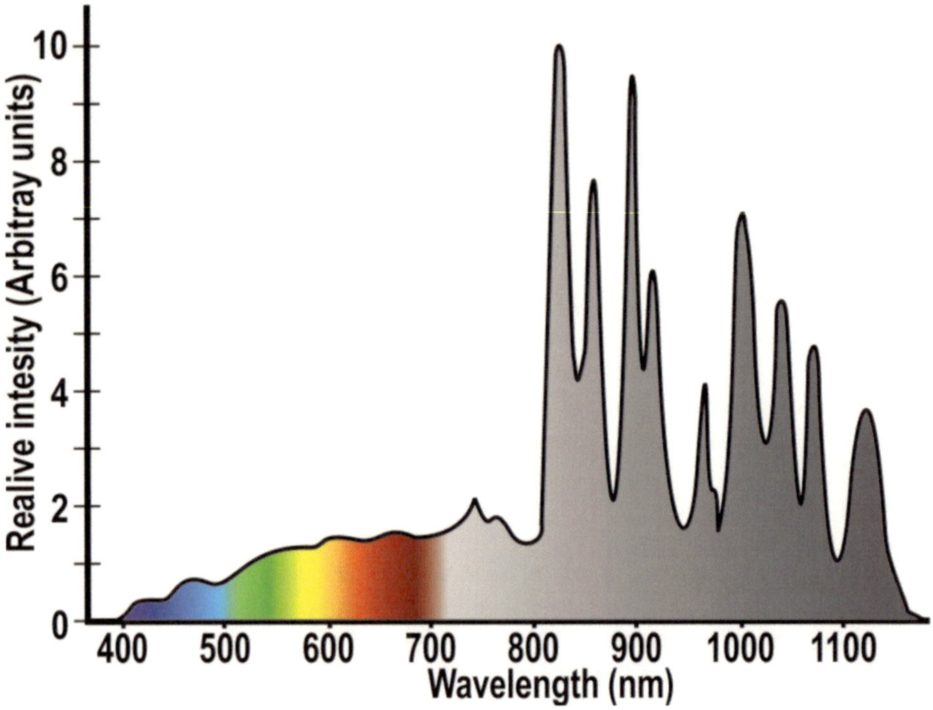

Figure 4. Approximate representation of the polychromatic spectral spread of a typical unfiltered continuous operation xenon lamp. The envelope of the lamp contains an ultraviolet filter to remove potentially harmful UV wavelengths. The majority of the output lies in the near-IR (from approximately 700 nm upwards). Some lamps apply the full spectrum in therapeutic practice. Others use cut-off filters to cut out the unwanted shorter wavelengths. However, all longer wavelengths are still delivered up to the cut-off point, that is, still polychromatic light, unless a cut-on filter is also applied to remove the unwanted longer wavelengths.

and then Calderhead to investigate the potential of the use of low incident levels of light energy for first pain attenuation, and then wound healing. Ohshiro had established a pain clinic in his Tokyo Clinic, and, in addition to the HeNe laser, he first looked at the 1064 nm wavelength of the continuous wave Nd:YAG laser, chosen because of its deeper penetration than 632.8 nm, and comparatively low absorption in melanin and blood. In addition, the HeNe laser tended to be rather low-powered, necessitating longer treatment times to achieve good results.

By defocusing the usual output of his CW Nd:YAG laser, delivered by a selectable variety of larger spot sizes, extremely practical and very low incident irradiances of less than 1 W/cm^2 could be delivered with good efficacy for pain attenuation of both acute and chronic pain. To compare the Nd:YAG with the HeNe, to produce a useful incident dose or energy density of 15 J/cm^2, an approximately 20 s exposure with the Nd:YAG was needed: over 15 min treatment was needed to get the same dose with a 15 mW/cm^2 HeNe.

The defocused CO_2 laser as a pain attenuation and wound healing device also attracted some attention in the late 1980s and early 1990s, but like the Nd:YAG system, they are large and expensive devices, and need a great deal of ancillary equipment and adaptation for regular use as phototherapy systems. Furthermore, technology advanced rapidly so that CW Nd:YAG lasers were quickly supplanted by more adaptable and versatile Q-switched and long-pulsed systems, and CW CO_2 lasers lost favor in the face of the much more precise superpulsed and ultrapulsed systems, followed by the fractionated approach. Having said that, small CW CO_2 lasers still occasionally attract attention in the literature for wound healing applications [7], although there have been no reports for defocused CO_2 laser systems for skin rejuvenation.

3.3. Laser diode-based therapeutic systems

As mentioned, Ohshiro's Nd:YAG laser was a large and expensive piece of equipment, so he worked with an electronics company in Tokyo to develop a much smaller, dedicated semiconductor-based laser therapy system for phototherapy. First tried was the gallium arsenide (GaAs) diode, but it could not be run at continuous wave without severely overheating, so finally the gallium aluminum arsenide diode was developed and found to be ideal. The first system to be trialled was a battery-operated 15 mW GaAlAs system, delivering around 500 mW/cm^2, and a controlled study on pain attenuation was published in 1981 comparing the efficacy of the GaAlAs diode system with the defocused CW Nd:YAG system in pain entity and age-matched patients at the same dose. Despite its small size, the diode laser proved to be at least as effective as the Nd:YAG system [8].

The first commercial laser therapy system was jointly developed by Ohshiro and Matsushita Electronics (National Panasonic,) and launched as the first of the 830 nm Panalas® systems in 1981. Ohshiro did not stop thinking about improving both systems and treatment techniques, as well as looking at underlying mechanisms. In 1988, Ohshiro launched a new GaAlAs diode laser based system, delivering 60 mW, the OhLase-3D1®, and that has evolved to the present day. Also in 1988, Ohshiro and Calderhead put all of their thoughts together in having the volume already mentioned above, 'Low-Level Laser Therapy: A Practical Introduction' published by John Wiley and Sons. In the same year, the journal *Laser Therapy* was announced by John Wiley of Chichester, and the International Laser Therapy Association (ILTA) was formed, all championing Low-Level Laser Therapy. LLLT was well and truly born and has continued to grow and develop up till today. The agreed MeSH term may be photobiomodulation, but if 'LLLT' is entered into PubMed as a search term, the reader will find over 4400 entries! A very large percentage of them are actually on clinical or research facets of LLLT and phototherapy, rather than any other laser-associated aspect.

LLLT systems based on laser diodes (LDs) remain extremely popular and are manufactured by a number of reputable companies worldwide. Some of them have USA FDA and other national regulatory body clearances. Because of the beam geometry of LD chips, the treatment area is usually punctal in nature with a spot sizes ranging from less than 1 mm^2 to defocused systems offering 1 cm^2 or so, but not a lot larger than that. Treatment techniques are therefore based on point by point approaches. To cover a larger area, quite useful for treating larger wounds, for example, an array of LDs could be considered. In reality, GaAlAs diodes run quite hot, so good heat sink design is need to keep even single LDs running cool. Too much heat in the chip will cause a change in the rated wavelength, and that would not meet the criterion of precisely targeting wavelength-dependent chromophores. It is therefore difficult to run arrays of LDs without some form of aggressive cooling. Light-emitting diodes (LEDs), on the other hand, do not run so hot and are much easier to cool than LDs. For such planar arrays, LEDs are the answer, which leads us into the next subsection.

3.3.1. *Enter the light-emitting diode*

When LLLT was dependent on LDs for the light source, as in the many publications appearing in the late 1980s and early 1990s, LEDs were commercially available. However, although they were certainly cheap and cheerful, ideal for indicator lamps, traffic signals and Christmas trees, they were on the other hand totally inappropriate for medical application because of their low and unstable output powers, extreme divergence and wide bandwidths. As said already, we could source red LEDs, but not 633 nm LEDs (*cf* **Figure 2** above and legend). Very expensive superluminescent diodes (SLEDs) were available offering almost laser-like bandwidths, but even these proved significantly inferior to LD-LLLT systems when compared side by side in controlled animal studies and could still only be applied point by point [9]. All this changed in 1988, however, when Professor Harry Whelan and his NASA Space Medicine Colleagues succeeded in developing what became known as the 'NASA LED' [10]. These LEDs were many-fold more powerful than their older generation cousins, typically 5 orders of magnitude more powerful in fact; they had much narrower divergence offering high photon intensities; they were remarkably stable; and probably the most important development, they were quasimonochromatic, offering spectral outputs with more than 95% of the photons at the rated wavelength. In other words, although they were still noncoherent, non-laser light sources, they offered laser-like precision for targeting wavelength-specific chromophores in tissue, cellular and subcellular targets. Finally, a real breakthrough had been made to provide a practical, clinically useful new light source for phototherapy, capable of being mounted in large area planar arrays. Whelan and his colleagues went on in the following 2 years to demonstrate that their new near-IR wavelength LEDs were clinically viable in an in vivo wound healing model [11]. In the first few years of the New Millennium serious and scientifically proven, LED-based systems were developed first for hands-free large area PDT for non-melanoma skin cancers using the 633 nm wavelength [12], followed by LED-only acne treatment using the combination of the visible blue 415 and 633 nm wavelengths [13], skin rejuvenation and accompanying histochemical and ultrastructural extracellular matrix changes with 830 nm near-IR and 633 nm wavelengths [14], sports medicine and pain attenuation with the 830 nm wavelength [15], and so on. LED-LLLT was well and truly demonstrated to work, and work well. All of the above wavelengths, with the exception of the 415 nm wavelength, fell within Karu's phototherapeutic window for effective cellular photoactivation with visible and near infrared lights sources, laser or non-laser [16]. Thus, it is when the reader examines these 4400-plus PubMed results for LLLT, that he or she will find more and more very serious papers demonstrating a growing solid body of evidence for both clinical and basic research into LED-LLLT among the laser-based literature.

Figure 5 schematically illustrates the differences in the patterns of emission from lasers, laser diodes, light-emitting diodes and filtered non-coherent lamps as used in phototherapeutic indications, including the rejuvenation of photo- and chronologically aged skin. **Figure 6** shows examples of commercially available laser diode-based, lamp-based and light-emitting diode-based systems used worldwide for LLLT.

http://dx.doi.org/10.5772/intechopen.68723

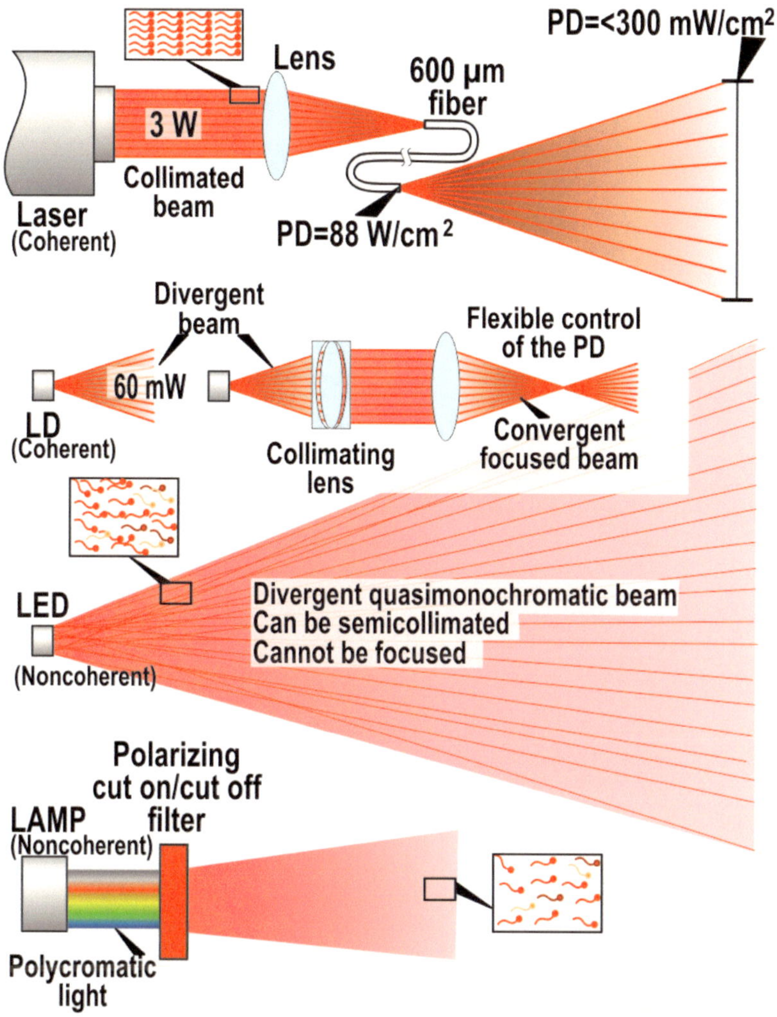

Figure 5. LLLT sources compared. Although not used these days, of historical interest is the defocused CW 1064 nm Nd:YAG. The optimum method was to couple the beam from the laser into an optical fiber. This could be any length, so the laser could be well away from the treatment room, and even several treatment rooms could be serviced with the one laser. The beam emerging from the distal end of the fiber is divergent and multimode, giving a uniform intensity across the beam. By using different beam sizes, the desired irradiance could be selected. Laser diodes (LDs) by their nature emit a defocused elliptical beam. The angle of divergence is high so it is normal to have the beam collimated (just like the ubiquitous laser pointer), because an LD is still a laser. The beam can then be focused within the handpiece of the system, so that either a convergent beam or a divergent beam can be used to give the ideal irradiance at the tissue, depending on the distance between the lens and the target tissue. The divergent beam is inherently safer. LEDs are also highly divergent, but emit noncoherent light. The better quality new generation LEDs are, however, quasimonochromatic, emitting all of their photon energy more or less at the rated wavelength, and no color filter is required. They can be semicollimated to decrease the angle of divergence and increase the irradiance, but they cannot be perfectly focused like a laser. They can be mounted in large planar arrays to irradiate a large area of tissue in a hands-free manner. The polychromatic lamp type system requires a filter to filter out (cut off) the unrequired shorter wavelengths, leaving only the wavelength wanted for treatment. To make this light output as similar as possible to an LED, the filter, however, needs to be very precise (i.e., narrow band), and it needs to have a cut on element to remove the unwanted longer heat-producing IR light. This means that the photon intensity at tissue is rather low, and longer exposures are required to give a reasonable dose.

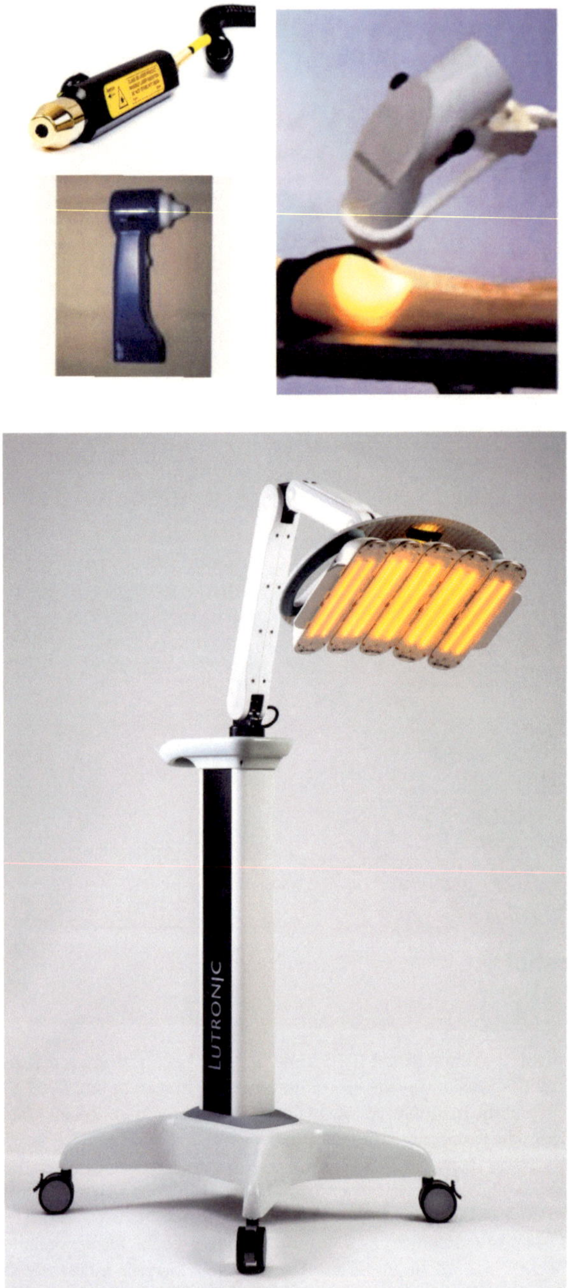

Figure 6. Examples of current phototherapy systems. Top left: laser diode (LD)-LLLT systems. The upper example shows a pen-type probe, near-IR system (Thor Probe, Thor Lasers, UK). This is connected a mains-operated control console. The lower example is a battery-operated 830 nm LD-LLLT system (OhLase-3D1 HT1, JMLL, Japan). In both cases, the treated area is very small, and the systems are used in a punctal fashion in contact mode, separating the treated points by a few millimeters or so. Top right: filtered polychromatic filtered lamp LLLT system (Bioptron, Switzerland). A larger area of tissue can be treated in a hands-free manner. The yellow cut-off filter is illustrated here. Bottom: free-standing 830 nm LED-LLLT system (HEALITE II, Lutronic, Korea). The large treatment head can be adjusted to treat anybody contour from the back, to the face, to an arm or leg, again in a hands-free manner.

4. Wavelength: the prime parameter in phototherapy

The first law of photobiology states that absorption must occur before there can be any reaction. This might appear to be self-evident, but what actually governs absorption of light in a target, and indeed, what decides the chromophore, or target, for that light? The reader would be excused for thinking it is the output power of the light source, but it is in fact the wavelength. This is particularly critical in phototherapy. Photons travel through space in straight lines, but with a sinusoidal waveform. Wavelength is a measurement of how far a photon will travel in one complete cycle, and is measured in nanometers (nm), one billionth of a meter, or fractions and multiples thereof. Light energy comprises a very small section of the very extensive electromagnetic spectrum which runs from ultrashort cosmic rays in femtometers and below all the way to wavelengths of kilometers for electrical energy (**Figure 7**). Knowing the wavelength of an LLLT system lets us understand if we can see the light it emits or not (visible or invisible light), and if we can see it, what color it is.

Figure 8 is a composite of three main concepts centered around wavelength. In the central part of **Figure 8**, the visible spectrum (400–700 nm) and a portion of the invisible near-IR spectrum can be seen (700–1010 nm), as part of a photospectrographic data set captured from polychromatic 'white' light which had been shone through a human hand in vivo [17]. The wavelength is indicated on the x-axis in nanometers (nm), and the optical density (OD) ranges from 3 to 8.5 (logarithmic units) on the y-axis. The higher the OD, the more dense the target is to specific wavelengths of the incident light. The upper portion of **Figure 8** schematically represents the relative penetration of selected wavelengths into skin, based on the OD findings of the central portion. The shorter wavelength visible light at blue (415 nm), green (532 nm) and yellow (590 nm) offers poor penetration into skin in vivo. From 590 nm yellow, it is only 43 nm to 633 nm red, but penetration increases by almost 3.5 orders of magnitude, more than 1000 times better than yellow. That is a critical difference in penetration which is highly wavelength dependent. Deepest penetration is achieved around 830 nm in the near infrared. In general, as wavelength increases, tissue penetration also increases.

The lower section of **Figure 8** offers an explanation as to why these wavelength-mediated differences in penetration exist. Here are shown the absorption spectra of three of the biological chromophores in living skin: melanin normally in the epidermis; blood (oxy- and deoxy-hemoglobin) in the dermis and water throughout the skin. From this, the strong affinity of the shorter visible wavelengths for blood and melanin precludes light at these wavelengths reaching much beyond the superficial papillary dermis. If the target for the phototherapy is, for example, fibroblasts, then these wavelengths will not reach the target ... no absorption, no reaction. Red light at 633 nm penetrates much better because it has much less absorption in both blood and melanin, and even less so at 830 nm. Beyond 830 nm, water starts to become of interest as a chromophore, and penetration into tissue starts to fall off quite rapidly after 1000 nm. This is why, apart from the now more or less extinct defocused 1064 nm beam of the CW Nd:YAG or the very occasional use of defocused CW CO_2 energy, no phototherapeutic light source is reported with a wavelength over 1000 nm.

The blue 415 nm is at the peak of the Soret band and is not only highly absorbed in melanin and blood, and it is right at the peak of the absorption spectrum of porphyrin. This wavelength is

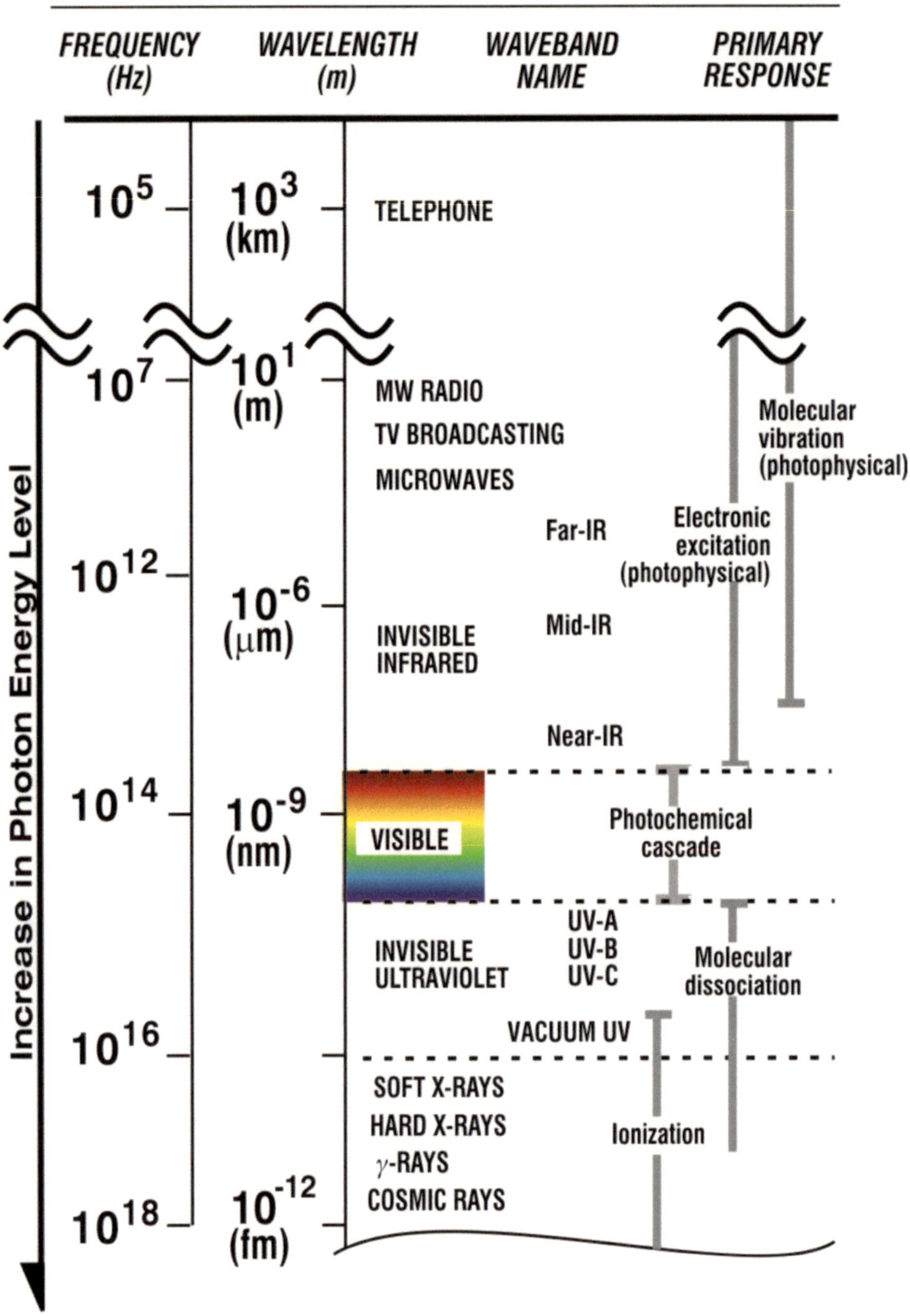

Figure 7. The electromagnetic spectrum (EM) covers a vast range of energy radiation types extending from the shortest cosmic waves (wavelengths measured in femtometers [fm] or shorter), through ultraviolet and visible radiation (nm), infrared radiation (μm) to the broadcasting waveband (m) and even mains current and wired telephone transmission (km).

http://dx.doi.org/10.5772/intechopen.68723

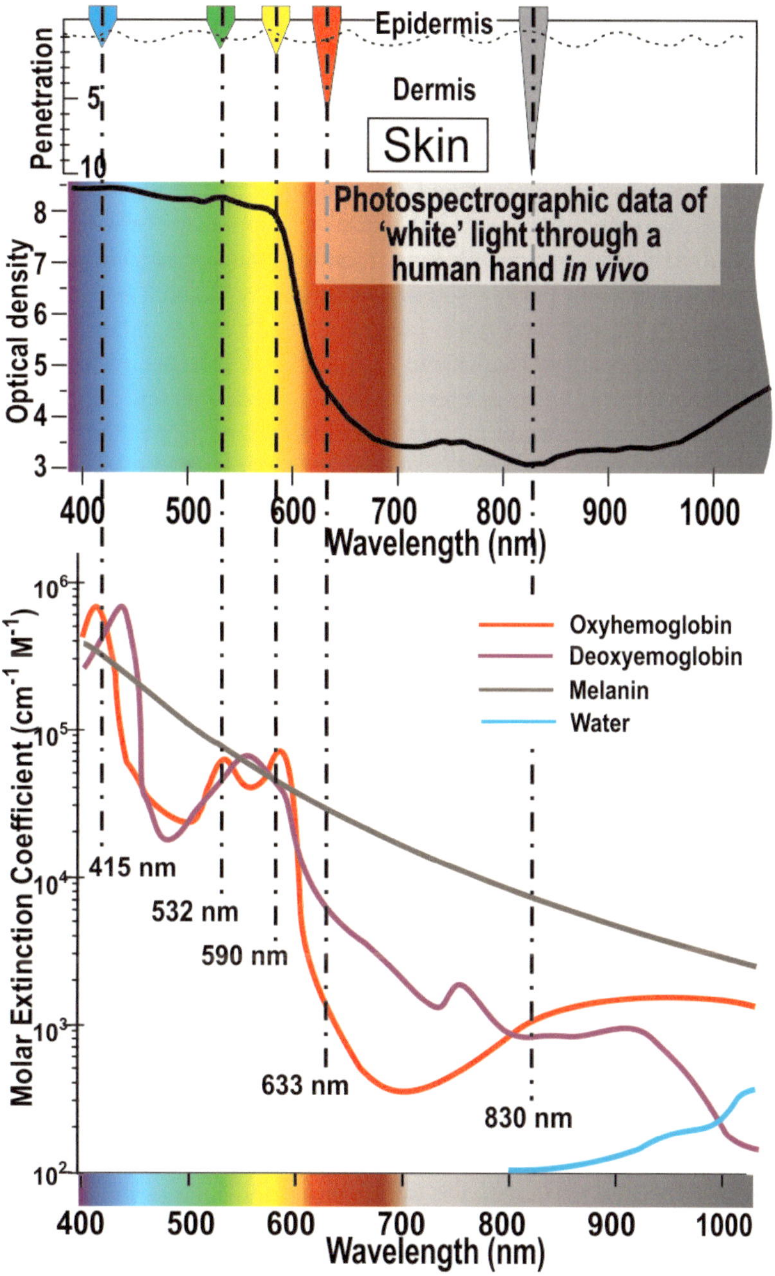

Figure 8. Several aspects illustrating the importance of wavelength in phototherapy. The central image shows photospectrometric data measured from penetration through a human hand in vivo. Based on the computer-derived trace on that part of the figure, the upper section illustrates relative penetration of selected wavelengths into the skin. Coupled with these, the lower section shows the absorption spectra of some biological chromophores, or targets, namely melanin, blood and water. Note the wavelength selectivity in these chromophores, and how that helps to determine the depth of penetration of different wavelengths into a living target as well as determining the target itself. Please see the text for further details.

popular as part of combination blue and red light (or near-IR) treatment of active inflammatory acne vulgaris [18]. The causative bacterium, *Propionibacterium acnes,* is known to harbor protoporphyrin IX (PpIX) and coproporphyrin III when it is active. By selectively targeting these porphyrins with light at 415 nm through endogenous photodynamic therapy (PDT), reactive oxygen species are rapidly generated within the *P. acnes,* and they are forced into apoptosis through oxidative stress [19]. With *P. acnes* damaged and destroyed, the inflammatory cycle of acne vulgaris is partially broken. No other wavelength is therefore appropriate for targeting the endogenous porphyrins in *P. acnes*. However, acne is recognized as a multifactorial disease with a strong inflammatory component, only partly associated with *P. acnes*, and both visible red (e.g., 633 nm) and near-IR light (e.g., 830 nm) have powerful antiinflammatory properties [20, 21]. If either of these wavelength therefore follows the 415 nm treatment some 48 h later, the remaining causes of the inflammation are targeted with deep penetration into the dermis, and an all-round approach to treating acne with blue and red (or infrared) light has been developed and well-reported [13, 22]. Here is an example where only a particular wavelength, or wavelengths, can affect a particular target, and in a multi-targeted disease a combination of wavelengths is therefore effective.

It can thus be stated that, in LLLT, wavelength governs both absorption, and penetration. However there is one other important factor which is connected with these two and that is intensity, consider **Figure 9a**. Two wavelength-specific targets exist in the upper dermis. An LLLT system, but with the incorrect wavelength, tries to treat target 1. The wavelength is incorrect, there is no absorption, and therefore, there is no reaction. Target 2 is irradiated with the correct wavelength, absorption occurs, and a reaction is successfully elicited. This is what the discussion above has been saying. Now look at **Figure 9b**: the targets are the same, but they are in the deeper dermis. An LLLT system irradiates the area over target 3, and the operator knows that the wavelength is correct. Unfortunately, there is insufficient photon intensity to get enough photons down through the dermis to the target: there is no absorption, hence no reaction. The operator therefore takes an LLLT system with a higher photon intensity and treats the area. The photons now reach the target 4 and are absorbed, and the desired reaction is achieved. So, although wavelength is key, if there is insufficient photon intensity from the light source giving low irradiance, or a too high angle of divergence diluting the irradiance, then the photon intensity at the target will not be sufficient to get the optimum reaction. In theory, one photon can activate one cell, but in practice, the cell needs to be bombarded with several photons, that is, multiphoton absorption, before the optimum level of reaction is reached. Sometimes having the right wavelength is just not enough.

This problem is associated more with LEDs than with LDs, because the photon intensity of LDs is many times higher than LEDs, given that LDs are coherent with all photons exactly the same wavelength, and in phase, exactly in step in temporally and spatially, like a regiment of identically clad soldiers marching in perfect time. The disadvantage of LD-LLLT is that it needs to be applied manually, point by point, in the contact mode, whereas LED systems have planar arrays which can cover large areas. Another way to ensure that as large a volume of tissue is involved is to maximize the scattering effect in tissue, and wavelength determines how well the light will scatter. Longer wavelengths scatter much better than shorter ones, in other words 830 nm scatters better than 640 which scatters better than 530 nm: **Figure 10** compares the penetration and scattering power of a 530 laser pointer (5 mW) with that of a

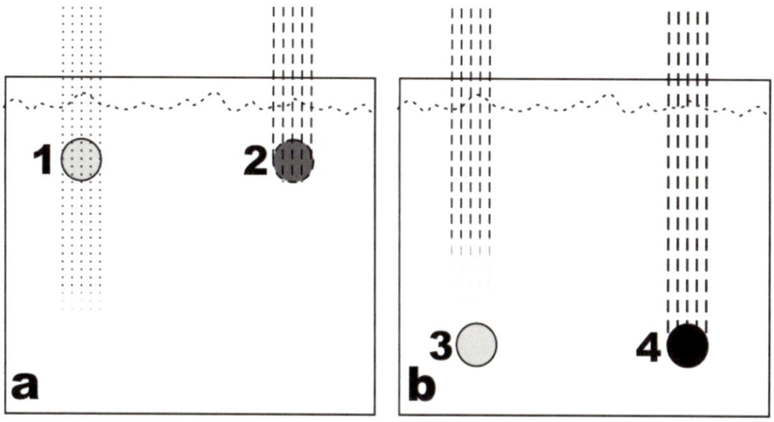

Figure 9. (a) The wavelength of light irradiating target 1 is inappropriate resulting in no absorption, therefore no reaction. On the other hand, target 2 is irradiated with an appropriate wavelength, and absorption occurs with a reaction. (b) The same targets are now deeper in the dermis. The same light source is used again, but the intensity is insufficient so not enough photons reach the target: no reaction. When the same light source is used at a higher intensity, the target is reached and a reaction is achieved.

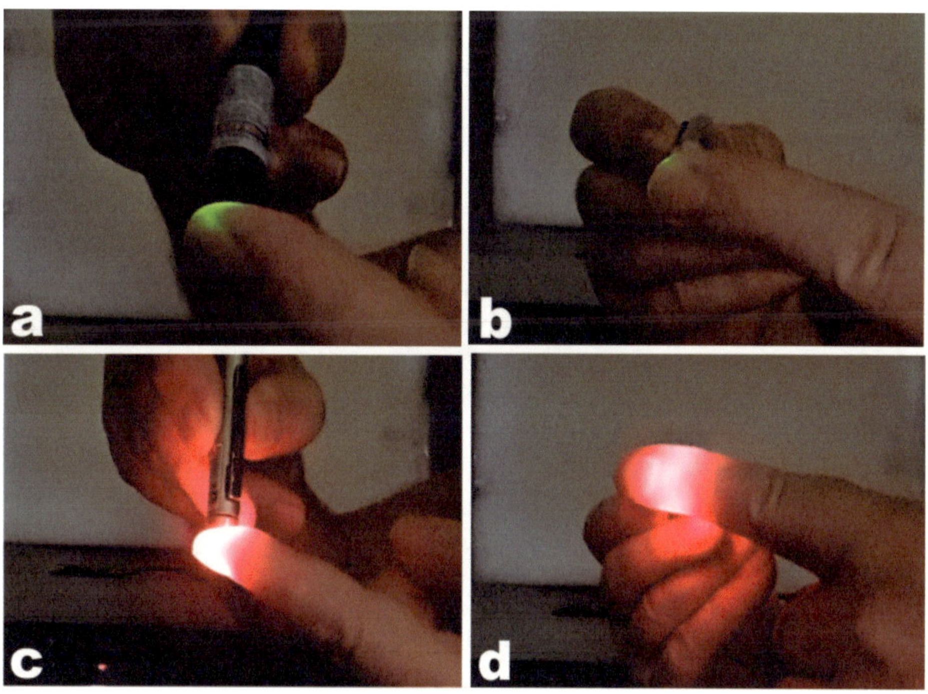

Figure 10. A green 530 nm 5 mW laser pointer compared with a red 640 nm 3 mW pointer. (a and b). Proof that green light, even laser energy, at 530 nm from a laser pointer neither penetrates deeply into a living finger nor does it scatter, even when placed near the thinner part of the fingertip. (c and d) On the other hand, the less powerful red laser light penetrates right through the finger and out the other side, even when placed a little bit further down the finger where there is bone as well (d). Note the scattering effect, transilluminating the whole lateral width of the finger. Note also the red light seen on the hand holding the pointer: that is illustrating powerful backscatter from the irradiated tissue.

640 nm laser pointer (3 mW). That figure illustrates very well that red light around 633 nm is capable of penetrating into living tissue deeper than 1 cm … the thickness of the author's (RGC) finger!

Scattering occurs when photons encounter different optical characteristics in the target and are pushed off their straight trajectory. They can be scattered forwards, laterally and backwards: actually, with enough photon intensity, it's a mixture of all three, and it is an excellent way to ensure that the largest possible area of tissue is affected by the incident light. In the case of laser energy, it is well understood that larger spot sizes minimize lateral and back scattering outside of the beam path in tissue and therefore get deeper absorption with more photons. Of course, the intrinsic absorption depth depends above everything else on the wavelength, but we can make science work for us to maximize that depth, and ensure multiphoton absorption in the target.

5. Light and tissue interaction

Unlike the situation in laser surgery, at the incident photon intensities associated with LLLT, there is no photothermally mediated effect. All effects take place at athermal, or almost athermal levels, and with no damage to cells or their organelles, or surrounding tissue. The key to the efficacy of LLLT in redressing the skin damage cause by the combination of photoaging and chronological aging lies in how the target cells, and other tissues, use the energy which is delivered to them by the incident photons, following absorption. As stressed in the previous section, there has to be absorption so that the little packet of energy carried by each photon is passed on to the energy pool of the target cells. The interaction between incident light and tissue is therefore at both the subcellular, cellular and tissue levels.

It was mentioned in passing in the previous section on wavelength that visible light and near-IR light actually have different primary mechanisms of action when absorption occurs in the target tissues. On referring back to **Figure 7**, there is a column titled 'Primary response.' For neither visible nor infrared light is photobiomodulation actually the primary response, but is rather the end result of the effect following the intermediate reactions associated with the primary response. As Karu has postulated [16], the basic stages of the LLLT-mediated reaction can be described as follows:

- Absorption (photoreception) occurs (by necessity … no absorption, no reaction) leading to the primary response.
- This induces the second stage, signal transduction and amplification.
- And leads to the ultimate stage of photobiomodulation (the photoresponse).

5.1. Visible light: primary photochemical reaction

For visible light, the primary response is photochemical in nature, with the main photoreceptor being the end terminal enzyme of the respiratory chain of the cellular mitochondria, cytochrome c oxidase, CCO, well demonstrated by Karu [16, 23]. The mitochondrion is arguably the most essential organelle for the cell, indeed for the entire organism, as its function is to act as the energy factory for the cell and surrounding tissue. The nucleus may be the heart and soul of a cell, but hearts and souls need energy to function, and that's the task of the mitochondrion. Mitochondrial CCO has an action spectrum which runs from the yellow through the red waveband (580–700 nm) with the peak around 630–635 nm. This made the helium neon (HeNe) laser at 632.8 nm an ideal phototherapy research tool, and almost all of Karu's and others' research on photobiomodulation in the 1970s to the end of the 1990s centered on the HeNe as the light source of choice. Now with quasimonochromatic LEDs available as a clinically useful light source, photoeffects of the 633 nm LED have also been well reported. The energy released by absorption of the incident photons in the CCO starts a photochemical cascade, resulting in the creation of adenosine triphosphate (ATP), simply described as follows: ATP synthase (ATPsy) with the coenzyme nicotinamide adenine dinucleotide (NAD) is triggered to combine inorganic phosphate (Pi) with adenosine diphosphate (ADP) to synthesize adenosine triphosphate (ATP). ATP is the fuel of the cell, and the organism. As part of this process, minute amounts of nitric oxide (NO) are released, NO being a powerful signaling compound with beneficial properties in tissues. In addition, calcium ions (Ca^{2+}) and protons (H^+) are also released into the cytosol, two very powerful additional signaling compounds. As the levels of these signaling compounds increase in the cytosol, the membrane transport mechanisms, in particular the sodium-potassium pump (Na^+K^+-ATPase), are stimulated into action resulting in interexchange of materials between the cellular cytosol and the extracellular fluid. At the same time, the message reaches the nucleus, and the final stage of photoresponse is reached: the cell is fully photoactivated. Photoactivated cells, if damaged or compromised, can repair themselves or be repaired; photoaged skin and wounded skin are examples of tissues with damaged or compromised cells. If the cells have a function to perform, for example, macrophages or fibroblasts, they will perform their job better and faster. If more of the cells are required, mitosis will be stimulated, or others will be recruited in. One, two or all three of these things can happen in photoactivated tissues. It is a powerful process.

On the other hand, light energy at 830 nm in the near-IR induces a completely different primary response, which is photophysical in nature rather than photochemical, as pointed out by Smith [2]. This comprises vibrational and rotational changes in the electrons of the atoms making up the molecules of the membranes of the target cells. This instantly activates the membrane transport mechanisms and intra- and extracellular exchange begins. The cellular energy requirements for this are very high, so the mitochondria are swiftly co-opted into action: at the same time, not only the cellular membranes, but also the membranes of the cellular organelles including the mitochondria are activated by near-IR wavelengths, so a secondary chemical ATP cascade is swiftly induced. Rather than being the primary photoresponse as with visible light, it therefore becomes part of the second stage of signal transduction and amplification with near-IR light, but the end result is exactly the same as for visible light: a photoactivated cell. The same three possible responses exist: repair, functional improvement or cell recruitment. Regarding the particularly interesting effect of LLLT at both visible and near-IR wavelengths on compromised or damaged cells, they actually and surprisingly respond many times better to LLLT than normal cells do, as has been commented on by many researchers [24]. As the cells found in photoaged skin are in various states of damage and are compromised to at least some degree, this aspect of the reaction to LLLT is of great interest in the photorejuvenation process in all affected cell types and extracellular matrix components. **Figure 11** schematically summarizes the effect of visible and near-IR LLLT on target cells. **Figure 12** takes us beyond the photoresponse, the endpoint achieved by both visible and near-IR light, and with a flow chart takes us through the various processes and complex interactions which have already been elicited and which lead to wound healing, as dealt with in a later section together with the antiinflammatory response [25]. The chart also shows the steps to pain attenuation which is also something that LLLT can achieve, but out with the scope of this chapter although it may be of interest to the reader.

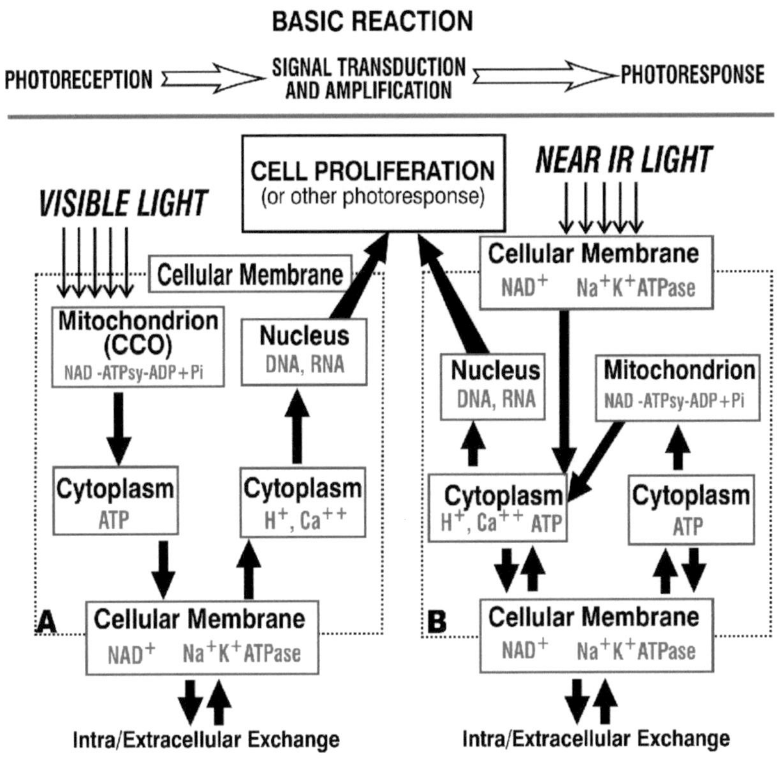

Figure 11. Primary and secondary photoresponse of target cells to visible and near-IR light. (A) Visible light penetrates through the cell membrane and is absorbed in cytochrome c oxidase in the mitochondrion respiratory chain, initiating a photochemical cascade with production of adenosine triphosphate. (B) Near-IR light, on the other hand, is mostly absorbed by the membrane itself, immediately initiating the membrane transfer mechanisms through a photophysical reaction. This leads to a secondary chemical cascade. See the text for further details (CCO, cytochrome c oxidase; NAD, nicotinamide adenine dinucleotide; NAD^+, oxidized form of NAD; ATP, adenosine triphosphate; ATPsy, ATP synthase; ADP, adenosine diphosphate; Pi, inorganic phosphorus; Ca^{2+}, calcium ion; H^+, proton; Na^+K^+ATPase, sodium-potassium pump [cell transport mechanism]).

http://dx.doi.org/10.5772/intechopen.68723

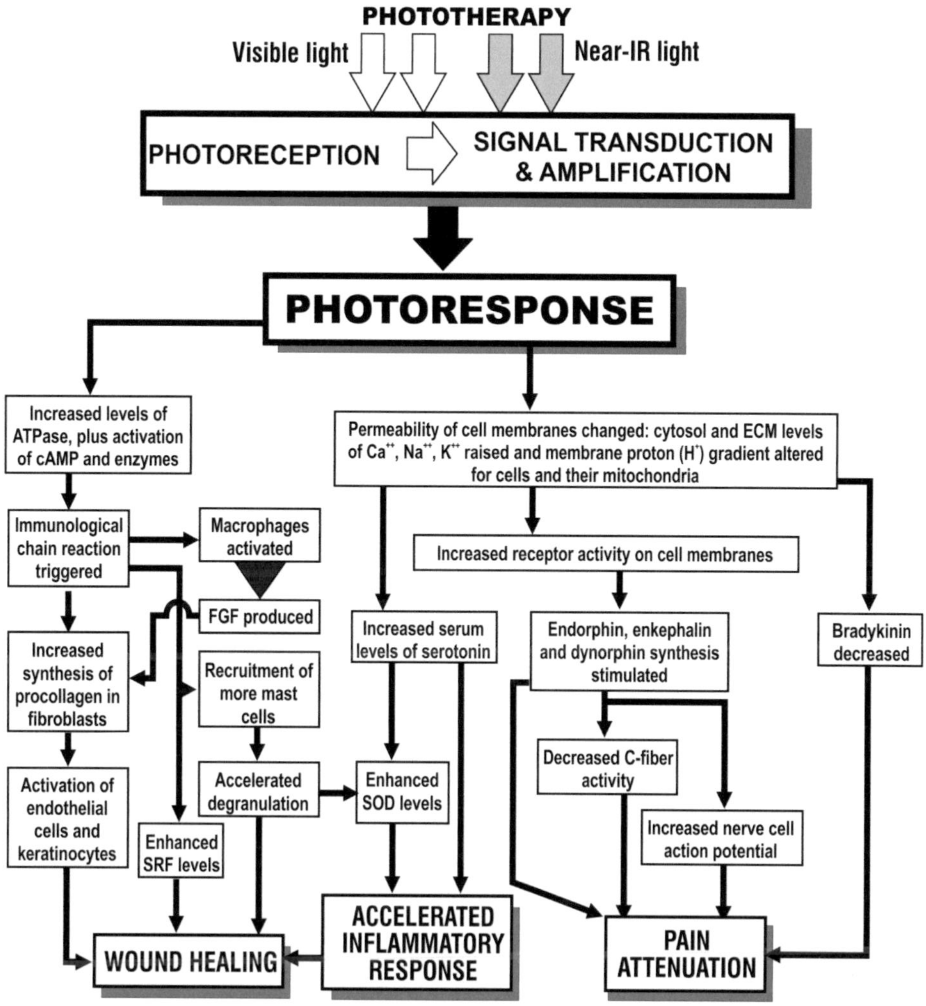

Figure 12. What happens after the photoresponse has been achieved and the target cells are photoactivated? This flowchart explores the already elicited steps on the pathway to wound healing, including the antiinflammatory effect of LLLT. These effects are mostly elicited with 830 nm (from Refs. [25, 26]. Used with permission of the publishers). ATPase, adenosine triphosphatase; cAMP, cyclic adenosine monophosphate; ECM, extracellular matrix; Ca^{2+}, calcium ion; K^{2+}, potassium ion; H^{+}, proton; FGF, fibroblast growth factor; SOD, superoxide dismutase; SRF, serum response factor.

5.1.1. Parameters involved in this interaction

The critical parameter has already been discussed above, namely the wavelength. What wavelength is required will depend largely on what targets are to be treated. In the case of rejuvenation of photoaged skin, the major target will be the cells in the epidermis and dermis whose function is to maintain the integrity of these structures. The next section will look at these cells in some detail, with a note regarding which wavelength or wavelengths have been examined for efficacy in achieving photomodulation in these cells. The other two parameters, which are also important, are the irradiance or power density measured in W/cm^2, and the dose or energy density, measured in J/cm^2.

The power density (PD) describes the actual power incident on the tissue per unit area. The output power on its own is a good guide to what the system is capable of delivering, but it does not become meaningful until the unit area the energy is irradiating is also brought into the equation: the area targeted by any system is called the spot size, from which the irradiated area can be calculated. For LD-LLLT systems, the spot size can be rather small with the diameter measured in mm, although there are some systems that deliver a defocused spot of 1 cm in diameter or more using an optical fiber delivery system. Typical output powers for these systems range from a few mW up to 1000 mW, 1 W. The irradiation pattern for LDs is an ellipse, with a longer and a shorter axis, so measuring the area is not as simple as that of a circular spot for which the area is calculated using the formula pi (π, 3.142) times the square of the radius (r) of the spot in centimeters, written as πr^2, expressed in cm^2. It is important to remember to use the radius, one-half of the diameter, rather than the diameter itself. To calculate the PD, the output power in watts is divided by the irradiated area in cm^2, giving W/cm^2, or mW/cm^2. In the following example, an LD-LLLT system delivers 1000 mW with a spot size of 1 cm: the power is thus 1.0 W and the radius is 5 mm, 0.5 cm, which when squared becomes 0.25 multiplied by 3.142, to give the area as 0.786 cm^2. Dividing the power by the area gives us the PD, 1.27 W/cm^2 in this example. The typical range of power densities can be from 15 mW/cm^2 or lower, up to as high as 5 W/cm^2 or even higher. It is possible to go up to a PD of 10 W/cm^2 without seeing any appreciable rise in the temperature of the irradiated tissue, but the exposure time becomes much shorter as will be discussed under energy density below. For elliptical spot sizes treated with an LD-based system, the area of an ellipse is calculated by πab, where a is the radius of the longer axis and b the radius of the shorter axis (expressed in cm). If the spot size is 2 mm x 1 mm, then the area will be $(3.142 \times 0.1 \times 0.05) = 0$ .0157 cm^2. A 60 mW LD-LLLT system with that spot size would thus have a power density of 3.82 W/cm^2. These examples give PDs (irradiances) on the high side, but which are still valid power densities to achieve athermal LLLT.

Having worked out the power density, the next consideration is how long will this be incident on the target tissue, referred to as the exposure time and measured in seconds (s). By multiplying the PD by the exposure time, the energy density (ED) or dose is calculated in J/cm^2. Quite often the energy of a system is stated in J. One joule is 1 W for 1 s, but without the unit area irradiated by that energy, the value is totally useless for anyone trying to replicate the experiment. The correct way to report any such LLLT experiment is to give all of the parameters, namely output power, spot size or irradiated area and the exposure time. Both the PD and the ED can then be calculated, and the same parameters can be replicated by anyone wishing to conduct the same treatment, with hopefully the same result. Once an ideal dose in J/cm^2 has been determined, then the irradiation time necessary to achieve that dose can be calculated for any system once the PD is known, by dividing the ED in J/cm^2 by the PD expressed in W. If 60 J/cm^2 is determined to be the optimum dose, then for an LLLT system delivering 100 mW/cm^2, the treatment time will be $60 \div 0.1 = 600$ s = 10 min. The higher the PD of the system, the shorter the irradiation time to achieve the same dose: a 500 mW/cm^2 system will take 2 min, and a 3 W/cm^2 system will take only 20 s to deliver 60 J/cm^2. However, caution is required when only the dose (ED) is considered without thinking of the PD. When a dose of 60 J/cm^2 is achieved over 30 ms with a PD of 2000 W/cm^2, the effect will be photosurgical, with heat and damage occurring in the tissue. On the other hand, if the same dose (60 J/cm^2) is delivered with a PD of 100 mW/cm^2 over 10 min, the effect will ne athermal and atraumatic, in other words LLLT, but the dose is the same. If we use a pharmaceutical analogy, the PD is the medicine, and the ED is the dose. As any pharmacist will tell you, if the medicine is not correct, there is no use in playing around with the dose.

In the case of LED-based systems, or the filtered lamp type of system, we are often at the mercy of the manufacturer regarding the rated irradiance of their system unless we have access to the sophisticated type of integrating sphere power meter needed to measure this output. In both types of system, a divergent cone of light is delivered: LEDs by their very nature emit a divergent ellipse-like cone, whereas the light from the lamp filter is a simple divergent cone. This means that the area irradiated by the light will increase as the light source is drawn away from the target, thereby reducing the incident PD by an inverse square ratio. This is illustrated in **Figure 13** comparing a single collimated LD, a single LED an LED panel and several panels in an articulated array, ideal for treating contoured biological targets, for example, the face, to give uniform intensity over the entire surface. It is therefore important to ascertain at what distance the manufacturer has calculated the irradiance (almost always in mW/cm^2). One of the advantages of LED systems, but which make calculation of the PD extremely difficult without actual measurement with a suitable power meter, is the fact that the intersecting LED beams create a phenomenon known as photon interference. **Figure 13** shows this schematically. A greater photon intensity is delivered at a distance from the surface of the LEDs in the array than actually at the surface of the array, that is, directly in front of the LEDs with no distance between them and the target tissue. For this reason, those LED mask-type facial photorejuvenation systems available on the market, and some hand-held systems designed to be used in contact with the target tissue, are not maximizing the effect of the LEDs mounted in the mask or applicator, because the full potential of the LEDs is not being realized by not creating a distance between the LEDs and the target tissue. This is not to say that these direct contact systems will not have any effect: there will be some absorption, therefore there will be a reaction, but it will not be as effective clinically as when the LED array is some centimeters from the target tissue. A recent study measured the irradiance of a commercially available 830 nm LED-LLLT system at various points from adjacent to the LEDs themselves to several cm away [26]. At some 10 cm away from the arrays, the actual irradiance in mW/cm^2 had gradually increased to be significantly higher than that measured at the LEDs themselves, because of the photon interference phenomenon, and remained high up to 17 cm from the panels before there was any noticeable drop off in intensity. Interestingly in this study, at 20 cm the measured irradiance was equal to that at 3 cm distance. The photon intensity of LED planar arrays is a function of the total area of the active array and the placing of the LEDs. From a certain distance between the array and the tissue: the array is not seen by the tissue as individual LEDs, but as a fairly homogeneous single irradiator.

When the benefit of photon interference is combined with the powerful scattering effect of red and particularly near-IR light in tissue (*cf* the scattering power of red *vs* green in **Figure 10**),

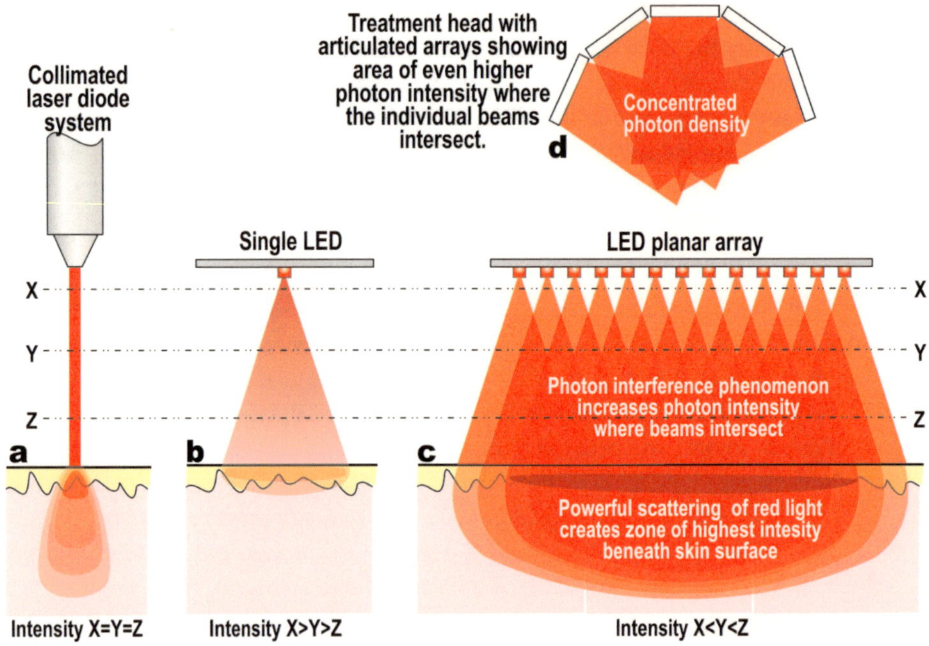

Figure 13. Different beam patterns above and in tissue compared among an LD and LEDs. (a) LD-based LLLT system showing a collimated, coherent beam without too much loss of intensity. Deep penetration is achieved in tissue because of the coherent nature of the beam and high photon intensity. Good scattering causes concentrated intensity in the target tissue just beneath the skin surface. (b) A single LED with a noncoherent divergent beam, losing in intensity as the beam diverges. Poor penetration is achieved with extremely low photon intensity in very superficial skin. (c) An array of LEDs showing intersection of each beam causing the photon interference phenomenon, increasing the photon intensity as the beams show multiple intersection as they near the tissue. Deeper penetration is achieved in the target because of the enhanced photon intensity, with scattering of the red light causing the zone of highest intensity in the target tissue beneath the skin surface. (d) Treatment head comprising 5 LED panels, articulated to allow adjustment to follow the contour of a curved target, for example, the face. Where the beams from all the panels intersect, a zone of even higher photon intensity is created to enhance treatment efficacy.

an interesting phenomenon has been noted whereby the highest photon intensity in the target tissue is actually beneath the surface, exactly where it is required, as the cellular targets for LED-LLLT lie at the stratum basale in the epidermis and in the dermal matrix. The same phenomenon of photon interference does not occur with the filtered light sources as many of these incorporate a polarizer in the lens, and therefore, a highly significant drop-off in intensity occurs concomitantly with the increasing distance between the lamp/filter and the target tissue, similar to the single LED seen in **Figure 12b**.

5.2. Cellular targets for light-tissue interaction

The following **Table 1** summarizes the main cellular targets for LLLT, and all can participate in some way to help to turn back the skin aging clock during the process of LLLT photorejuvenation.

The majority of these cells are the key players in the wound healing process. What has the wound healing process to do with photorejuvenation of skin? The answer is … everything, and that will be made clear in the next section.

http://dx.doi.org/10.5772/intechopen.68723

Cell	Location/function	Effective wavelength(s)	Photobiomodulation-boosted activity
Keratinocytes [27]	Epidermis: Stratum basale Germinative cells ('mother keratinocytes'), producing constantly upward-moving daughter keratinocytes making up the stratum spinosum. Also known for plentiful cytokine synthesis	590 nm 633 nm 830 nm	590 nm and 633 nm: target CCO in the abundant keratinocyte mitochondria to boost intra-and extracellular ATP, $Ca2+$ and $H+$. Improve tight cell adhesion in stratum spinosum and enhance cellularity of daughter keratinocytes. Improve quality of epidermis through efficient daughter keratinocyte production by mother keratinocytes. Synthesize multiple pro- and antiinflammatory cytokines, some of which drop down into the dermis and react with fibroblasts, macrophages and mast cells 830 nm: act on keratinocyte function via photophysical interaction with membrane. End result same as for 590 nm and 633 nm End result: a fresh-looking and plump epidermis, an essential component in skin photorejuvenation
Melanocytes [28–30]	Epidermis: Stratum basale Melanin-producing dendritic cells (in melanosomes), with pigment-darkening as melanosomes proceed out along dendrites for incorporation in daughter keratinocytes as granules	633 nm 830 nm 415 nm	Both 633 nm and 830 nm have been shown to regulate the tyrosine-tyrosinase oxidation process, reduce excess amounts of pigment-darkening tyrosinase and quantities of tyrosinase-related proteins (TyRPs) 1 & 2. Normalization of dopa and dopamine, associated with over- and underactivity of tyrosinase. Some reports on 830 nm repigmentation of systemic vitiligo lesions 415 nm has shown the potential to help with repigmentation of depigmented areas through action on the melanocyte End result: can be normalization of any abnormal pigment synthesis and over-darkening activity as well as the potential to repigment depigmented areas
Fibroblasts [14, 30–32]	All layers of the dermis Most important cells for producing and monitoring structural components of the extracellular matrix (ECM, collagen and elastin fibers). Also produce and regulate the ECM lubricating ground substance	590 nm* 633 nm 830 nm	633 nm, 830 nm: LLLT-irradiated fibroblasts produce better quality collagen (mostly type I), better elastin and replenish the ground substance. Photoactivated fibroblasts also more efficiently keep homeostasis of the dermal extracellular matrix through balancing levels of lytic enzymes (matrix metalloproteinases, MMPs) and protective enzymes (tissue inhibitors of MMPs, TIMPs). LLLT-treated facial skin showed plump, fibroplasic fibroblasts with good collagen bundles compared with unirradiated and sham-irradiated skin End result: much better structured ECM with plump, well-oriented collagen bundles (better sheer strength), and new elastic fibers (better ability for skin to reform after deformation)
Mast cells [30, 33, 34]	Exist throughout the ECM, usually found clustered around blood vessels Basophilic granulocytes which play a role during allergic and wound repair activity through release of pro- and antiinflammatory granules, cellular chemotactic agents, trophic factors and superoxide dismutase (SOD), a powerful endogenous antioxidant	830 nm 633 nm (lesser extent)	When irradiated during LLLT with 830 nm in particular, mast cells are stimulated to release their granules in several stages into the ECM, which normally only happens following wounding or as part of an allergic response. First stage is proinflammatory, which peaks and then quenches the inflammatory stage of wound healing. Second stage is antiinflammatory to hasten movement from the inflammatory stage into proliferative stage, and release of chemotactic factors to recruit more reparative cells, plus release of trophic factors to support these cells. Finally mast cells release SOD which remains in the ECM and acts as a protective agent against future oxidative stress, for example, UV radiation-mediated as part of the extrinsic aging process End result: mast cell degranulation accelerate the usual wound healing phases, allowing a quicker interphase transition between inflammation and proliferation, thus the remodeling stage starts earlier and works more efficiently to give good alignment and better orientation of new fibers, especially in the Grenz zone just under the dermoepidermal junction

Cell	Location/function	Effective wavelength(s)	Photobiomodulation-boosted activity
Macrophages [35–38]	Free-floating in the ECM throughout all layers of the dermis Phagocytic cells whose task is to maintain the cleanliness of the ECM by removing all detritus, such as denatured fibrous fragments, cellular and other debris. An important point si that during phagocytic action, they release fibroblast growth factor (FGF), ideal for fibroblasts during the proliferative stage of wound healing	830 nm 633 nm (lesser extent)	LLLT with 830 nm in particular, although 633 nm has also been trialled, has been shown to photoactivate macrophages to work harder and faster through more efficient target identification and chemotaxis, to internalize their collected debris better and return to their task faster. When photoactivated, macrophages were shown to release at least an order of magnitude more FGF, thus making the ECM a better and more favorable environment for fibroblasts during the proliferative stage End result: with a cleaner and clearer ECM, the skin condition is maintained better. Fibroblasts are able to do their job in a more favorable environment thanks to the presence of trophic factors
Neutrophils [39–42]	White blood cells (granulocytes, part of the polymorphonuclear cell family) found when required anywhere in the dermis First line of defense by the immune system against invading pathogens. They engulf their target and kill it through oxidative stress via the release of singlet oxygen species. Associated with trophic factor release, particularly transforming growth factor (TGF) α and β	830 nm	Neutrophils are normally associated with an attack by invading pathogens or as prophylactic protection immediately after wounding. When irradiated with 830 nm, neutrophils are recruited into normal skin. Even although there are no pathogens for them to kill, they still release trophic factors beneficial to the wound healing process as a whole End result: more trophic factors added to the ECM to assist other cells during either the wound healing process or as part of their normal duties

CCO, cytochrome c oxidase.

*Only from in vitro studies, but very limited in vivo by extremely poor penetration.

Table 1. Target cells for phototherapy, their biological location, the wavelength(s) to which they respond best and a description of their activity when photoactivated.

5.3. Blood supply as a target for LLLT photorejuvenation

There is no point in encouraging the skin cells to thrum along nicely unless these cells are receiving nutrition and oxygen and that is the function of the dermal vasculature. Both 633 and 830 nm have been associated with supportive activity for the blood vessels in the dermis [42–47]. The interaction between blood vessels and LLLT is therefore of equal importance to the interaction between LLLT and the skin cells. Because of its deeper penetration, and possibly because it delivers a photophysical primary response to the endothelial cells, 830 nm has a good body of literature supporting a strong interaction with the blood supply, delivering a higher flow rate and volume and thus bring oxygenation and nutrition to the ECM. In addition, where there have been circulatory problems, LLLT has restored circulation such as in ischemia animal models, and Raynaud's patients [47, 48]. It has been suggested that the LLLT acts directly on the vessel walls, but there is also a reaction involving the parasympathetic system, inducing further extended vasodilation. In one study involving patients with the athetotic type of cerebral palsy, patients in a state of sympathetic hypertension with very poor blood supply to the peripheral circulation as assessed by real-time fine plate thermography received one single 830 nm LLLT session on acupuncture points on the chest. Within 5 min, thermography revealed increasing body warming which remained highly significant in the extremities at 90 min after the single treatment [49].

This effect on the parasympathetic system, our 'rest and digest' or 'rest and relax' nervous system is important as a destressor, as stress is also a contributory factor to the aging of the skin. In particular with the 830 nm LED-LLLT system, it is often noted that patients quickly fall asleep during photorejuvenation sessions and wake up feeling refreshed. Within 5–10 min, a gentle warming of the face is also felt as the microvasculature brings more blood to the superficial dermis through vasodilation. The latter is without a doubt a physical beneficial phenomenon, whereas the former is more of a psychosomatic benefit. However, if patients feel more relaxed, and in fact, their faces have been treated with LLLT photorejuvenation; the importance of the psychosomatic benefits cannot be ignored, mostly due to the improved vascular supply following parasympathetic system stimulation by, in particular, 830 nm LLLT.

6. Wound healing: the basis of photorejuvenation

As stated above, the wound healing process underpins good skin rejuvenation. When the photoaged and intrinsically aged skin is studied carefully, the onslaught from environmental factors such as air pollution, ultraviolet-related oxidative stress, smoking for those who smoke, or even for those who are forced to exist in a smoky atmosphere, nutritional factors and even the water in which we wash our skin and drink takes an enormous toll on the ordered structures of the extracellular matrix and the level of activity of the cells populating it. Photoaged skin is every bit as compromised as wounded skin, and so one of the optimum and most elegant ways to fight this skin damage, most of which is due to sunlight, is to use the beneficial side of light through application of LLLT: in other words, apply photorejuvenation.

When the aims of photorejuvenation are considered carefully, the reader will see clearly that the end results of the wound healing process and photorejuvenation are synonymous. We need new and well-organized collagen fibers and bundles, efficiently remodeled to give optimum orientation, body and strength to the skin including a nicely linearly oriented Grenz zone coursing under the dermoepidermal junction, and adding support to the epidermal appearance. We need the degraded elastotic elastic fibers replaced with newly synthesized elastin forming new, viable elastic fibers to return the reforming and tightening properties to sagging photoaged skin. We need fresh and well-hydrated ground substance, to lubricate and oxygenate the components of the ECM. We need toned up and active fibroblasts to deliver all three of these goals just mentioned, and to regulate the homeostasis of the ECM supported by hard-working macrophages to maintain ECM health through keeping it free of clogging debris. Furthermore, above this restored and youthful ECM, we need a clear, luminous epidermis, with good basement membrane function to support and nourish the activities of the germinative and other cells in the stratum basale; well-convoluted papillary processes are also needed to give as large a supporting area as possible at the dermoepidermal junction, and above the epidermis, we need a well-ordered stratum corneum to provide good skin barrier function without excess sebum. With application of LLLT, all of these can be achieved through the athermal and atraumatic action of LLLT on the target cells, particularly if LLLT is used in combination with moisturizing and nutrifying creams and sera with the added protection of a daily regimen using a good UVA/B sunscreen.

The wound healing cells have been introduced in **Table 1**, namely, the mast cells, macrophages and neutrophils during the immediately post-wound inflammatory process; the fibroblasts and endotheliocytes (to repair damaged blood vessels or for neovascularization) during the proliferative stage; and the transformational cells during the long remodeling stage, fibroblast to myofibroblast transformation and fibroblast to fibrocyte dedifferentiation. All these cells occur at their different stages, and in different numbers. If we can marry LLLT with these potential targets, then we can get more efficient wound healing, and faster, without compromising the process in any way. The wavelengths which have shown efficacy for each cell type are listed in **Table 1**. In general, 830 nm near-IR is the favorite, followed by 633 nm visible red, and LED-based systems are in the ascendency compared with LD-based systems, simply because the LED systems are capable of irradiating a large area in a hands-free manner. If we can get efficient wound healing, then we can most certainly extrapolate the same benefits to the indication of phototherapy for photorejuvenation of the aging skin.

A PubMed search using 'LLLT' and 'Wound healing' brings up over 700 titles in a vast range of wound types, and surgical specialities. That is an impressive number. How does LLLT affect frank wound healing? In a study by Trelles and colleagues on the application of LED-LLLT after full face ablative resurfacing with the Er:YAG and CO_2 laser in 50 patients, 25 received LLLT after their resurfacing procedure, and 25 received sham treatment [50]. In the LLLT group, healing (as defined by full reepithelization and resolution of edema and erythema) occurred in an average of 6.1 days compared with 13.2 days in the non-LLLT group. In addition, all the usual side effects associated with full-face ablative resurfacing, edema, erythema, bruising and pain were significantly reduced in the LLLT group, with better than 92% of the LLLT patients being extremely satisfied with the procedure compared with 55%

of the sham-LLLT group. A recent study by Min and Goo examined 830 nm LED-LLLT for a variety of skin wounds which had proved recalcitrant to normal healing, including severe inflammation, bacterial infection, viral infection, and Bell's palsy [51]. All cleared up in from 1 to 5 weeks with no visible scar formation, even in one case of a severe ischemic ulcer with a large defect. In a case report on contact irritant dermatitis caused by a home-use alpha-hydroxy peel, corticosteroids failed to reduce the inflammation for more than 5 weeks: 830 nm LED-LLLT in three sessions, 3 days apart, completely controlled it [25]. Moreover, 830 nm LED-LLLT has shown significant prophylaxis against hypertrophic scar formation postthyroidectomy in a controlled study [52]. To summarize, it can be argued that LLLT not only speeds up the wound healing process, but ensures that good quality wound healing is achieved, with prophylaxis against unwanted scar formation.

7. Clinical indications of phototherapy in skin rejuvenation

So, finally, having looked at some of the science and technology behind phototherapy, what about LLLT for photorejuvenation of the aging and aged skin? First the methods available need to be considered. Discussed earlier in this chapter were LD-based systems, LED-based systems, and filtered lamp-based systems. It has to be said that LD-based systems deliver higher photon intensities than LEDs, which in turn are in general much more intense than filtered lamp systems. LDs deliver coherent light at a precise wavelength. LEDs deliver non-coherent light, but with more than 95% of the photons at the rated wavelength, quasimonochromaticity, and with clinically useful photon intensity thanks to their treatment head design and photon interference among the LED beams. Filtered lamps deliver polarized light at a slightly broader bandwidth than LEDs because of the filter technology, but with rather low intensities requiring longer exposure times. Almost all LD-based systems require manual application in a point-by-point mode, and even those with some form of stand-based applicator can cover only a small area at a time. LED-based systems have large-areas planar arrays, the better systems having multiple articulated panels to enable uniform irradiation of curved areas of the body, such as the face: these are applied in a completely hands-free manner, covering large areas of the body in one session. Filtered lamp systems are also available with stands to hold the lamp in a hands-free manner, but have a smaller treatment area than LED systems, and cannot cover curved areas with uniform irradiance.

Based on the statements above, the authors therefore feel that, given the rise of popularity of LED-based phototherapy systems in the clinical world and also given the increasing body of LED-based evidence in the peer-reviewed literature [25, 53], the optimum phototherapy system for photorejuvenation should thus be the large array LED-based system. The wavelengths which have achieved the largest coverage in the literature are as follows: 415 nm, but only as part of acne phototherapy, so perhaps cannot be included in photorejuvenation; 633 nm visible red; and 830 nm. Of the latter two, several articles have examined the use of the wavelengths in sequential combination for photorejuvenation, with very good results. [14, 54, 55]. The regimen as it evolved called for the near-IR 830 nm to be applied first, then 2–3 days later the 633 nm visible red head was applied. This was repeated over 4 weeks. The dose for the 830 nm component was usually 60 J/cm^2, and for the 633 nm was over the 100 J/cm^2 mark. All three studies had a follow-up period, ranging between 8 and 12 weeks during which no further treatment was given, subjects being allowed only to wash their faces with hypoallergenic soap without any other skin care preparation. In all studies, steady improvement was noted in the skin condition in the weeks after the final treatment. The ultimate study in photorejuvenation with LED-LLLT was that by Lee and colleagues [32], in which she compared 633 used on its own with 830 used on its own, the 830/633 nm combination and a sham treated control group. All subjects had only one-half of their faces treated. Lee not only took clinical photography, she also conducted histological, profilometric, ultrastructural and immunohistochemical assays to examine what was happening underpinning the very good results of her study at 12 weeks after the final treatment session. All the LED-treated groups were statistically significantly better than the sham group, and the treated sides were improved compared with the untreated sides: in the sham-irradiated group, there was no real improvement between the sides. It was anticipated that the combination group would show the best results, but in fact it was the 830 nm group who led in most of the assays. Skin elasticity at 2 weeks after the final treatment was significantly better for the 830 nm group, as was neocollagenesis and elastinogenesis. A strong Grenz zone was seen under a plumper and better organized epidermis, and fibroblasts in transmission electron microscopy were active and fibroplasic, surrounded by bundles of good quality collagen fibers. At 2 weeks after the final treatment, tissue inhibitors of matrix metalloproteinases (TIMPs) 1 and 2 were seen, suggesting a photoprotective effect, which was not seen in the sham or unirradiated specimens. The major finding for the subjects themselves was assessed via patient satisfaction. In all the treated groups, this grew significantly from immediately after the final session to 12 weeks after the session. The combination 830/633 nm group was significantly superior to the 633 nm only group. However, the most surprising finding was the much earlier and better satisfaction recorded by the 830 nm group.

So how does LED-LLLT help with rejuvenating the photoaged face? In short, LED-LLLT stimulates all phases of the wound healing process, but without causing any wound. It was shown that 830 nm LED in a human subject study in vivo recruited significantly more mast cells, macrophages and neutrophils into irradiated tissue 48 h after a single irradiation of one arm in all 8 subjects in the study, compared with the unirradiated arms [34]. Moreover, at 48 h the mast cells had mostly degranulated, compared with no degranulation at all seen in the contralateral untreated arm. Similar findings have also been observed in the mouse tongue model, although with 633 nm rather than 830 nm [33]. Additionally, ultrastructural assessment with transmission electron microscopy showed that the ECM in all the treated tissue specimens was in what appeared to be an inflammatory state with abundant interstitial spaces and the clear presence of perivascular edema. The findings resembled those after a wound, but there was no wound.

The authors surmised that the swift degranulation of the mast cells very soon after 830 nm LED-LLLT had dumped a slew of proinflammatory cytokines into the normal tissue during the first stage of excellulation of granules which had induced a wound-like response. More mast cells and macrophages were then recruited in via chemotactic signals released by the granules, together with neutrophils, none of the latter being found in any of the fields in the specimens from the unirradiated arms. In other words, a quasi-wound had been formed with a strong inflammatory response, but without heat or damage, and with no grossly visible aspects of any of the traditional signs of wounding, calor, rubor or dolor. The wound healing process teaches us that, after inflammation, comes proliferation, followed by remodeling. The authors concluded that the action of the 830 nm LED-LLLT on mast cells had elucidated the first stage toward photorejuvenation by creating the inflammatory response.

It could therefore be argued, based on the findings in the Lee study referenced above, and the speedy wound healing in other studies, that the continued regimen of LED LLLT, twice weekly over 4 weeks, accelerated the wound healing process underpinning the rejuvenation of both the ECM and the epidermis in a stepwise manner, enhancing the fibroblast activity in the proliferative stage, and allowing the remodeling stage to be entered earlier. That continued improvement seen in the Lee study following the end of the actual treatment in all three treatment groups, but particularly in the 830 nm group, was the visible result of the remodeling process working on the newly laid down collagen fibers in the dermis during the proliferative stage, supported by the fresh elastinogenesis. On the other hand, it took time, 12 weeks in fact, to see the optimum results. This shows how important it is to prepare patients to be patient when planning photorejuvenation with low level light therapy. LED-LLLT certainly works, but it works from the inside out and takes time. However, concomitant use of good skin care preparations and establishment of a daily UVA/B sunscreen regimen would accelerate results and quite possibly maintain them even longer.

As to the optimum wavelength, in a review on the efficacy of LED-LLLT, Kim and Calderhead came down firmly in favor of the 830 nm wavelength [25]. Calderhead and colleagues reviewed 830 nm LED-LLLT both in stand-alone and in adjunctive indications and came to the same conclusion [56]. In a recent invited review for *Clinics in Plastic Surgery*, Calderhead and Vasily examined the efficacy of LED-LLLT in the aging face, and again pointed to the overall efficacy of the 830 nm wavelength [57]. Having said that, 633 nm has shown interesting results on induction of fibroplasia in fibroblasts in a human in vivo model, so cannot be discounted [32]. As long as there is absorption there will be reaction, and remember that the key to absorption to achieve effective photorejuvenation is primarily wavelength.

8. Innovations in photorejuvenation

The previous sections in this chapter have dealt mostly with very narrow-band light sources in photorejuvenation as part of photomedicine, concentrated on non-coherent but quasimonochromatic LEDs and coherent LDs at specific wavelengths. However, one of this chapter's authors (YT) has recently launched exploration into a new concept of potentially phototherapeutic light having built up an impressively large body of evidence. Tanaka offers an innovative approach to photorejuvenation, namely comparatively broad band near-IR with a cut-on/cut-off water filter to exclude certain wavelengths in that IR waveband.

A specific band of near-IR energy (1100–1800 nm together with a water-filter that excludes wavelengths 1400–1500 nm) has been demonstrated by Tanaka to induce various biological effects through a broad range of clinical, histological, and biochemical investigations [58–72]. Tanaka reported that water-filtered broad-spectrum near-IR can promote up-regulation of genes related to type I collagen synthesis, including LARP6 and COL1A1, which achieves skin tightening and skin rejuvenation [72]. This exciting development of a specific broad-band IR waveband is also associated with deep penetration of the water-filtered waveband into the dermal ECM, targeting both cells, subcellular components and the vascular plexus.

Tanaka also reported that water-filtered broad-spectrum near-IR induces long-lasting vasodilation that may prevent vasospasm and be beneficial for ischemic disorders [65]. Near-IR also relaxes and weakens dystonic and hypertrophic muscles to reduce wrinkles and myalgia [60, 61]. The ability of LLLT at 830 nm to activate the parasympathetic system and counteract sympathetic hypertension was noted above as reported by Asagai and colleagues [49], so this new approach pioneered by Tanaka may also have far-reaching benefits in the treatment of athetotic tonic spasm in profoundly affected cerebral palsy quadriplegic patients. Near-IR is an essential tool in cancer detection and imaging and induces drastic non-thermal DNA damage of mitotic cells, which may be beneficial for treating cancer [66, 67]. Activation of stem cells by near-IR energy may be useful in regenerative medicine [62, 68, 70, 73].

Although the underlying mechanisms of various biological effects by water-filtered broad-spectrum near-IR have not been clearly elucidated, the potential of this innovative approach may be also significant, and the range of its applications in the medical field is expected to be wide [70]. Therefore, further studies in this area are needed to more accurately investigate the biological effects of water-filtered broad-spectrum near-IR phototherapy and photorejuvenation, and to evaluate its potentially large contribution as a new component in the low level light therapy armamentarium.

9. Conclusions

The authors of the present chapter are of the clear opinion that LLLT is a valuable tool for the aesthetic clinician in rejuvenating the photoaged face, but it is only one such tool. We further believe that LED-based systems are the best way to go because of their ease of use and hands-free delivery, compared with LD-based devices. We finally believe that 830 nm offers very interesting properties compared with other wavelengths, making it the wavelength of choice because of its superior depth of penetration, and larger number of cells and targets it has been shown to photoactivate. However, the novel indication of Tanaka's broad-band water-filtered near-IR must also be watched extremely closely, since this waveband penetrates well into the ECM and beyond and has been proved to target and photoactivate wound healing cells and the vascular plexi.

A great deal of work remains in exploring the exact mechanisms of LLLT action, although many pathways at subcellular and genetic levels have been and are being explored. The TGF-β/Smad signaling pathway is the latest to be explored in the collagen synthesis chain of events [74], coupled with up-regulation of genes related to type I collagen synthesis, including LARP6 and COL1A1 [72], and more will doubtless be uncovered. The more that is known, the better can we use LLLT to target the correct pathways to help turn back the skin's aging clock in photorejuvenation, from the inside out … fighting photodamage with reparative phototherapy. However, 'No man is an island, entire of itself' (*1624 Meditation 17*, from *Devotions Upon Emergent Occasions*, John Donne, 1573–1631): in the same way LLLT photorejuvenation cannot possible accomplish everything. Combination is without a doubt the key, and whereas LLLT as a stand-alone modality has a lot of promise in rejuvenating the not-so aged face, when we come to treat the seriously aged face, then LLLT will be an excellent adjunctive modality to the more aggressive laser and energy-based device treatments.

Just to leave the reader with a teasing thought, the authors have often seen the term 'photoantiaging' bandied about, when what people are really talking about is photorejuvenation, the central subject of this chapter. But what about 'true photoantiaging'? Suppose we clinicians and researchers start to apply pure LLLT, either with near-IR LEDs or broad-band water-filtered near-IR in younger patients in their late teens, for example … would that give us true 'photoantiaging' and remove or at least postpone the necessity for photorejuvenation later in life? It is an intriguing thought.

Finally, a group of authors, writing almost 10 years ago in *Lasers in Medical Science* on their years of experience in the use of light in facial rejuvenation, concluded that no single modality could accomplish all the complex events required for effective skin rejuvenation, and suggested that combination phototherapy was the best approach, amalgamated with other conventional modalities, and with an adjunctive epidermal care regimen [75]. There is indeed, nothing new under the sun.

Author details

Robert Glen Calderhead[1]* and Yohei Tanaka[2]

*Address all correspondence to: docrgc1213@gmail.com

1 Clinique L Dermatology, Goyang, South Korea

2 Clinica Tanaka Plastic and Reconstructive Surgery and Anti-aging Center, Nagano, Japan

References

[1] Ohshiro T, Calderhead RG. Low Level Laser Therapy: A Practical Introduction. Chichester, UK: John Wiley and Sons; 1988

[2] Smith KC. Laser (and LED) therapy is phototherapy. Photomedicine and Laser Surgery. 2005;**23**:78–80

[3] Maiman TH. Stimulated optical radiation in ruby. Nature. 1960;**187**:493–494

[4] http://www.nobelprize.org/nobel_prizes/medicine/laureates/1903/finsen-bio.html

[5] Mester E, Spiry T, Szende B, Tota JG. Effect of laser rays on wound healing. The American Journal of Surgery. 1971;**122**:532–535

[6] Mester AF, Mester A. Wound-healing. Laser Therapy, 1989;**1**:7–15

[7] Zand N, Fateh M, Ataie-Fashtami L, Djavid GE, Fatemi SM, et al. Promoting wound healing in minor recurrent aphthous stomatitis by non-thermal, non-ablative CO_2 laser therapy: A pilot study. Photomedicine and Laser Surgery. 2012;**30**:719–723

[8] Calderhead RG, Ohshiro T, Nakajima N. The Nd:YAG and GaAlAs lasers: A comparative analysis in pain therapy. In: Atsumi K, Nimsakul N, editors. Laser Tokyo '81. Tokyo: Japan Society for Laser Medicine; 1981. p. 1. Section 21.

[9] Kubota J, Ohshiro T. The effects of diode laser low reactive-level laser therapy (LLLT) on flap survival in a rat model. Laser Therapy. 1989;**1**:127–135

[10] Whelan HT, Houle JM, Whelan NT, Donohoe DL, et al. The NASA light-emitting diode medical program—progress in space flight and terrestrial applications. Space Tech & App Int'l. Forum; 2000;**504**:37–43

[11] Whelan HT, Smits RL Jr, Buchman EV, Whelan NT, et al. Effect of NASA light-emitting diode (LED) irradiation on wound healing. Journal of Clinical Laser Medicine & Surgery. 2001;**19**:305–314

[12] Szeimies RM, Morton CA, Sidoroff A, Braathen LR. Photodynamic therapy for non-melanoma skin cancer. Acta Dermato-Venereologica. 2005;**85**:483–490

[13] Lee SY, You CE, and Park MY. Blue and red light combination LED phototherapy for acne vulgaris in patients with skin phototype IV. Lasers in Surgery and Medicine. 2007;**39**:180–188

[14] Lee SY, Park KH, Choi JW, Kwon JK, et al. A prospective, randomized, placebo-controlled, double-blinded, and split-face clinical study on LED phototherapy for skin rejuvenation: Clinical, profilometric, histologic, ultrastructural, and biochemical evaluations and comparison of three different treatment settings. Journal of Photochemistry and Photobiology B, 2007;**88**:51–67. (available online as Epub ahead of print)

[15] Baxter GD, Bleakley C, Glasgow P, Calderhead RG. A near-infrared LED-based rehabilitation system: Initial clinical experience. Laser Therapy. 2005:**14**:29–36

[16] Karu T. Primary and secondary mechanisms of action of visible to near-IR radiation on cells. Journal of Photochemistry and Photobiology B. 1999:**49**:1–17

[17] Smith KC. The Science of Photobiology. New York, USA: Plenum Press; 1977

[18] Papageorgiou P, Katsambas A, Chu A. Phototherapy with blue (415 nm) and red (660 nm) light in the treatment of acne vulgaris. British Journal of Dermatology, 2000;**142**:973–978

[19] Nitzan Y, Kauffman M. Endogenous porphyrin production in bacteria by δ-aminolevulinic acid and subsequent bacterial photoeradication. Lasers in Medical Science. 1999;**14**:269–277

[20] Lim W, Choi H, Kim J, Kim S, Jeon S, et al. Anti-inflammatory effect of 635 nm irradiations on in vitro direct/indirect irradiation model. Journal of Oral Pathology & Medicine. 2015;**44**:94–102

[21] Fukuda TY, Tanji MM, Silva SR, Sato MN, Plapler H: Infrared low-level diode laser on inflammatory process modulation in mice: Pro- and anti-inflammatory cytokines. Lasers in Medical Science. 2013;28:1305–1313

[22] Goldberg DG, Russell B. Combination blue (415 nm) and red (633 nm) LED phototherapy in the treatment of mild to severe acne vulgaris. Journal of Cosmetic and Laser Therapy. 2004;**8**:71–75

[23] Karu T. The identification of photacceptor molecules. In: Karu T, editor. Ten Lectures on Basic Science of Laser Phototherapy. Grangesberg: Prima Books AB; 2007. pp. 115–142

[24] Tafur J, Mills PJ. Low-intensity light therapy: Exploring the role of redox mechanisms. Photomedicine and Laser Surgery. 2008;**26**:323–328

[25] Kim WS, Calderhead RG. Is light-emitting diode low level light therapy (LED-LLLT) really effective? Laser Therapy. 2011;**20**:205–215

[26] Park MK, Kim BJ, Kim MN, Mun SK, Hong HK, et al. The measurement of optimal power distance in LEDs. Korean Journal of Dermatology. 2011;**49**: 125–130. (in Korean, abstract in English)

[27] Samoilova KA, Bogacheva ON, Obolenskaya KD, Blinova MI, et al. Enhancement of the blood growth promoting activity after exposure of volunteers to visible and infrared polarized light. Part I: Stimulation of human keratinocyte proliferation in vitro. Photochemical & Photobiological Sciences. 2004;**3**(1):96–101. Epub 2003 Sep 1

[28] Ohshiro T. Practical LLLT in the treatment of naevi. In Ohshiro T, editor. Laser Treatment for Naevi. Chichester, UK: John Wiley & Sons; 1995. pp. 203–205

[29] AlGhamdi KM, Kumar A, Ashour AE, AlGhamdi AA. A comparative study of the effects of different low-level lasers on the proliferation, viability, and migration of human melanocytes in vitro. Lasers in Medical Science. 2015;**30**:1541–1551

[30] Avci P, Gupta A, Sadasivam M, Vecchio D, Pam Z, et al. Low-level laser (light) therapy (LLLT) in skin: Stimulating, healing, restoring. Seminars in Cutaneous Medicine and Surgery. 2013;**32**:41–52

[31] Rigau J, Trelles MA, Calderhead RG, and Mayayo E. Changes in fibroblast proliferation and metabolism following in vitro helium-neon laser irradiation. Laser Therapy. 1991;**3**:25–34

[32] Takezaki S, Omi T, Sato S, Kawana S. Ultrastructural observations of human skin following irradiation with visible red light-emitting diodes (LEDs): A preliminary in vivo report. Laser Therapy. 2005;**14**:153–160

[33] Trelles MA, Rigau J, Velez M. LLLT in vivo effects on mast cells. In Simunovic Z, Editor. Lasers in Medicine and Dentistry (Part 1). Switzerland:LaserMedico; 2002. pp. 169–186

[34] Calderhead RG, Kubota J, Trelles MA, Ohshiro T. One mechanism behind LED phototherapy for wound healing and skin rejuvenation: Key role of the mast cell. Laser Therapy. 2008;**17**:141–148

[35] Young S, Bolton P, Dyson M, Harvey W, Diamantopoulos C. Macrophage responsiveness to light therapy. Lasers in Surgery and Medicine. 1989;**9**:497–505

[36] Bolton P, Dyson M, Young S. The effect of polarized light on the release of growth factors from the u-937 macrophage-like cell line. Laser Therapy. 1992;**4**:33–37

[37] Bolton PA, Young S, Dyson M. macrophage responsiveness to light therapy—a dose response study. Laser Therapy. 2004;**14**:23–28

[38] Souza NH, Ferrari RA, Silva DF, Nunes FD, Bussadori SK, Fernandes KP. Effect of low-level laser therapy on the modulation of the mitochondrial activity of macrophages. Brazilian Journal of Physical Therapy. 2014;**18**:308–314

[39] Osanai T, Shiroto C, Mikami Y, Kudou E, et al. Measurement of GaAlAs diode laser action on phagocytic activity of human neutrophils as a possible therapeutic dosimetry determinant. Laser Therapy. 1990;**2**:123–134

[40] Dima VF, Suzuki K, Liu Q, Koie T, et al. Laser and neutrophil serum opsonic activity. Roumanian Archives of Microbiology and Immunology. 1996;**55**:277–283

[41] Fujimaki Y, Shimoyama T, Liu Q, Umeda T, Nakaji S, Sugawara K. Low-level laser irradiation attenuates production of reactive oxygen species by human neutrophils. Journal of Clinical Laser Medicine & Surgery. 2003;**21**:165–170

[42] Cerdeira CD, Lima Brigagão MR, Carli ML, de Souza Ferreira C, de Oliveira Isac Moraes G, et al. Low-level laser therapy stimulates the oxidative burst in human neutrophils and increases their fungicidal capacity. Journal of Biophotonics. 2016 May 31. [Epub ahead of print]

[43] Kubota J. Effects of diode laser therapy on blood flow in axial pattern flaps in the rat model. Lasers in Medical Science. 2002;**17**:146–153

[44] Saito S, Katagiri T, Ogawa M, Matsumoto S, Kubota J, et al. Effects of diode laser irradiation on superficial blood flow in college sumo wrestlers: A preliminary study. Laser Therapy. 2005;**14**:83–86

[45] Asagai Y, Sujaritpong T, Tranvan L, Ohshiro T. Assessment of changes in carotid blood flow following LLLT of the neck. Laser Therapy. 2007;**16**:127–132

[46] Larkin KA, Martin JS, Zeanah EH, True JM, Braith RW, Borsa PA. Limb blood flow after class 4 laser therapy. Journal of Athletic Training. 2012;**47**:178–183

[47] Zaidi M, Krolikowki JG, Jones DW, Pritchard KA Jr, Struve J, et al. Transient repetitive exposure to low level light therapy enhances collateral blood vessel growth in the ischemic hindlimb of the tight skin mouse. Photochemistry and Photobiology. 2013;**89**:709–713

[48] Hirschl M, Katzenschlager R, Francesconi C, Kundi M. Low level laser therapy in primary Raynaud's phenomenon—results of a placebo controlled, double blind intervention study. The Journal of Rheumatology. 2004;**31**:2408–2412

[49] Asagai Y, Ueno R, Miura Y, Ohshiro T. Application of low reactive-level laser therapy (LLLT) in patients with cerebral palsy of the adult tension athetosis type. Laser Therapy. 1995;**7**:113–118

[50] Trelles MA, Allones I, Mayo E. Combined visible light and infrared light-emitting diode (LED) therapy enhances wound healing after laser ablative resurfacing of photodamaged facial skin. Medical Laser Application. 2006;**21**:165–175

[51] Min PK, Goo BCL. 830 nm light-emitting diode low level light therapy (LED-LLLT) enhances wound healing: A preliminary study. Laser Therapy. 2013;**22**:43–49

[52] Park YJ, Kim SJ, Song HS, Kim SK, Lee JH, et al. Prevention of thyroidectomy scars in Asian adults with low-level light therapy. Dermatologic Surgery. 2015:**42**:526–534

[53] Trelles MA. Phototherapy in anti-aging and its photobiologic basics: A new approach to skin rejuvenation. Journal of Cosmetic Dermatology. 2006;**5**:87–91

[54] Russell BA, Kellett N, Reilly LR. A study to determine the efficacy of combination LED light therapy (633 nm and 830 nm) in facial skin rejuvenation. Journal of Cosmetic and Laser Therapy. 2005;**7**:196–200

[55] Goldberg DJ, Amin S, Russell BA, Phelps R, et al. Combined 633-nm and 830-nm led treatment of photoaging skin. Journal of Drugs in Dermatology. 2006;**5**:748–753

[56] Calderhead RG, Kim WS, Ohshiro T, Trelles MA, and Vasily DB. Adjunctive 830 nm light-emitting diode therapy can improve the results following aesthetic procedures. Laser Therapy. 2015;**23**:277–289

[57] Calderhead RG, Vasily DB. Low level light therapy with light-emitting diodes for the aging face. Clinics in Plastic Surgery. 2016;**43**:541–550. Epub 2016 May 6

[58] Tanaka Y, Matsuo K, Yuzuriha S, Shinohara H. Differential long-term stimulation of type I versus type III collagen after infrared irradiation. Dermatologic Surgery. 2009;**35**:1099–1104

[59] Tanaka Y, Matsuo K, Yuzuriha S. Long-term evaluation of collagen and elastin following infrared (1000 to 1800 nm) irradiation. Journal of Drugs in Dermatology. 2009;**8**:708–712

[60] Tanaka Y, Matsuo K, Yuzuriha S. Long-lasting muscle thinning induced by infrared irradiation specialized with wavelengths and contact cooling: A preliminary report. ePlasty. 2010;**10**:e40:327–335

[61] Tanaka Y, Matsuo K, Yuzuriha S. Long-lasting relaxation of corrugator supercilii muscle contraction induced by infrared irradiation. ePlasty. 2010;**11**:e6:42–49

[62] Tanaka Y, Matsuo K, Yuzuriha S. Near-infrared irradiation non-thermally affects subcutaneous adipocytes and bone. ePlasty. 2010;**11**:e12:97–105